GENERAL MICROBIOLOGY

GENERAL MICROBIOLOGY

Dr. K. Rajeshwar Reddy
M.Sc. (Med. Micro); M.Ed; PGDEM; PGDCA; Ph.D.
Associate Professor
Department of Microbiology
Prathima Institute of Medical Sciences
Nagunur, Karim Nagar, AP-505417

PUBLISHING FOR ONE WORLD

NEW AGE INTERNATIONAL (P) LIMITED, PUBLISHERS

New Delhi • Bangalore • Chennai • Cochin • Guwahati • Hyderabad
Jalandhar • Kolkata • Lucknow • Mumbai • Ranchi

Visit us at **www.newagepublishers.com**

Published by New Age International (P) Ltd., Publishers
Frist Edition: 2009

Branches:

- 36, Malikarjuna Temple Street, Opp. ICWA, Basavanagudi, **Bangalore**. ✆ (080) 26677815
- 26, Damodaran Street, T. Nagar, **Chennai**. ✆ (044) 24353401
- Hemsen Complex, Mohd. Shah Road, Paltan Bazar, Near Starline Hotel, **Guwahati**. ✆ (0361) 2543669
- No. 105, 1st Floor, Madhiray Kaveri Tower, 3-2-19, Azam Jahi Road, Nimboliadda, **Hyderabad**. ✆ (040) 24652456
- RDB Chambers (Formerly Lotus Cinema) 106A,1st Floor, S.N. Banerjee Road, **Kolkata**. ✆ (033) 22275247
- 16-A, Jopling Road, **Lucknow**. ✆ (0522) 2209578
- 142C, Victor House, Ground Floor, N.M. Joshi Marg, Lower Parel, **Mumbai**. ✆ (022) 24927869
- 22, Golden House, Daryaganj, **New Delhi**. ✆ (011) 23262370, 23262368

ISBN: 978-81-224-2671-7

Rs. 250.00

C-09-03-3485

Printed in Ramprintographs, Delhi.
Typeset at Kalyani Computer Services, Delhi.

PUBLISHING FOR ONE WORLD
NEW AGE INTERNATIONAL (P) LIMITED, PUBLISHERS
4835/24, Ansari Road, Daryaganj, New Delhi-110002
Visit us at **www.newagepublishers.com**

Dedicated to

My Great Grand Parents
Late Sri Raji Reddy
Late Smt. Laxmamma

and

My Grand Parents
Late Sri Narsa Reddy
Late Smt. Venkamma

PREFACE

This book has originated from my lecture notes which have been compiled over the last 20 years of my teaching Microbiology. Microbiology is an exceptionally broad discipline encompassing several specialities. This book titled "General Microbiology" is primarily intended for both undergraduate and postgraduate microbiology students in the fields of Basic Sciences, Biological and Life Sciences, Biotechnology, Genetics, Agriculture, Medicine and Veterinary Sciences.

Undertaking this job was an incredible task, because any textbook to remain useful, must keep up with advances in knowledge and with changes in teaching patterns. The contents were reorganised to expand the scope of the book. Therefore, this book will also be immensely useful for Microbiology teachers.

I request the readers to give their constructive criticism and valuable suggestions to improve this book further.

KASARLA RAJESHWAR REDDY

CONTENTS

1

History of Microbiology

- *Antony Van Leeuwenhoek*
- *The theory of spontaneous generation (abiogenesis)*
- *La Zaro Spallanzani and Biogenesis*
- *Edward Jenner*
- *Louis Pasteur*
- *Robert Koch/ Koch's Postulates*
- *Joseph Lister*
- *Iwanowsky*
- *Metchnikoff*
- *Alexander Flemming*
- *Paul Ehrlich*
- *Mac Farlane Burnet*

ANTONY VAN LEEUWENHOEK (1632–1723)

He was the first Person, who invented the microscope and discovered the microbial world. He was a draper (Merchant) from Delft, Holland. He used to grind lenses and made microscopes as a hobby. The microscopes of Leeuwenhoek could magnify objects about 200-300 times.

With his microscopes, Leeuwenhoek observed a variety of things like rain water, pond water and scrapings from his own teeth. He saw minute moving objects and called them as "**Little animalcules**", which we now know them as protozoa, yeasts and bacteria. He made accurate sketches and communicated his findings to "Royal Society of London".

Thus, Leeuwenhoek was the first person to discover microscope and the presence of bacteria and spirochetes in mouth.

THE THEORY OF SPONTANEOUS GENERATION (ABIOGENESIS)

After the discovery of microorganisms by Leeuwenhoek, scientists began investigations about the origin of microbes. Since organic matter decomposes quickly outside the living body, it was assumed that microorganisms were arising by spontaneous generation. John Needham (1749), an Irish priest, observed the appearance of microorganisms in putrefying meat and interpreted this as spontaneous generation.

LA ZARO SPALLANZANI (1729–1799) - THEORY OF BIOGENESIS

Spallanzani, an Italian priest, boiled beef broth for an hour, sealed the flasks and observed no appearance of microorganisms and disproved the theory of spontaneous generation or abiotic origin of life and proposed the theory of biogenesis. He said that every form of life takes its origin from their parents, germ cells or seeds. This theory of biogenesis was later proved and supported by Louis Pasteur.

EDWARD JENNER (1749–1823)

Jenner was an English country physician, who discovered a safe and efficient vaccination against small pox. which ultimately led to the eradication of small pox (**Variola**).

Jenner observed that dairy workers, exposed to occupational cowpox infection were immune to small pox. He proved experimentally that resistance to small pox can be induced by injecting cow pox material (**Vaccinia**) from disease pustules into man (in 1796).

Pasteur gave the general term "Vaccine" (Vacca = cow) in honour of Jenner's cow pox vaccine, to various materials used to induce active immunity. Jenner published his findings in 1798 in a pamphlet "*An inquiry into the cause and effect of variole vaccine*".

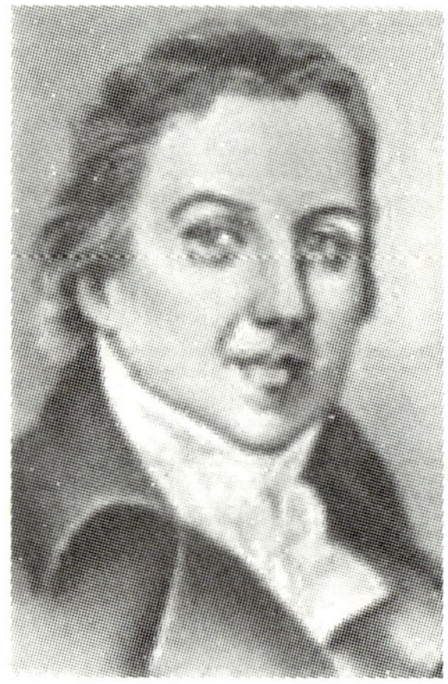

Fig. 1.1 Edward Jenner (1749–1823)

LOUIS PASTEUR (1822–1895)

He was a Professor of Chemistry at the University of Lille, France. He is considered as "**Father of Microbiology**", as his contribution led to the development of Microbiology as a separate scientific discipline.

He proved the theory of "Biogenesis" and disproved the "Theory of spontaneous generation" (Abiogenesis), experimentally by using swan-necked flasks.

He worked on souring of wine and beer and found that this alcohol spoilage is due to the growth of undesirable organisms, while the desirable microorganisms produce alcohol by a chemical process called "**Fermentation**". He showed that wine did not spoil, if it is heated to 50-60°C for a few minutes. This method is called **"Pasteurization"**, now widely used in dairy units, to kill pathogenic microorganisms in milk.

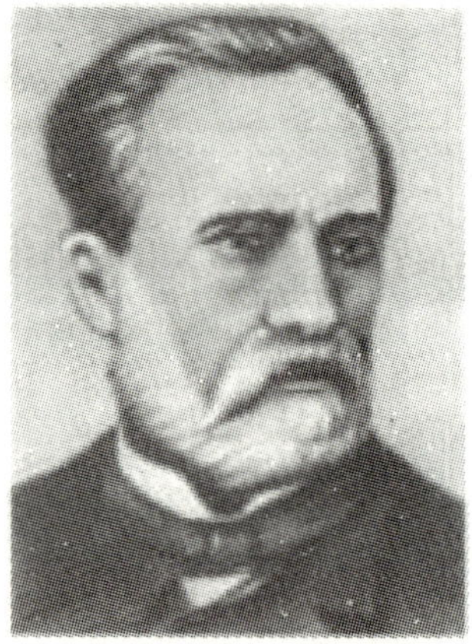

Fig. 1.2 Louis Pasteur (1822–1895)

He is a founder of **"Germ theory of disease"** as he visualized that diseases are caused by microorganisms.

In course of his research, he discovered the importance of sterilization and discovered steam sterilizer, autoclave and hot air oven. He also established the importance of cotton wool plugs for protection of culture media from aerial contamination.

He differentiated between aerobic and anaerobic bacteria and coined the term "anaerobic" to refer to the organisms that do not require oxygen for growth.

He worked on "Pebrine", a silk-worm disease caused by a protozoan and showed that infection can be controlled by choosing worms free from the parasite for breeding.

He developed the process of **"attenuation"** during his work on "chicken cholera" in fowls. He found that cultures which had been stored in the laboratory for sometime would not kill the animals as fresh cultures did. This attenuation is now used in protective vaccination against diseases.

Pasteur showed that the anthrax disease in cattle and sheep is caused by a bacterium. He cultivated anthrax organisms in sterile yeast water, and showed that these cultures can produce disease when inoculated into healthy animals. He developed a live attenuated **anthrax vaccine**, by incubation at 40-42°C, which proved to be useful in protecting animals against anthrax. He also worked on swine erysipelas.

Pasteur developed a vaccine against rabies (Hydrophobia), which made a greatest impact in medicine. He obtained the causative agent of rabies by serial intracerebral passage in rabbits and the vaccine was prepared by drying pieces of spinal chord. In 1888, Pasteur institute was established for mass antirabic treatment.

Pasteur gave the general term "**Vaccine**" (Vacca=cow) in honour of Jenner's cow pox vaccine, to various materials used to induce active immunity.

ROBERT KOCH (1843–1912)/KOCH'S POSTULATES

He was a German country Doctor who later became the Professor of hygiene and Director of institute of infective diseases at Berlin. He perfected many bacteriological techniques and known as "Father of Practical Bacteriology".

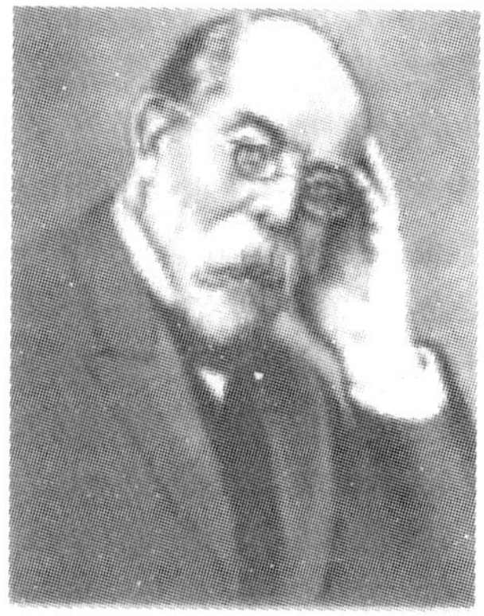

Fig. 1.3 Robert Koch (1843–1912)

He discovered rod shaped organisms in the blood of animals, that died of anthrax. He experimentally obtained the anthrax organisms in pure culture on a depression slide by inoculation of infected blood into the aqueous humour of a bullock's eye. He observed multiplication of bacteria and spore formation. He injected these spores into mice and reproduced the disease.

He found that in certain conditions, the anthrax bacillus forms spores, that can survive on earth for years. He passed anthrax bacilli, from the blood of an infected animal, from one mouse to another through twenty generations, and found that they bred true. He worked out its life-history.

He introduced staining techniques. He prepared dried bacterial films (Smears) on glass slides and stained them with aniline dyes for producing a better contrast under microscope. He discovered tubercle bacillus (*Mycobacterium tuberculosis*) which is popularly called as Koch's bacillus. He injected tubercle bacilli into laboratory animals and reproduced the disease, satisfying all Koch's postulates.

He discovered *Vibrio cholerae*, the causative agent of cholera disease.

He developed pure culture techniques by introducing **solid media**. The use of agar-agar obtained from dried sea weeds (*Gelidium* Sp.) in the preparation of solid bacteriological media was first suggested by Frau Hesse, the wife of Koch' student. This agar-agar is totally inert with no nutritive value, solidifies at 45°C and melts at 90°C, and was found to be most suitable solidifying agent in the preparation of culture media. Koch isolated bacteria in pure cultures on these solid media. It revolutionized bacteriology.

He discovered "**Old Tuberculin**". Koch noted that when tubercle bacilli or its protein extract was injected into a Guinea-pig already infected with the bacillus, an exaggerated reaction took place and the reaction remain localized. This is popularly called **"Koch Phenomenon"** and it is a demostration of cell mediated immunity. The tuberculin test is based on Koch's phenomenon. He erroneously thought that protein extracted from tubercle bacilli, called "Old tuberculin", could be used in the treatment of tuberculosis. Koch did a series of experiments to fulfill the criteria laid by his teacher, Henle to establish the causative role between a particular microorganism and a particular disease. They are popularly known as **Koch's postulates** (Henle-Koch's Posulates). They are:

1. A specific organism should be found constantly in association with the disease.
2. The organism should be isolated and grown in a pure culture in the laboratory.
3. The pure culture when inoculated into a healthy susceptible animal should produce symptoms/ lesions of the same disease.
4. From the inoculated animal, the microorganism should be isolated in pure culture.
5. An additional criterion introduced is that specific anitbodies to the causative organism should be demonstrable in patient's serum.

JOSEPH LISTER (1827–1912)

He is popularly known as **"Father of antiseptic surgery".** He was a professor of surgey at University of Glasgow and Edinburg and later at King's College, London.

He was deeply interested in the prevention of post-operative sepsis. He was attracted by Pasteur's germ theory of disease and concluded that sepsis or wound infection may be due to microbial growth, derived from the atmosphere.

He successfully prevented post-operative sepsis by introducing antiseptic techniques. He chose carbolic acid (Phenol) and used as spray on the wound or during surgery. He applied dressings soaked in carbolic acid on wounds. As a result, there was a marked reduction of post-operative sepsis, wound inflammation and suppuraton. It saved millions of lives from the jaws of death due to wound infections.

Lister's antiseptic surgery later led to the development of aseptic surgery. He suffered many criticism but never lose courage and followed his own ideas and revolutionized the science of surgery by introducing antiseptic system in 1867.

IWANOWSKY (1892)

Dmitri Iwanowsky, a Russian botanist, occupies a pivotal position in the history of virology.

In 1866, Adeolf E. Meyer, a Dutch agricultural chemist described a disease of tobacco called "Mosaic" and showed that the disease could be transmitted to healthy plants through the sap of the diseased plant.

Iwanowsky (1892) demonstrated that this disease was caused by an agent which could pass through the filter, which withholds bacteria. He obtained the sap from infected leaves and passed it through a bacterial filter, called chamberland candle filter, which retained all bacteria and the filtered sap still retained infectivity when applied to healthy leaves.

Beijerinck (1898), a Dutch Microbiologist, showed that this infectious agent could diffuse through an agar gel and that it was a non-corpuscular "*Contagion vivum fluidum*" which he called "**Virus**".

Stanley (1935), a British Mycologist was able to obtain the infectious agent of tobacco mosaic in a crystalline form.

METCHNIKOFF (1845-1916)

Elie Metchnikoff, the Russian-French biologist, discovered the phenomenon of **phagocytosis**, the cellular concept of immunity.

In Italy, where he had gone on a research visit, he studied the transparent larvae of starfish and noticed some of their cells could engulf and digest foreign protein particles. These cell eaters are called "**Phagocytes**".

He continued his work on phagocytic action, at Pasteur Institute, Paris and found that in human blood a large proportion of the leucocytes (White blood cells) are phagocytic and attack invading bacteria. This, in turn, results in increased numbers of leucocytes in the infected areas followed by the inflamed area becoming hot, red, swelled and painful due to dead phagocytes forming pus.

He spent his last two decades on the study of human aging, since he believed that phagocytes eventually begin to digest that host cells aided by the effects of intestinal bacteria and that effectively combating them would increase the life span of human being.

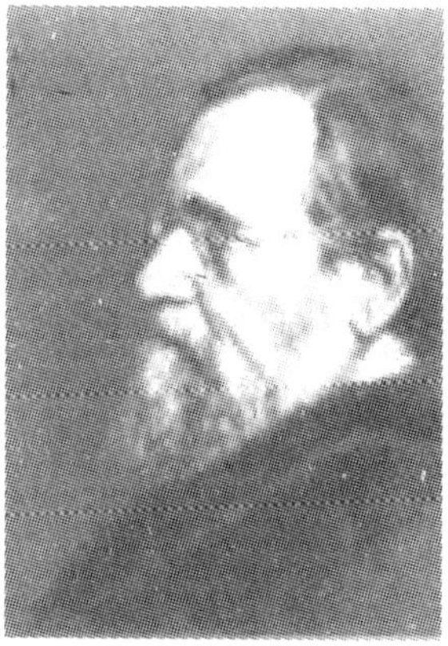

Fig. 1.4 Elie Metchnikoff (1845–1916)

ALEXANDER FLEMMING (1881–1955)

He was an English scientist worked at St. Mary's hospital in London.

Flemming was associated with two major discoveries-lysozyme and penicillin. In 1922, he discovered **lysozyme** by demonstrating that the nasal secretion has the power of dissolving or lysing certain kinds of bacteria. Subsequently, he showed that lysozyme was present in many tissues of the body.

In 1929, Flemming made an accidental discovery that the fungus *Penicillium notatum* produces an antibacterial substance which he called penicillin. Flemming was culturing Staphylococci in petridishes and some of his cultures were contaminated with a mold, subsquently identified as *Penicillium notatum*. Around the mold colony, there were clear zones, where Staphylococci disappeared. Flemming attributed this to the production of an anti-bacterial susbstance by the mold. Flemming cultured the fungus *Penicilium notatum* in broth cultures, filtered the fungal mat and obtained the **penicillin** in soluble form in the culture filtrate.

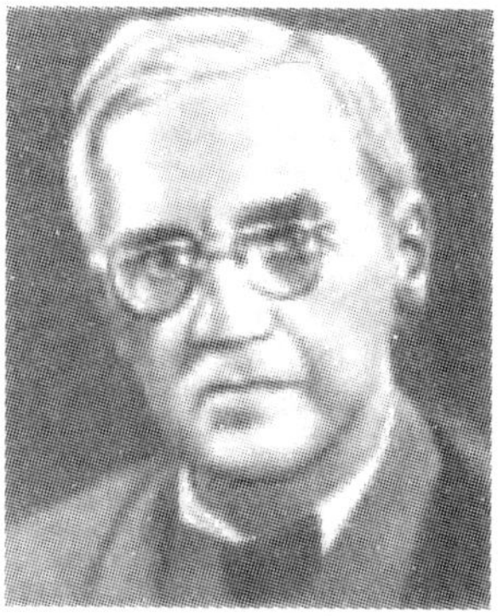

Fig. 1.5 Sir Alexander Fleming (1881–1955)

In 1940, Howard Florey and Ernst Chain demonstrated its antibacterial action *in vivo*. Working in U.S.A., they were able to produce large quantities of penicillin in pure form. In 1945, Flemming, Florey and Chain shared the nobel prize in physiology and medicine for the discovery of penicillin.

PAUL EHRLICH (1854–1915)

He was a German Bacteriologist, who pioneered the technique of chemotheraphy in medicine.

From his discovery that certain tissues have a specific affinity, he reasoned that organisms causing diseases could be selectively killed with chemical drugs. This led him to produce "arsphenamine" (an arsenic compound), the first synthetic drug, which destroyed the syphilis microbe in the body.

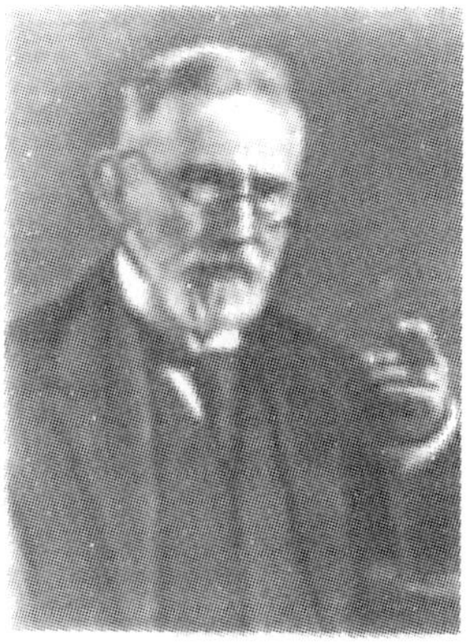

Fig. 1.6 Paul Ehrlich (1854–1915)

Ehrlich observed that organic arsenicals killed trypanosomes in an infected animal, but, if smaller doses were administered, the trypanosomes acquired tolerance to the drug. Therefore, he aimed at "*therapia magna sterilans*" *i.e.,* the introduction into the blood of a single dose of chemotherapeutic agent sufficient to kill the parasite. He also observed that drug would undergo certain changes in the body after it would produce the desired action.

SIR FRANK MAC FARLANE BURNET (1967)

Burnet is an Australian scientist, won nobel prize for the discovery of acquired immunological tolerance. He proposed clonal selection theory to explain antibody synthesis.

His work on bacteriophages and method for culturing some viruses in live chick embryo, led him to the view that an animal's ability is not inborn, but is developed during fetal life.

Burnet (1967) developed concept of **"immunological surveillance".** According to which the primary function of the immune system is to preserve the integrity of the body, seeking and destroying all "foreign" antigens, whether autogenous or external in origin.

Burnet's work also included the mode of action and the epidemiology of influenza virus, polio, Q fever and the cholera vibrio.

QUESTIONS

Short Notes

1. Louis Pasteur.
2. Robert Koch.
3. Koch's Postulates.
4. Burnet.
5. Iwanowsky.
6. Joseph Lister.
7. Leeuwenhoek.
8. Jenner.
9. Flemming.
10. Metchnikoff.
11. Paul Ehrlich.

2

Microscopy

- *Introduction*
- *Compound microscope*
- *Magnification*
- *Numerical aperture*
- *Resolution/Resolving power*
- *Definition and Aberrations*
- *Objectives*
- *Oil-immersion objective*
- *Eye-pieces (oculars)*
- *Condensers*
- *Care and use of microscope*
- *Phase-contrast microscope*
- *Dark-field microscope*
- *Interference microscope (Stereo micro scope)- NDIC microscope*
- *Fluorescent (UV) microscope*
- *Electron microscope*
  - *– Transmission electron microscope (TEM)*
  - *– Scanning electron microscope (SEM)*
  - *– Scanning tunneling microscope*
  - *– Immune electron microscopy*
- *Polarising microscope*
- *Micrometry*
- *Photomicrography*

INTRODUCTION

Microscope is an optical instrument used to magnify (enlarge) minute objects or microorganisms which cannot be seen by naked eye.

The morphological study of bacteria requires the use of microscopes. It provides the magnification which enables one to see the organism and structures invisible to the naked eye. A microscope, therefore, is the most important tool for a microbiologist. Microscopes are of several types:

COMPOUND MICROSCOPE/LIGHT MICROSCOPE/BRIGHT-FIELD MICROSCOPE

The microscope essentially consists of following parts:

1. The supporting system in the form of a base, body and stage.
2. The illuminating system consists of a plano-concave mirror and condenser with the iris diaphragm.
3. The magnifying system consists of optical lenses. The objectives on the rotating nose piece, the mechanical tube and the ocular or eye-piece.

4. The adjustment system consists of coarse and fine adjustment knobs and the rack and pinion system on the stage to move slide either laterally or forward or backward.

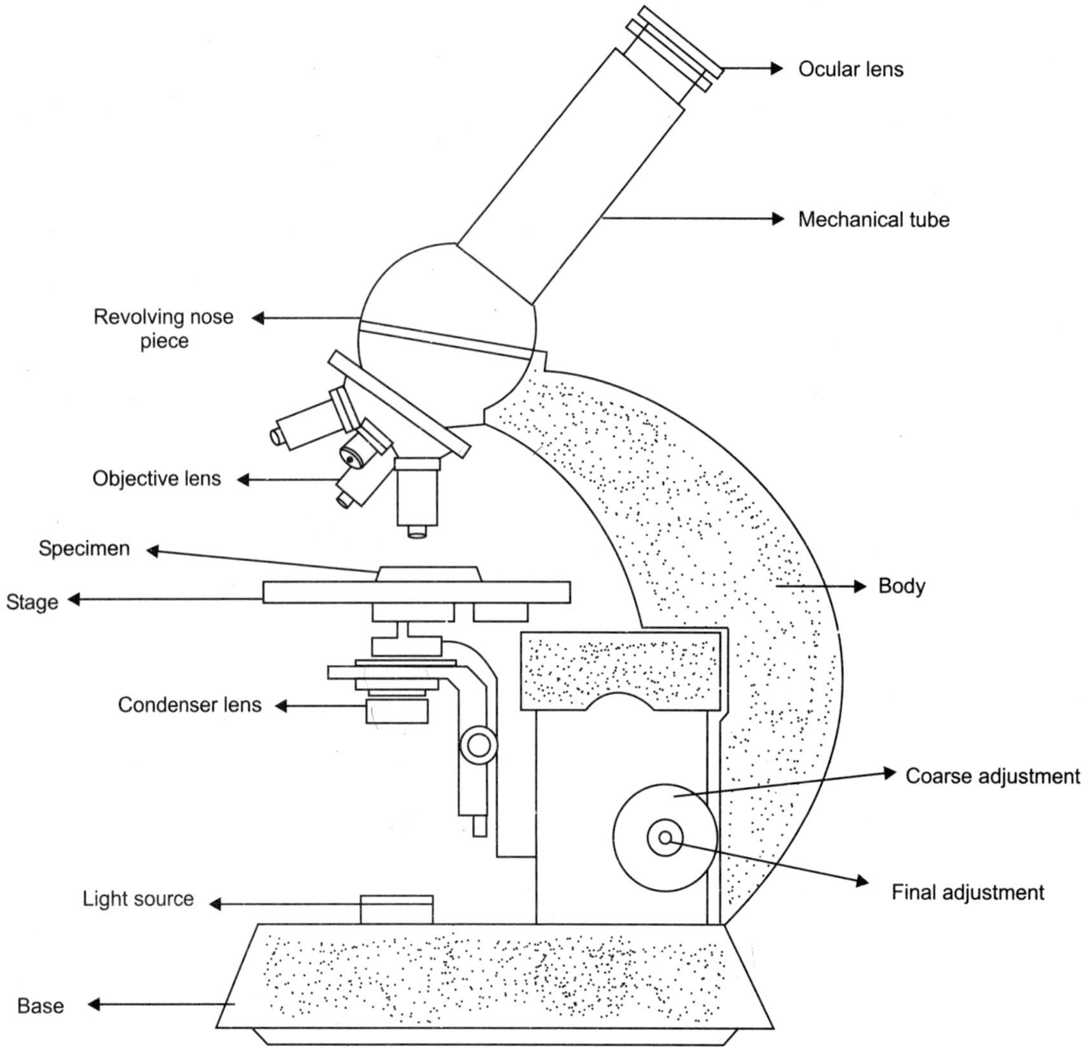

Fig. 2.1 The Compound microscope

MAGNIFICATION

Magnification is defined as the degree of enlargement of object achieved by a microscope. Magnification through a microscope is achieved by a series of two lens systems. The lens system nearest the object called **"objective"** magnifies the specimen and produces a **"real image"** inside the mechanical tube. The eye-piece lens system magnifies the real image further yielding **"virtual image"** which is seen by the eye.

Hence, there is magnification at two levels. The final magnification achieved by a microscope is a product of the magnifying power of the eye-piece and the magnifying power of the objectives.

The total magnification of microscope = Objective magnification × Eye-piece magnification

The magnification of a microscope depends on the following factors:

1. Mechanical tube length
2. Focal length of the objective
3. The magnifying power of eye-piece.

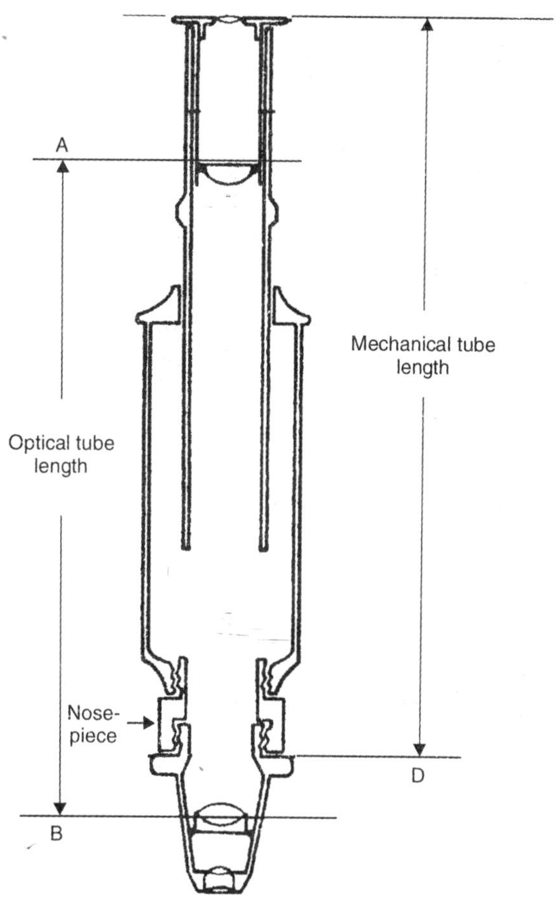

Fig. 2.2 Mechanical tube length and optical tube length.

The **mechanical tube length** is the distance between the point where the objective fits into the lower end of the body or the nose-piece and eye lens of the eye-piece; a measurement easily made with a ruler. Most modern microscopes have a mechanical tube length of 160 mm; but a few manufacturers employ 170 mm.

$$\text{The magnification of an objective} = \frac{\text{Mechanical tube length}}{\text{Focal length of objective}}$$

The magnification of eye piece is clearly engraved on the mount.

Since the total magnification of the compound microscope is the product of the magnification of the two lens systems, one might expect that the total magnification would be indefinitely increased by the use of additional lenses. However, this is not so, owing to the property of the lenses called **"Resolving power"**.

NUMERICAL APERTURE (NA)

The numerical aperture may be defined as the ratio of the diameter of the lens to its focal length. In other words, NA is the product of the refractive index of the medium between the object and objective lens, and sine of half of the angle formed by the light rays entering the lens from a point on the object.

NA is expressed mathematically as follows:

$$NA = n \sin U$$

Where n = Refractive index of the medium between object and objective (1.0 for air, 1.5 for cedar wood oil)

U = angle of aperture *i.e.*, the angle formed by the two extreme rays of light, which starting from the centre of the object, reach the eye of the observer. Theoretical limit of 2U = 180°.

NA of dry lens is 0.65; of oil immersion lens is 1.28 or 1.3 (highest 1.4 in apochromatic objective). Objectives may have equal focal lengths, but different numerical apertures depending on the diameter of the front lens.

NA indicates the amount of right which enters an objective from a point in the microscopic field. It is a function of the effective diameter of the objective in relation to its focal length and the light bending power on refracactive index of the medium between the specimen and objective.

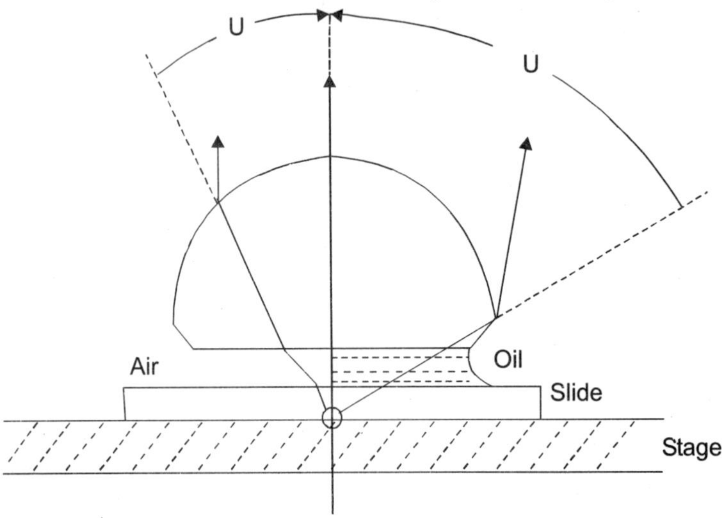

Fig. 2.3 Numerical Aperture (NA) shows the gain in NA by oil immersion (right) as compared with a dry objective (left).

RESOLUTION/RESOLVING POWER

The resolving power of a microscope is its ability to reveal closely adjacent structural details as separate and distinct. Expressed, quantitatively, resolution is its capacity to distinguish two neighboring points as separate entities. For example, the human eye has a resolving power of 0.25 mm, which means that two dots placed 0.25 mm apart can be distinguished as two separate dots. If the distance between the two dots is less than 0.25 mm, only one dot will be seen. Thus, the **"limit of resolution"** may be defined as the shortest distance between two objects, where they can be distinguished as two separate entities.

$$\text{Resolution (R)} = \frac{0.61 \times \lambda}{NA}$$

Where, λ = Wavelength of light used for illumination

NA = Numerical aperture

Therefore, resolving power of a microscope depends upon two factors:

1. Wavelength of light used for illumination
2. Numerical aperture.

The shortest wavelength of light will give the maximum resolution. Similarly, the higher the numerical aperture, the finer will be the detail (high resolution) revealed by the objective.

Resolving power of normal eye = 0.25 mm

Resolving power of compound microscope = 0.25 μm

Resolving power of electron microscope = 5 Å.

DEFINITION AND ABERRATIONS

"Definition" is the capacity of an objective to render the outline of the image of the object clear and distinct.

Lens systems are made up of lenses having spherical surfaces, and such surfaces do not form perfect images. This is because of inequalities of refraction and focus by peripheral portions of the objective lenses. This phenomenon is known as **"Aberrations".** They are of two types:

Spherical aberration: It is due to light rays passing through the edge of lens will never be brought to same focus as those passing nearer the center, resulting in serious distortion of the image.

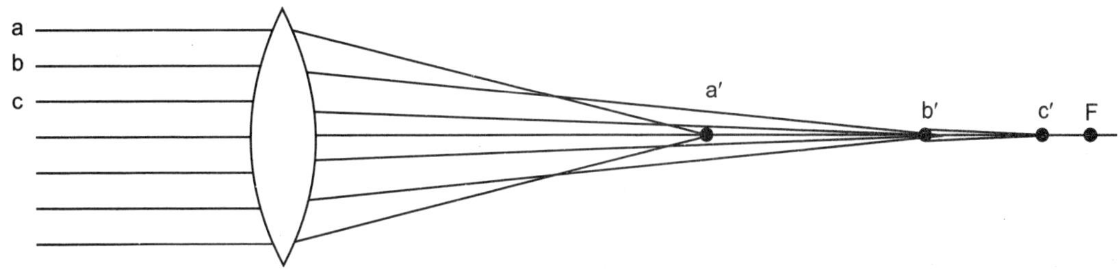

Fig. 2.4 Light entering a convex lens is brought to a focus at point F. Light rays a, b, c refracted to different degrees to reach the focus point a′, b′ and c′, which are situated at points apart from each other.

Chromatic aberration. White light while passing through a lens is diffracted as it would be in a prism, to its various component colors, each with its own wavelength. The light rays of different wavelengths are refracted by the lens to varying extents and may not be recombined in the same focus, resulting in a hazy image fringed with colors of the spectrum.

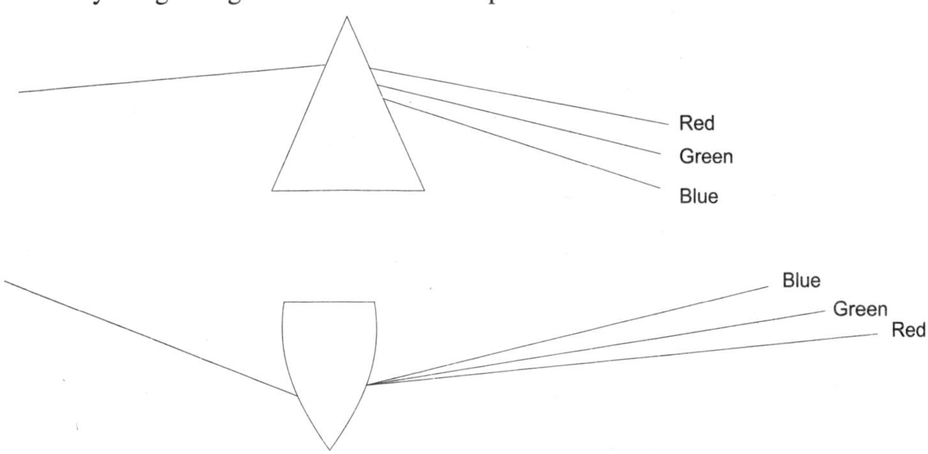

Fig. 2.5 Chromatic aberration

OBJECTIVES

The objective is the most important lens in a microscope. The main functions of objective lens are:

1. to gather light rays coming from any point of the object
2. to unite the light rays in a point of the image
3. to magnify the image.

An objective capable of utilizing a large angular cone of light coming from the specimen will have better resolving power than an objective limited to a smaller cone of light. Objecitves may be of several types:

Achromatic objectives are the simplest in construction and least expensive. They are perfectly satisfactory for all routine work and much research work.

Apochromatic objectives are very expensive and used for special purposes such as photomicrography. In apochromatic objectives, the light of atleast three different wavelengths (colors) may be united, the aberrations are less, and the NA is usually higher. The lenses are made up of mineral fluorite which gives brilliance and crispness to the image. Apochromatic objectives must always be used with compensating eye-pieces and a properly centered condenser.

Semiapochromatic objectives are those in which certain amount of fluorite is present and are intermediate between apochromatic and achromatic objectives.

In microbiology, three objectives are generally adequate, 1. low power (10X), 2. high dry power (45X), 3. oil immersion objective (100X). If we employ 10X ocular, we get magnifications of 100, 450, 1000 times respectively.

OIL IMMERSION OBJECTIVES

Oil immersion objectives are most frequently used in microbiology, because of their greater magnification and resolution. It is so named because the medium between slide (object) and objective is occupied by oil.

When a dry objective is used, the space between objective and object is occupied by air (refractive index 1.0). When light rays pass from a dense medium (glass of slide and cover slip; Refractive index 1.5) to a less dense medium (air; Refractive index 1.0) are refracted obliquely outwards so that many light rays cannot enter the objective lens. Since the brightness of the image depends upon the amount of light entering the objective, and the resolution depends on the effective numerical aperture, this refraction of light outwards diminishes brightness and clarity of the image.

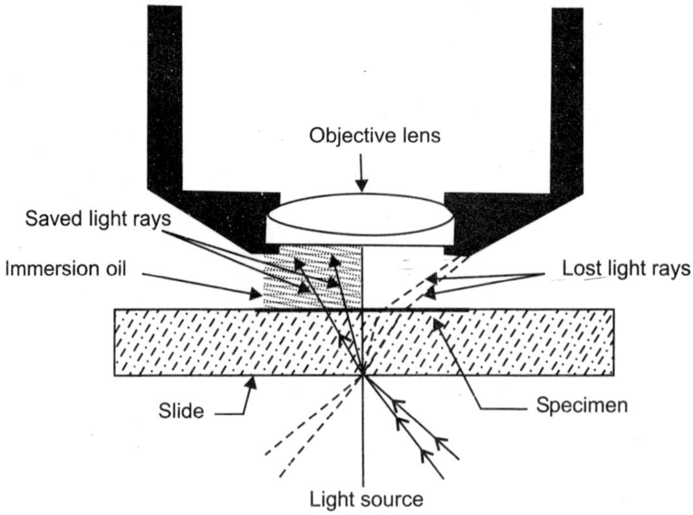

Fig. 2.6 How the oil immersion objective increases the amount of light passing from the specimen into the objective lens.

If the space between slide (object) and objective is filled with some transparent oil, with same refractive index as glass, then the light rays do not undergo refraction and pass directly into the objective. Usually cedar wood oil (R.I. = 1.515) is used. Castor oil can also be used. As a result, the NA of the lens is increased. The lens can be brought much closer to the object, admitting most of divergent rays into the objective lens, and thus resolution is increased.

EYE-PIECES (OCULARS)

Eye-piece is a short tube consisting of two lenses and fits into the upper part of the mechanical tube. Eye-pieces are available with 5X, 10X, 15X magnifications, engraved on the mount. The functions of the eye-pieces are:

1. the magnification of the real image
2. the formation of a virtual image of the real image produced by the objective
3. carries markers, measurement scales, cross-hairs etc.

There are different types of eye-pieces:

Huygenian eye-pieces are constructed with the plane surface of the two lenses facing upwards and the diaphragm is situated between them. Huygenian eye-pieces are sometimes described as "**negative oculars**", because the focus occurs within the eye-piece.

Ramsden or positive eye-pieces are constructed with the convex surface of both lenses facing inwards, and the diaphragm is placed externally below the lower lens. They are suitable for micrometry and give more accurate results than huygenian eye-pieces.

Hyperplane eye-pieces give flatter fields and are known as flat-field eye-pieces.

Compensating eye-pieces consist of an achromatic triplet combination of lenses.

They are designed specially for use with apochromatic objectives.

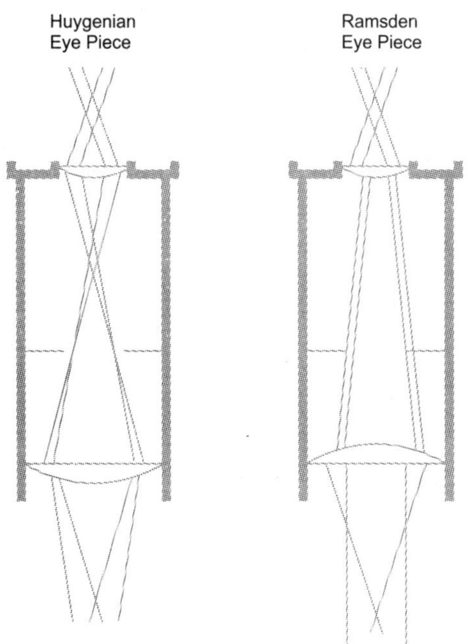

Fig. 2.7

CONDENSERS

A condenser may be defined as a series of lenses for illuminating the object; located under the stage of the microscope, hence, referred to as substage condenser. There are several types of condensers.

Abbe condensers consists of two lenses, both of which are not corrected for spherical and chromatic aberrations. Because of its simplicity and good light gathering ability, it is extensively used for general microscopy.

Aplanatic condensers contain a third or middle lens, which is corrected for spherical aberration, but not for chromatic aberration. It gives good results when used with monochromatic light.

Achromatic condensers are corrected for both chromatic and spherical aberrations and therefore recommended for research and color photomicrography, where a high degree of perfection in the image is required. The NA of the condenser generally equals that of the objective.

Variable-focus condenser is a two lens system in which the upper lens is fixed and the lower lens focusable. This condenser is basically similar to the Abbe condenser when the lower lens is raised to its top position.

CARE AND USE OF A MICROSCOPE

Clean the microscope with a clean soft cloth. The objectives and eye-pieces must be cleaned with a lens paper and xylol or benzol. Alcohol and acetone should not be used as it dissolves cement that binds the lenses. Set up the microscope in a convenient position, facing the source of light. Place the object (slide with smear) on the stage and adjust the mirror to the illuminant. Always tilt the mirror towards blue sky, if artificial light is not available. Direct sunlight should not fall on the mirror. For prolonged work, it is advisable to use artificial light of a particular wavelength.

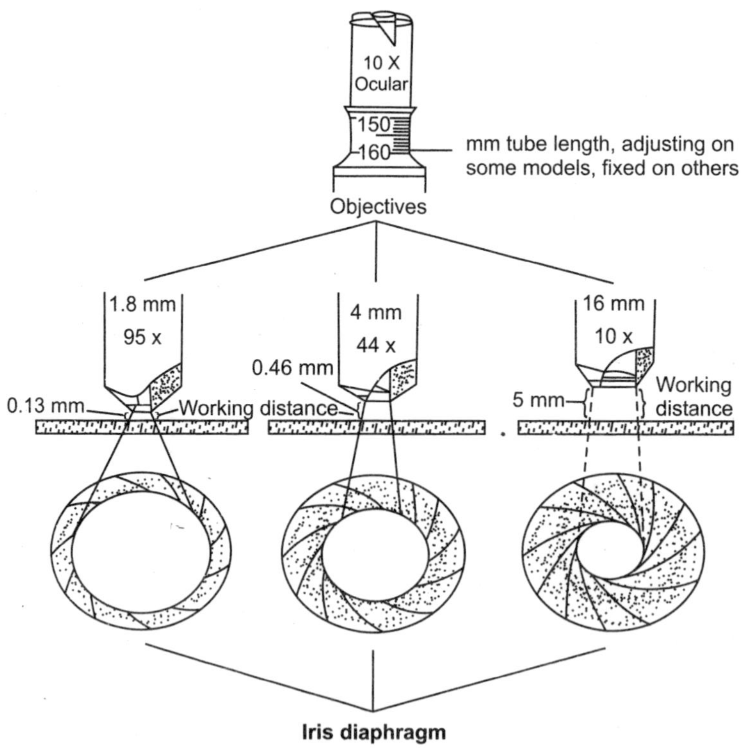

Fig. 2.8 Relationship between working distance of objective lens and adjustment of iris diaphragm. The shorter the working distance, the more open the diaphragm. The shorter the focal length of the objective, the shorter is the working distance of the lens.

Low power (10X) and high dry power (45X) objectives are used for examination of wet films or hanging drop preparations. The oil immersion (100X) objective is used for stained smears or sections only.

For the examination of unstained preparations under low power or high dry power objectives, following adjustments have to be made:

1. Lower the condenser.
2. Close the iris diaphragm partially to reduce the light intensity.
3. Use concave mirror.
4. Lower the objective to near about the working distance by looking from the side. Never attempt to bring the object into focus by lowering the body tube while looking through the eye-piece.
5. Focus under low power and then turn on to high dry power objective. Focussing is achieved by movement of coarse or fine adjustment slightly.

For the examination of stained smears under oil-immersion objective, following adjustments have to be made (Fig. 2.8):

1. Raise the condenser fully.
2. Open the iris diaphragm fully to allow maximum light.
3. Use plane mirror.
4. Place a drop of oil on the smear.
5. Looking from the side, rack the objective down until the tip of objective lens touches the oil. Then focus the object with fine adjustment by looking through ocular.
6. After use remove the oil from the objective and object with a soft cloth dipped in xylol or tissue paper.
7. After use, keep the low power lens in focussing position and condenser lowered down.

PHASE-CONTRAST MICROSCOPE

It was originally developed by Frederick Zernike (1953), hence known as Zernike Microscope.

Phase contrast microscope is used to enhance contrast to study unstained microorganisms in living state. The light rays pass through the specimen and are partially deflected by different densities or thickness or refractive indices of the microbial cells or cell structures in the specimen. The greater the refractive index of an object, the more the light beam is slowed, resulting in decreased light intensity. These differences in light intensity translate into differences that provide contrast (phase contrast). As a result, some structures appear darker or dark-grey against a bright background.

Phase contrast microscopy requires special optical system – a **"phase contrast objective"** and a **"phase contrast condenser".** With this system, it is possible to observe unstained structures within cells, based only on their refractive indices or thickness.

The light rays while passing through the object/specimen on slide, will emerge in different phases as direct and diffracted beams, which are passed through different thicknesses in phase plate (a disk of glass with a circular trough etched in it) in the back focal plane of the objective, which retards the diffracted rays one quarter of a wavelength with respect to the direct rays. These phase differences are converted into differences in light intensity, and therefore, the objects appear darker or dark-grey against a bright background.

The special phase condenser consists of annular diaphragms on a rotating disk fitted to the bottom of the condenser. A different size of annulus is required for use with each objective of different NA.

Phase contrast microscope is more valuable in general biology. It is useful

1. to study unstained living cells
2. to differentiate internal structures in living cells
3. to study flagellar movements and motility of bacteria and protozoans
4. to study intestinal and other live protozoa such as amoebae and *Trichomonas*
5. to examine fungi grown in culture.

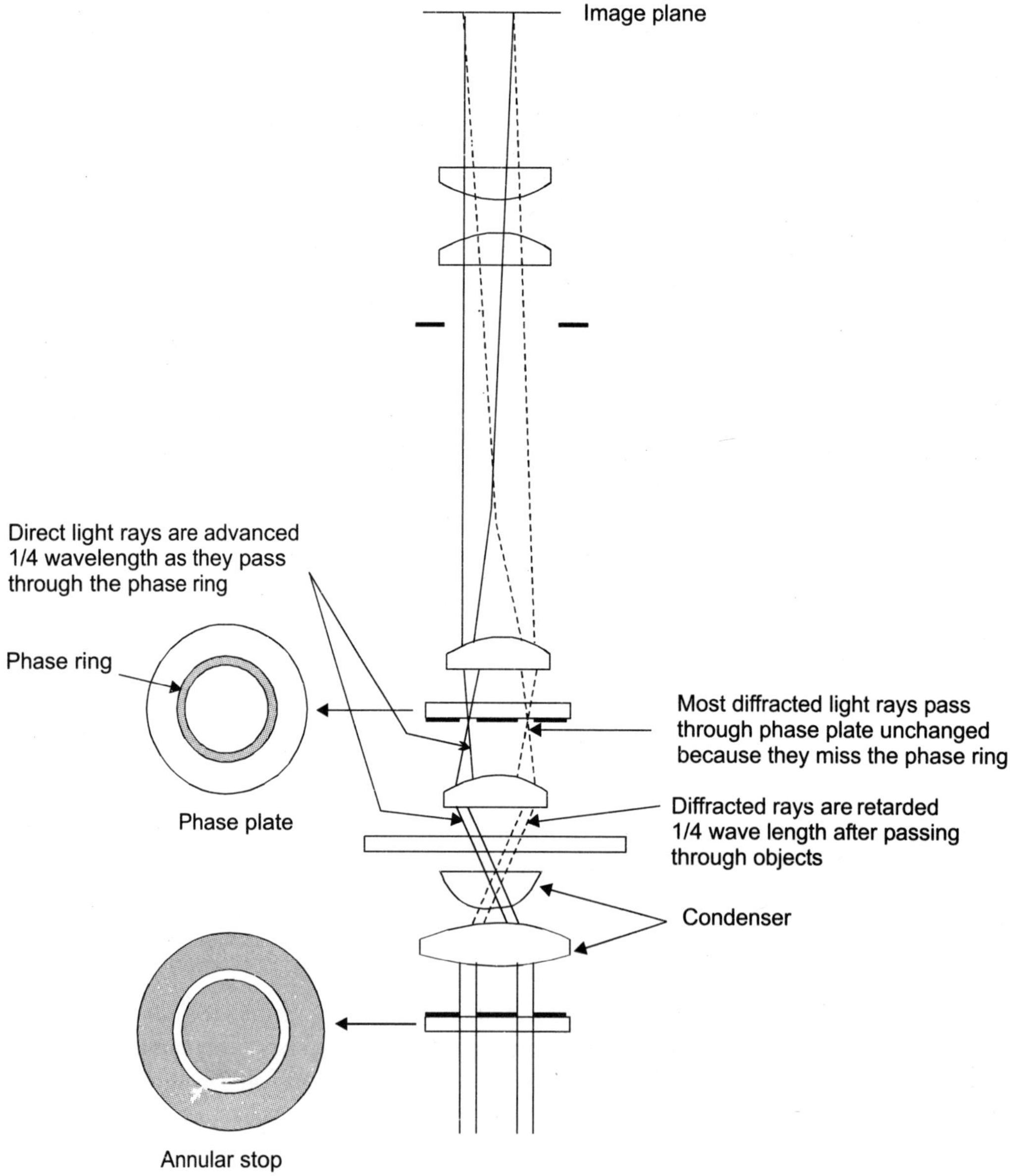

Fig. 2.9 Phase-contrast microscope.

DARK-FIELD (GROUND) MICROSCOPE

In dark-field microscope, objects are seen brightly illuminated against a dark background. It gives an increased resolution and is used to observe microorganisms that cannot be resolved by ordinary microscope. It is used to observe very slender microorganisms such as spirochetes.

Dark field microscope is based on the principle that when a beam of light enters a dark room, it renders minute dust particles floating in the air, which cannot be seen ordinarily in a room with light.

In dark-field microscope, **reflected light** is used instead of transmitted light. A **dark-field condenser** with a **central circular stop** is an essential part of this microscope. By means of this "stop" central rays of light (usually eliminated) are prevented from passing upward, through the object to the eye. The peripheral rays (usually admitted) are refracted by the dark-field condenser to emerge so obliquely from the surface of the slide, so that they do not enter the objective and do not reach the eye when the field is devoid of any object. The field, therefore, appears dark (hence, dark field). When these oblique rays impinge on an object (*e.g.*, a spirochete, dust, bacterium) on the slide, they are reflected upward from the surface of the object into the objective lens. The object is then brightly outlined by the rays reflected from its surface.

Dark field microscope is used

1. to demonstrate *Treponema pallidium*, a causative agent of syphilis, in exudates from ulcers
2. to detect *Leptospira and Borrelia* in clinical materials
3. for *Treponema pallidium* immobilization test
4. as a method of rapid diagnosis of cholera by immobilization test using monospecific antibody
5. to detect thin cell organelles such as flagellae.

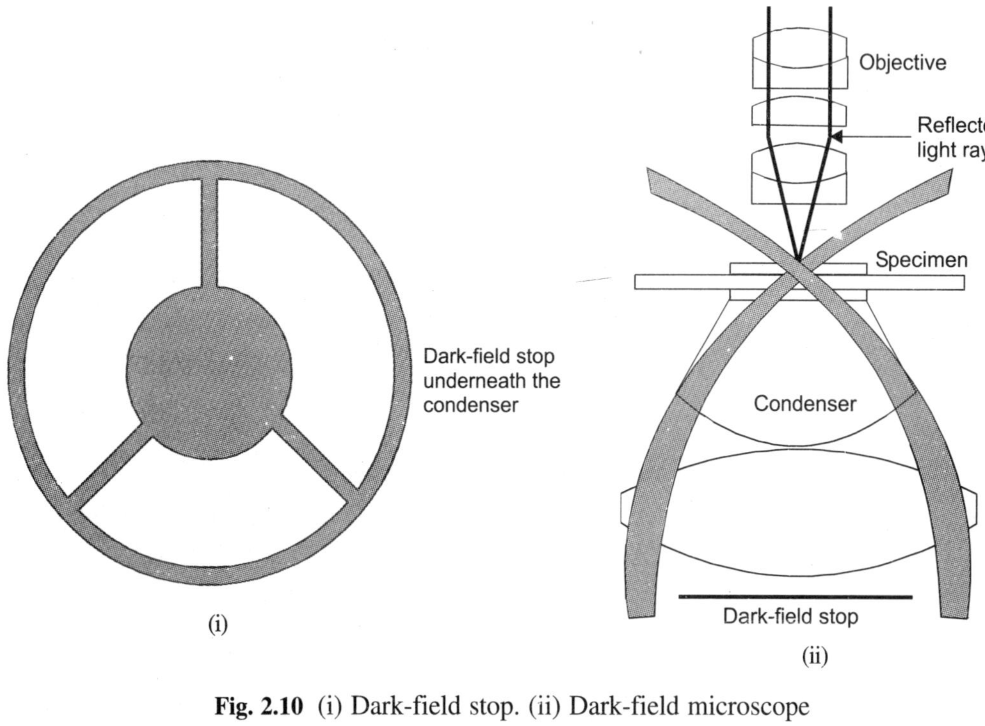

Fig. 2.10 (i) Dark-field stop. (ii) Dark-field microscope

INTERFERENCE MICROSCOPE, STEREO MICROSCOPE, NOMARSKI DIFFERENTIAL INTERFERENCE CONTRAST (NDIC) MICROSCOPE

Interference microscope is based on the same principle as that of phase contrast microscope. A single beam of light passing through the object is made use of in phase contrast microscope, whereas interference microscopes have two beams of light that combine after passing through the specimen. This produces an interference pattern. Interference microscopes are more versatile in comparison with phase contrast microscopes as they have objectives of higher NA and also use color to increase the contrast.

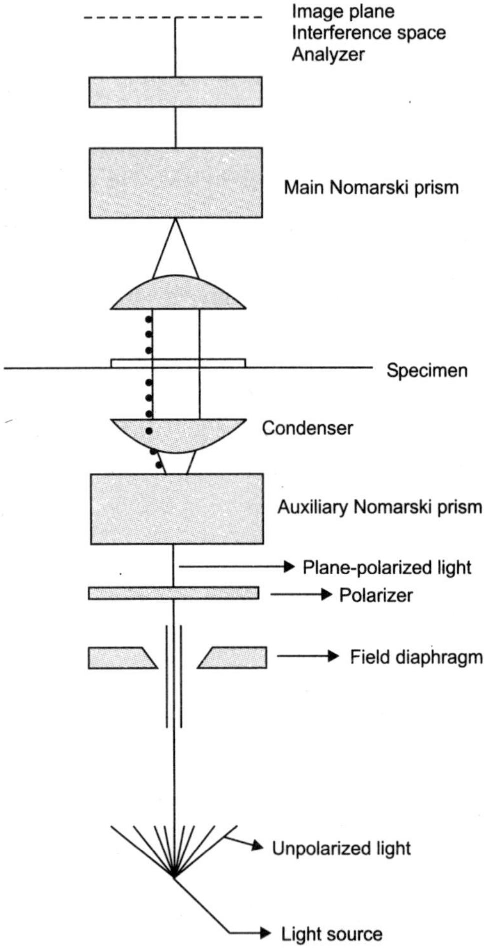

Fig. 2.11 The Nomarski interference microscope

The most frequently used interference microscope is a "**Nomarski Differential Interference Contrast** (NDIC) microscope" which can produce a high contrast, with almost three dimensional image of transparent objects. Different structures of microorganisms appear in different colors that are related to the phase changes in the light passing through each structure and images seen through the interference microscope are normally, brilliantly colored.

Interference microscopes are very useful for qualitative observations of unstained cells, because they produce images with high constrast and striking topographic effect.

FLUORESCENT MICROSCOPE (ULTRAVIOLET MICROSCOPE)

When certain dyes and minerals are exposed to invisible light such as ultra-violet or blue-violet light, they absorb radiant energy, and become excited and release their trapped energy as light, and so become luminous (fluorescent). This phenomenon is known as **Fluorescence,** and it provides a good contrast, which is exploited in fluorescence microscope.

In fluorescence microscope, the specimen is exposed to ultraviolet, violet or blue light and forms an image of the object with the resulting fluorescent light. A mercury vapour arc lamp produces an intense beam of UV light. A special infrared filter or heat filter filters out infrared rays produced by mercury lamp, which may generate heat. This filter does not prevent the transmission of UV and

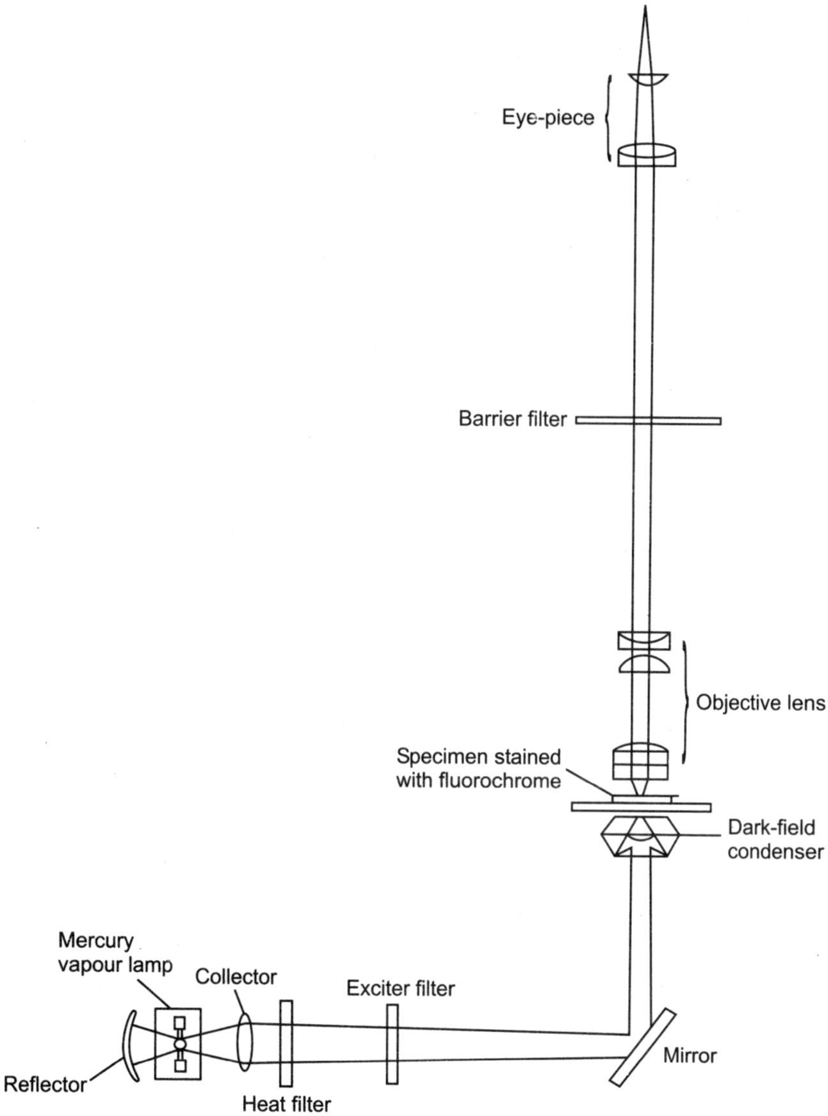

Fig. 2.12 Fluorescence microscopy.

visible rays. The light passes through an exciter filter that transmits only the desired (shorter) wave length by absorbing other light rays. A dark-field condenser provides a black background against which the fluorescent objects glow. A barrier filter, positioned after the objective lenses removes any remaining UV light, which could harm the viewer's eye; or blue and violet light, which would reduce the image's contrast.

The fluorescence microscope has become an essential tool in medical microbiology and microbial ecology. Staining techniques for fluorescent microscopy may be of two types.

1. ***Staining by fluorescent dyes/fluorochroming.*** If tissues, cells or bacteria are stained with a fluorescent dye and are examined under the microscope, with UV light instead of ordinary visible light, they become luminous and are seen as bright objects against a dark background. Moreover, these fluorescent dyes have a selective action for the various microorganisms and cells and for their constituents, which thus become readily recognized and identified. Dyes used for fluorescent staining are Auramine 'O', Acridine orange R, berberine sulphate, primulin, thioflavin S, trypaflavin, thiazo-yellow G, morin, fluorescein isothiocyanate, rhodamine etc. *e.g.,*
   (*i*) Detection of acid fast bacilli (AFB) such as *Mycobacterium tuberculosis* in sputum smears by staining with **Auramine 'O'**, which gives a yellow fluorescence. The procedure is similar to acid-fast stain, but substitutes Auramine 'O' for the carbol fuchsin.
   (*ii*) **Acridine orange R** has an affinity for nucleic acids, fluorescing orange red with RNA and yellow green with DNA, may be used to stain viral nucleic acids in infected cells and tissues.
2. ***Immunofluorescence (IF).*** It combines serology with fluorescent microscope. Fluorescent dyes are chemically combined/coupled/conjugated/labelled with antibodies (labelled antibodies), which can be used to detect antigens of bacteria, viruses, protozoa, fungi in tissue sections, as well as human tissue antigens. This application is known as immunofluorescence or fluorescent-antibody technique. It is of two types:
   (*i*) **Direct Immunofluorescence** or direct fluorescent antibody (FA) technique *e.g*, detection of Rabies antigen in brain impression smears in the diagnosis of rabies
   (*ii*) **Indirect Immunofluorescence** or indirect fluorescent antibody (IFA) technique *e.g.*, fluorescent treponemal antibody (FTA) test in the serodiagnosis of syphilis.

ELECTRON MICROSCOPE

Electron microscope was introduced by Ernst Ruska (1934). There are two basic types of electron microscopes.

1. ***Transmission electron microscope (TEM)*** gives a magnification thousand times greater than light microscope (one million times the actual size).
2. ***Scanning electron microscope (SEM).*** It uses moving electron beam to scan the specimen's surface, generating pictures with depth. Surface details of whole specimen in striking three dimensional way seen.

   Neither TEM nor SEM allows the observation of living specimens.

TRANSMISSION ELECTRON MICROSCOPE (TEM)

In electron microscope, an electron beam is used instead of light to visualize objects. Because of the relatively long wavelength of visible light (about 500 nm), objects than a certain distance (0.2 μm) apart cannot be differentiated (or resolved) by ordinary microscope. Electrons have a much shorter wavelength than ordinary light (about 0.5 nm). Therefore, a microscope utilising electron beams, instead of visible light has a much greater resolving power and is capable of giving distinct images at magnifications of 1,00,000 (one lakh) or more.

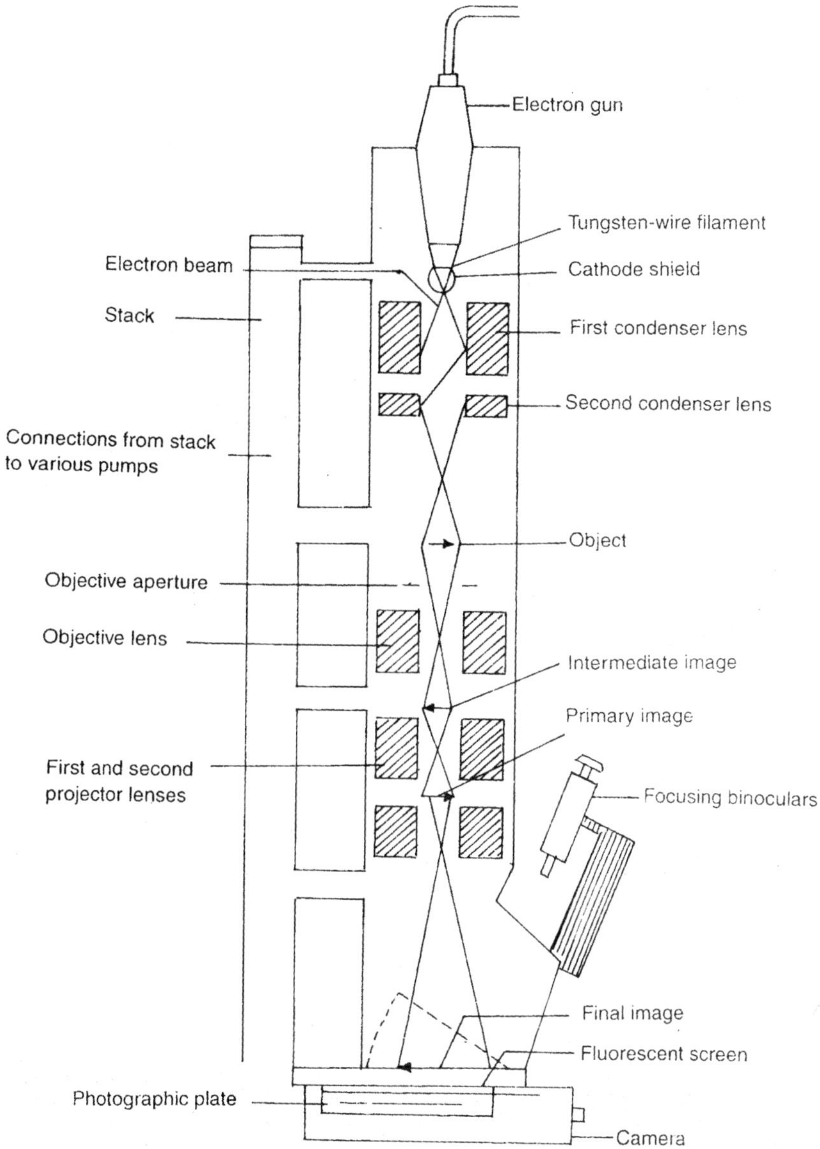

Fig. 2.13 Transmission electron microscope.

Electron source is a tungsten filament. The electrons are focused by circular electromagnets, which take the place of glass lenses, since glass is opaque to electrons. Electrons are focused by varying the strength of the magnetic fields. Three major magnet-lens systems are used, each having a function analogous to its counterpart in an ordinary microscope. The specimen to be examined is placed in a special holder and then introduced into electron microscope between the condenser and objective lenses. Because electron images are not directly visible to the eye, they are viewed on a fluorescent screen or are recorded on photographic plates. Like X-ray pictures, they are electron-shadow graphs (electron micrographs).

Since gas molecules scatter electrons, the interior of electron microscope must be maintained at vacuum. Electrons travel well only in a vacuum. Hence, living organisms cannot be examined; dead and dried objects can be examined.

Final magnifications over 10^5x are possible. Objects invisible with optical microscopes, such as viruses, and certain structures of bacteria etc. become visible by this means. Electron microscope enables the detailed study of bacteria, viruses, cells and tissues.

Specimens for electron microscopy can be stained by various methods:

1. ***Shadow casting with vaporised heavy metals*** produces good contrast and three dimensional effect and helps in studying the surface morphology of the organisms.
2. ***Negative staining with phosphotungstic acid*** helps in studying fine structure by providing a dark background.
3. ***Positive staining with high atomic weight metals*** enhances contrast in ultrathin sections of bacteria, protozoa, and other cells. They combine differently with different cell components and help in the identification of different parts.
4. ***Freeze-etching*** is a process to prepare sections of the specimen without resorting to chemical treatment. The specimen is embedded in a frozen ice block and sectioned. Carbon replicas of the cut surfaces are then prepared which reveal internal structures of the cell.
5. ***Autoradiography.*** A thin specimen exposed to radioactive substance and then coated with photographic emulsion and stored in the dark for some weeks or months. On developing the photographic plate, the image can be seen as grains of silver in the electron microscope to localize a particular celluiar constituent.

SCANNING ELECTRON MICROSCOPE (SEM)

SEM is useful in the study of surface architecture of viruses, bacteria, fungal spores etc. in great detail. However, the resolving power of SEM is much less that of the TEM. The SEM differs from other electron microscopes in producing an image from electrons emitted by an object's surface rather than from transmitted electrons.

Microorganisms are fixed, dehydrated, dried, mounted and coated with a thin layer of metal to prevent the buildup of an electrical charge on the surface and to give a better image.

The SEM scans a narrow, tapered electron beam back and forth over the specimen. Then the surface atoms discharge secondary electrons, which are trapped by a special detector, where they strike a scintillator and generate an electric signal. This signal is sent to a cathode ray tube (CRT) and produces an image like a television picture, which can be viewed or photographed. The image on CRT screen is three-dimensional with great depth of focus.

When the electron beam strikes a raised area, a large number of secondary electrons enter the detector; in contrast, fewer electrons escape a depression in the surface and reach the detector. Thus, raised areas appear lighter on the screen and depressions are darker.

SCANNING TUNNELING MICROSCOPE

It can achieve magnifications of 100 million and allow to view atoms on the surface of a solid. It has a needle like probe, which is lowered toward the specimen surface until its electron cloud just touches that of the surface atoms. If a small voltage is applied between the tip and specimen, electrons flows through a narrow channel in the electron cloud. This tunneling current is very sensitive to distance and will decrease about a thousand-fold if the probe is moved away by a distance equal to the diameter of atom. Therefore, the arrangement of atoms on the specimen surface is determined by moving the probe tip back and forth over the surface, while keeping it at constant height; its motion is recorded and analyzed by a computer to create an accurate three-dimensional image of the surface atoms. It is also used to directly view DNA.

This microscope can examine objects when they are immersed in water, hence useful in studying biological molecules.

It is discovered by Gerd Binning and Heinrich Rohrer (1986), who shared the noble prize.

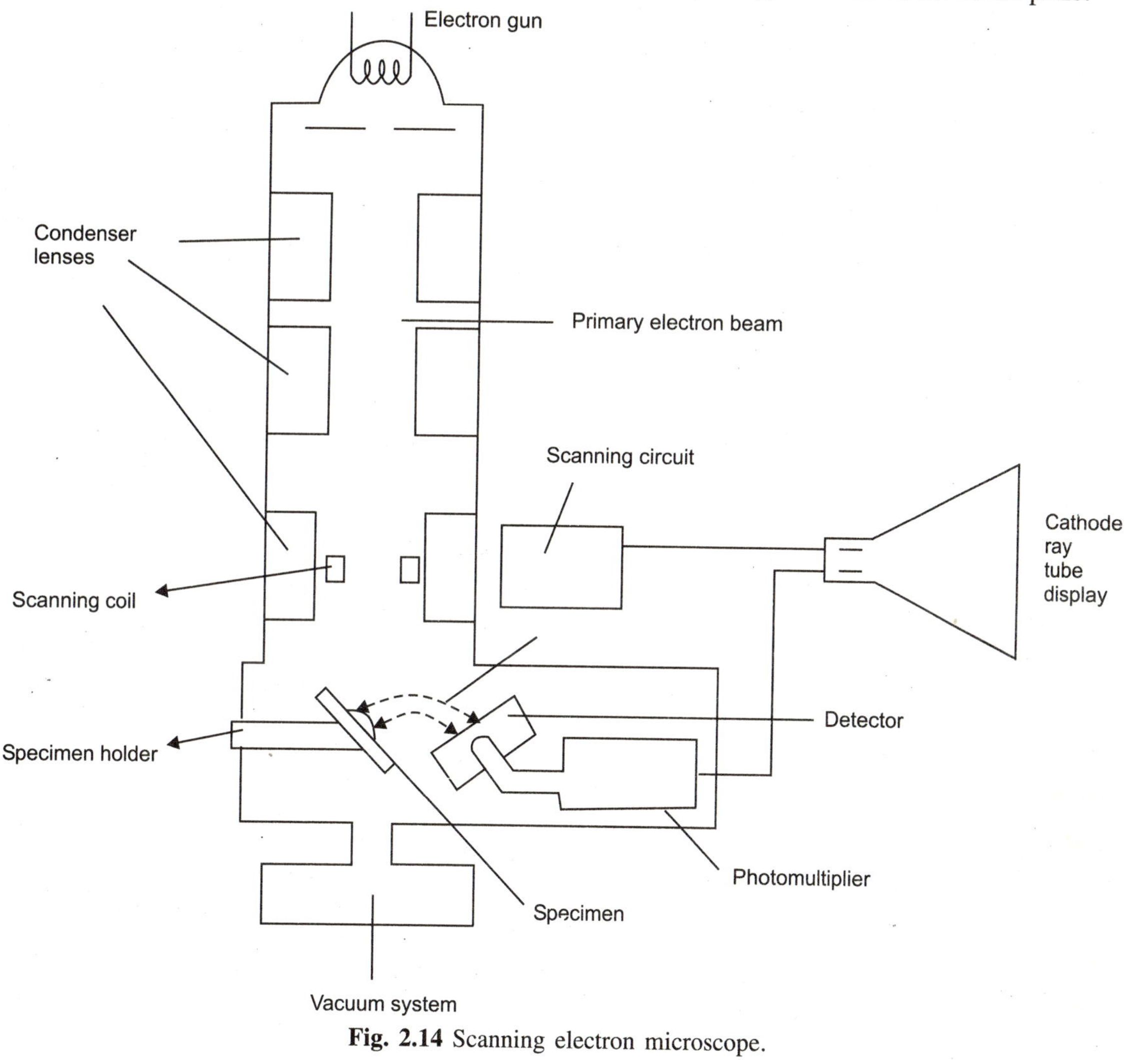

Fig. 2.14 Scanning electron microscope.

IMMUNE ELECTRON MICROSCOPY (IEM)

IEM is a powerful experimental tool available to study cellular structures and their functions. IEM exploits the specific interaction between antigen and antibody to identify and localize proteins via an electron dense label. The label can be either ferritin molecules or colloidal gold particles.

The antibodies, particularly IgG can be bound to the gold particles and used to stain the specimen processed for electron microscope, can be detected as dense or dark particles. These IgG bound gold or ferritin particles are called "immunolabels".

Protein-A from *Staphylococcus aureus*, which binds to Fc portion of the IgG fraction may be labelled with colloidal gold or ferritin molecules to localize the site of the target antigen.

"Pulse-chase" experiments in cellular trafficking of macromolecules can be studied by IEM, which would allow to map the synthetic and processing pathways.

POLARISING MICROSCOPE

Light is assumed to be due to a wave motion, to the upward and downward vibration of ether particles. They move at right angle to the direction of the light. Since, ether is supposed to be an homogenous medium, the particles can move in any direction at right angles to the path of light rays. But when the light rays passes through a Nicol's prism, it becomes polarized and the direction in which the particles move is known as the "optical path". Now, if another prism is introduced in the path of the light rays, it will pass unchanged, provided the optical path of the second prism is in alignment with the former and if the second prism is rotated through 90^0, so that the optical paths are crossed, then the light-rays will be totally reflected out of the second prism. Thus no light will pass through crossed prisms.

In the polarising microscope two prisms are used, one below the condenser and the other above the objective. When both are crossed no light will pass through the upper prism. If a birefringent object, such as cholesterol crystals are placed at the object plane, those light rays that pass through these crystals are absorbed by the upper prism. Because the prisms are no longer crossed for these light rays. The rays that do not pass through these crystals are absorbed by the upper prism. Thus, the crystals will be seen as bright objects against a black (dark) background.

MICROMETRY

Micrometry or microscopic measurements refer to measurement of microorganisms under light microscope. The standard unit in bacteriology is a micrometer or µm, which is 0.001 mm.

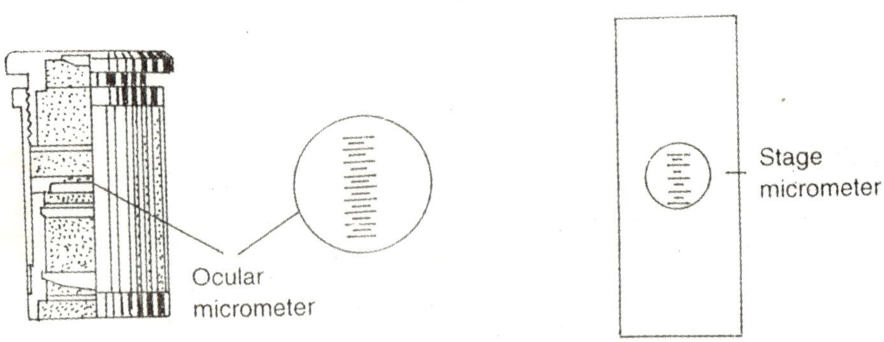

Fig. 2.15 (a) Microscopic measurements

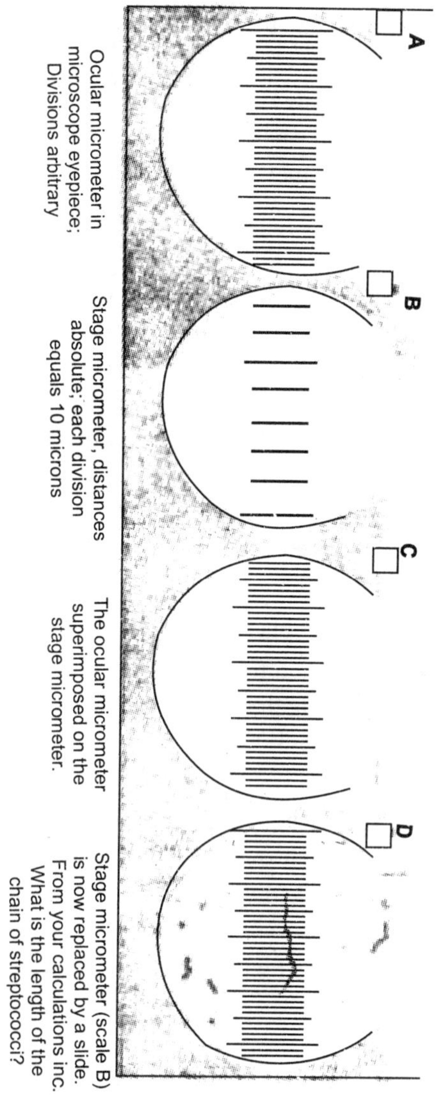

Fig. 2.15 (b) Microscopic measurements.

Standardization of the ocular micrometer and its use in measuring bacterial cells. In measuring a microscopic object an **ocular micrometer** serves as a scale or ruler. This is simply a disc of glass upon which are etched equally spaced divisions. When placed in the ocular, these ruled lines super-impose certain distance markers on the microscope field. The actual distance superimposed may be calibrated by using a stage micrometer at the focal plane of the microscopic field on which parallel lines exactly 0.01 mm apart are etched.

To measure microscopic objects ocular micrometer and stage micrometer are used in conjunction.

Ocular micrometer. It is a small, circular, glass disc on which a graduated scale is engraved. This scale is arbitrary and do not indicate any measurement of length. It usually contains 100 equally spaced divisions, marked 0 to 10 equally. This occular micrometer is placed inside the eye-piece, resting of the field stop.

Eye-piece micrometers may be purchased with the scale permanently in position. These are usually kellner eye-pieces which have a focal plane below their bottom lens. They give a sharp image on the scale and have a greater eye clearance.

Stage micrometer. It is a microscope slide bearing an engraved scale 1 mm in length and graduated at intervals of 0.01 mm (*i.e.*, 10 μm). Thus, each division of stage micrometer is equal to 10 μm.

Calibration. The scale of ocular micrometer is calibrated by comparison with stage micrometer, under different objectives:

1. Insert the ocular micrometer into eye-piece and focus the eye-piece scale.
2. Place the stage micrometer on the microscope stage and centre the scale in the field.
3. With the objective to be used for micrometry, focus the scale of the stage micrometer and move the stage so that the stage and eye-piece scales lie in parallel, side-by-side. When oil immersion objective is used, place oil directly on the stage-micrometer scale.
4. Count the number of divisions on the eye-piece scale that correspond to a definite number in the stage scale.

From knowledge, that each stage scale division is 0.01 mm (or 10 μm), calculate the length measured by an eye-piece scale division when used with the chosen objective.

Measurement

1. Remove the stage micrometer and replace it with a slide bearing the specimen to be studied.
2. Focus the specimen with the objective for which the calibration was done and count the number of divisions of the eye-piece scale that just cover the object to be measured. The tube length should not be altered between calibration and measurement.

Calculation

Calculate the measurement of the object as in the following example.

If with oil immersion objective 10 stage scale divisions (*i.e.*, 10 × 10 μm) are found equal to 91 eye-piece scale divisions, each eye-piece scale division will correspond to 100/90 μm *i.e.*, 1.1 μm, in the field of the oil immersion objective.

If then, the length of a bacterium viewed with the same eye-piece and objective is found to equal 3.5 eye-piece divisions, the length of the bacterium would be 3.5 × 1.1 μm = 3.85 μm.

PHOTOMICROGRAPHY

Photography of microorganisms under microscope is necessary for recording, teaching and for publications. In teaching, color photographs and color transparencies are invariably used. Photography is also used in micrometry to determine the size of cells or organisms under study.

There are many versions of photomicrographic apparatus in the market usually allowing routine microscopy to be undertaken with the camera in position. Modern photomicrographic apparatus contains a fixed photoelectric cell so that the light intensity can be measured and the exposure set automatically.

In photomicrography, following precautions have to be observed:

1. Smears/sections must be free of all fixation, cutting and staining artefacts.
2. Staining should be of good contrast for color photography. Contrast may be improved in black and white photomicrography by the use of contrast filters.

3. Flat-field apochromatic objectives and aplanatic condenser will give superior results.
4. The field should be evenly illuminated and the microscope should be accurately adjusted.
5. Tungsten light sources (run at the correct voltage) are preferred for color photography.

QUESTIONS

Essay Type Questions

1. Give a list of microscopes used in microbiology and explain with a neat sketch the working principle of fluorescence microscope.
2. Briefly describe the working principles of operation and importance of electron microscope.
3. Describe the working principles of light microscope and phase-contrast microscope.
4. Bring out the differences between the working principles of a light microscope and an electron microscope.
5. Describe the principles involved in the phase-contrast microscope and electron microscope.
6. Explain the principles of photography and its applications.
7. Describe the working principles of stereomicroscope and fluorescence microscope.

Short Notes

1. Compound microscope/bright-field microscope.
2. Magnification.
3. Numerical aperture/NA.
4. Resolution.
5. Limit of resolution.
6. Definition.
7. Aberrations.
8. Spherical aberration.
9. Chromatic aberration.
10. Oil immersion lens.
11. Care and use of a microscope.
12. Dark-field microscope.
13. NDIC microscope.
14. Transmission electron microscope (TEM).
15. Scanning electron microscope (SEM)
16. Immune electron microscope (IEM).
17. Polarising microscope.
18. Micrometry.
19. Phase contrast microscope.
20. Photomicrography.

3

Staining Methods

- *Introduction*
- *Examination of living bacteria in unstained condition*
  - *– Wet coverslip preparation*
  - *– Hanging drop experiment*
- *Terms used in staining*
- *Smear preparation*
- *Bacteriological staining methods (Examination of dead bacteria in stained condition)*
  - *– Simple staining*
  - *– Differential stains*
    - *– Gram's staining*
    - *– Acid-fast (Ziehl-Neelsen's) staining*
      - *– Kinyoun's modification*
      - *– Gabbet's (cold acid-fast) staining*
      - *– Cold acid-fast staining for Cryptosporidium*
      - *– Fluorochrome staining for tubercle bacilli*
  - *– Silver impregnation methods*
    - *– Negative staining (background staining)*
  - *– Stains to demonstrate volutin granules or to stain diphtheria bacilli*
    - *– Albert's stain*
    - *– Neisser's stain*
    - *– Ponder's stain*
    - *– Pugh's stain*
  - *– Staining of spores*
    - *– Modified acid-fast stain*
    - *– Malachite green stain*
    - *– Staining of capsules*
  - *– Negative staining*
    - *– Wet film India ink method*
    - *– Positive staining by dry-film method*
    - *– Hiss stain*
    - *– Capsule swelling (Quellung) reaction – Staining of flagellae*
    - *– Leifson method*
  - *– Vital staining and supravital staining*
  - *– Staining of fungi in wet mounts*
  - *– Lactophenol cotton blue stain.*

INTRODUCTION

The morphological features of an organism can be studied by examining them under microscope by using unstained and stained preparations.

EXAMINATION OF LIVING BACTERIA IN UNSTAINED CONDITION

The unstained preparations of living organisms can be studied by any one of the following methods:

1. Wet coverslip preparation
2. Hanging drop preparation
3. Phase contrast microscope
4. Dark ground microscope.

Wet coverslip preparation

A small drop of material to be examined is taken on a clear glass slide and covered with a coverslip, without allowing air bubbles to form. Examined under low and high dry power objectives.

Uses : 1. Examination of urinary sediment, cerebrospinal fluid (CSF), other body fluids etc., for pus cells, crystals, casts and bacteria.

2. Examination of vaginal secretions for presence of motile protozoan parasites like *Trichomonas vaginalis*.

3. Examination of feces in saline and iodine preparations for protozoans and helminthic eggs.

Hanging drop preparation

This experiment is done to demonstrate motility and to study morphology of bacteria.

***Requirements* :**
1. A clean cavity (depression) slide
2. A clean coverslip
3. Young broth culture
4. Wire loop
5. Bunsen burner/spirit lamp
6. Microscope.

***Procedure*:**

1. Apply a small amount of vaseline/grease on four corners of the coverslip.
2. Place drop of culture using the sterile wire loop on the centre of the coverslip.
3. Invert the cavity slide over the coverslip so that the drop of the culture is in the center of the cavity; press it lightly, so that the coverslip adheres to the vaseline ring.
4. Quickly and carefully turn the slide over, so that the coverslip is upper most, and a drop hanging from the coverslip into the cavity.
5. Focus the edge of the drop under dry low power objective, after reducing the light intensity (by partial closing of iris diaphragm), so that the edge of the drop is exactly in the center of the microscopic field. Then turnover to high dry power objective (45X) to observe the motility and morphology of bacteria. Their shape, approximate size and general structure can be observed (Fig. 3.1).

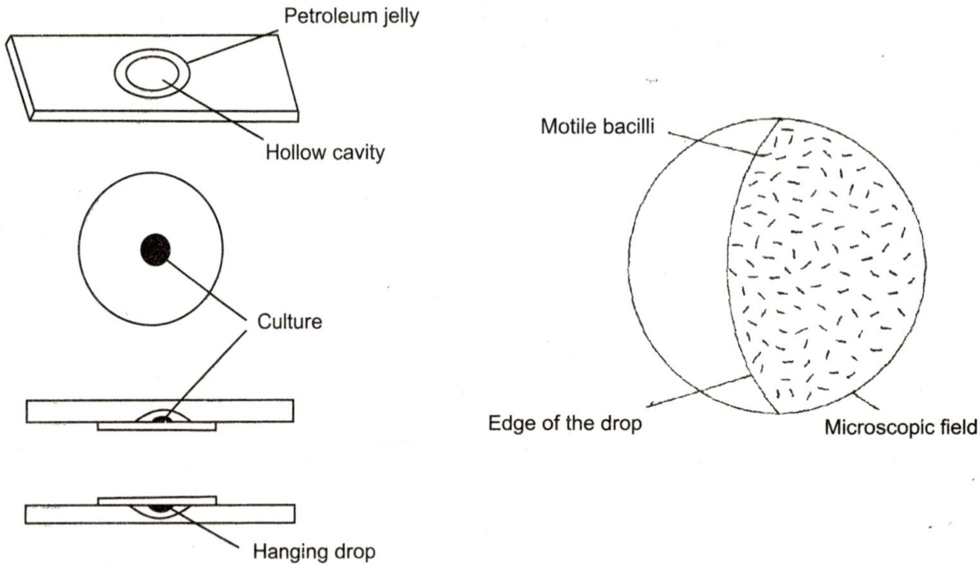

Fig. 3.1. (*a*) The hanging drop technique. (*b*) Hanging drop preparation.

The edge of the drop is focussed to observe motility and morphology for the following reasons:

1. The concentration of the organisms is more at the edge, because – (*a*) aerobic organisms tend to move towards the edge, (*b*) surface tension is less at the edge, hence the concentration of organism is more.

2. Density is less at the edge of the drop, hence the contrast is better, so that organisms are clearly visible. The differences in refractive index of light rays that pass through glass slide and liquid gives a better contrast at the edge.

It is essential to differentiate between true motility and false motility. In true motility, there is a displacement of position *i.e.,* the organism moves from one place to another in different directions. The false motility, also known as brownian movement is an oscillatory vibration, exhibited by both living and non-living bodies, due to water convection currents.

Apart from hanging drop experiment, motility can also be demonstrated by:

(*i*) Macroscopic methods:

1. Noting swarming growth on agar medium
2. Use of semi-solid agar (0.2 % agar) medium
3. Craigie's tube or 'U' shaped tube

(*ii*) Microscopic methods:

1. Dark ground microscopy
2. Phase contrast microscopy

(*iii*) Demonstration of flagellae.

Some organisms are motile at one temperature and nonmotile at another temperature *e.g.*,

1. *Yersinia enterocolitica* is motile at 22°C and non-motile at 37°C.
2. *Listeria monocytogenes* is motile at 25°C and non-motile at 37°C.

Table 3.1 Motile and non-motile organisms.

Motile	*Non-motile*
Camplylobacter jejuni	*Flavobacterium*
Enterobacter	*Klebsiella*
Escherichia coli	*Shigella*
Helicobacter pylori	*Yersinia pestis*
Legionella	
Proteus	
Pseudomonas	
Salmonella	(All cocci are non motile except
Serratia	*Rhodococcus*)
Spirillum	
Vibrio cholerae	
Yersinia enterocolitica	
Yersinia pseudotuberculosis	
Clostridium tetani	

TERMS USED IN STAINING

Direct or simple staining. The organism or tissue is stained by immersion in the stain.

Indirect staining. The organism or tissue is stained only with the aid of a mordant.

Primary stain. The initial stain used to stain the bacteria or the stain retained by bacteria after decolorisation.

Mordant. The link or anchor between organism (or tissue) and stain.

Some material will not stain until the combination of stain and mordant has formed a compound, which is capable of attaching itself firmly to the organism or tissue *e.g.,* Gention violet dye-Iodine complex in Gram's staining.

Decolorising agent. Decolorising agent is one which removes the dye from the bacterial cell wall *e.g.,* acetone, absolute alcohol or a mixture of acetone and alcohol.

Counter stain. It is a secondary stain used to stain decolorised bacteria (Gram negative bacteria) *e.g.,* Safranine, neutral red, dilute carbol fuchsin; or to provide a colored background as in ZN staining *e.g.,* Methylene blue, Malachite green, picric acid.

Fixative. Fixes the smear (film) to the slide. Fixative can be physical (heating gently) or chemical (methanol).

Specific stains. Stains which act only on certain constituents of cells or tissues leaving other remaining elements virtually unstained.

Accentuators. Substances which increase the staining power and selectivity of a stain. They differ from mordants as they do not combine with the dye.

SMEAR PREPARATION (or) METHODS OF MAKING FILM

Before staining, the material concerned must be suitably prepared. This involves making slides of films, smears or sections.

Slides. The slides and coverslips used should be clean and grease-free; they should be boiled in a detergent solution for 5 to 10 minutes, scrubbed, rinsed well and stored in alcohol until required.

Films/Smears. Films are made either by spreading a loopful of liquid (*e.g.,* broth culture, sputum, pus, urine etc.) thinly on a slide, or, if the sample is a bacterial culture on agar, by emulsifying a very small portion of the colony in a drop of water or physiological saline (normal saline) on the slide. It is important that films should be thin. They may be allowed to dry in air, or drying may be accelerated by holding the slides, high above a bunsen flame. The film should then be fixed by passing the slide, slowly through the flame 2 to 3 times.

Sections. The tissue is first fixed, then dehydrated by immersion in ethanol solution containing successively less amounts of water, and finally embedded in paraffin. Sections are cut, flattened on warm water, floated onto slides and allowed to dry.

BACTERIOLOGICAL STAINING METHODS (Examination of dead bacteria in stained condition)

Staining is usually effected by the application of an aqueous (watery) solution or an alcoholic solution of the dye.

The staining procedures are broadly divided into:

1. Simple staining
2. Differential staining
3. Negative staining or background staining
4. Fluorescent staining
5. Impregnation methods
6. Special stains.

1. Simple staining

A single stain is used in simple staining. Simple stains include basic aniline dyes such as methylene blue, gention violet, carbol fuchsin (basic fuchsin), safranine.

The bacterial suspension is smeared on the surface of the slide, fixed by gentle heating and flooded with a dye solution (*e.g.,* methylene blue) for about one minute. The dye is washed off with water and the slide blotted dry.

Simple stains shows the presence of microorganisms and the cells in exudates. But, different bacteria take up the same color, as a single dye is used for staining (Fig. 3.2).

Uses:

1. For the examination of cerebrospinal fluid (CSF) in the diagnosis of pyogenic meningitis *e.g., Hemophilus influenza* meningitis.

2. To demonstrate *Yersinia pestis* (plague bacillus) in pus or aspirated fluid.

***Advantages*:**

1. Simple to perform
2. Margins of bacteria are seen clearly in contrast to other stains.

***Disadvantages*:**

1. Morphology of the bacteria cannot be made out as same color is taken up by the bacteria.
2. Cannot differentiate between Gram positive and Gram negative bacteria and hence antibiotic sensitivity cannot be made out.

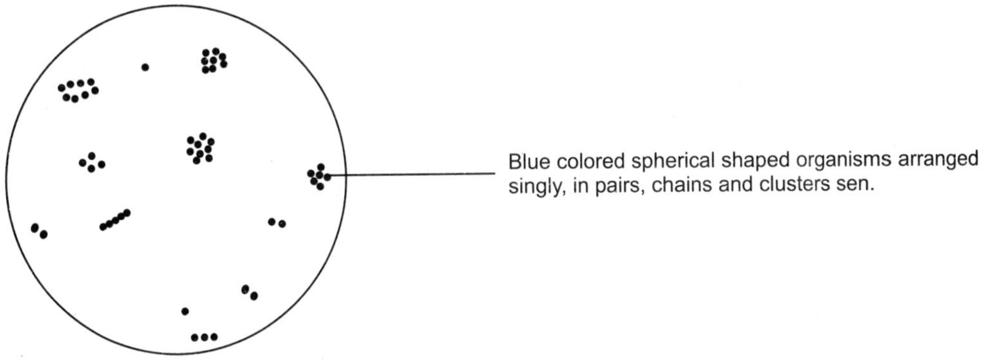

Fig. 3.2 Simple staining with methylene blue.

Loeffler's methylene blue. Of the many preparations of methylene blue dye, Loeffler's methylene blue is most useful. It is made of methylene blue solution saturated in alcohol, dissolved in KOH (0.01 % in distilled water). It shows the characteristic morphology of pus cells, lymphocytes and other cells more clearly than Gram's or ZN stainings. Hence, it is widely used as a counterstain in Acid-fast (ZN) staining.

Polychrome methylene blue. This stain is prepared by allowing Loeffler's methylene blue to "ripen" for 12 months in half-filled bottles by shaking and aeration, during which time, the methylene blue slowly oxidizes to give a purple compound, that gives the stain its polychrome properties. It may be ripened quickly by the addition of 1% potassium carbonate.

***Uses*:** The stain is used to demonstrate Mc Fadyean's reaction for the identification of anthrax bacilli in blood films.

2. Differential stains

Differential staining makes possible differentiating different types of bacteria or different parts of the same cell by differences in the staining pattern. Usually combinations of stains are used.

Differential stains are: Gram's staining, ZN staining.

***Gram's staining*.** Gram's staining is the most widely used differential staining in microbiology, first developed by Hans Christian Gram (1884), a Danish physician. Gram's stain differentiates bacteria into two broad groups – Gram positive bacteria and Gram negative bacteria.

***Procedure*:**

Though, there are several variations of the Gram's staining, the basic principle is the same.

1. Primary staining of the smear with an aniline dye such as Gention violet (crystal violet/methyl violet) for 1-2 minutes (Gention violet is a mixture of crystal violet and methyl violet dyes).

2. Pour off the excess stain, then wash off the rest with Gram's iodine.

Cover the smear with fresh Gram's iodine solution, and allow to act for 1 minute. Iodine acts as a mordant.

3. Pour off the iodine and hold the slide at a steep slope. Then pour decolorising agent, such as acetone or alcohol or a misxture of acetone and alcohal or aniline, slowly drop-wise from one end of the slide. The purple color starts running off. This decolorisation is carried on for a few seconds (2-3 seconds) only.

4. Counterstaining with a dye of contrasting color such as saffranine, dilute carbol fuchsin or neutral red for 30 seconds.

Gram positive bacteria are those that take up and retain Gention violet and resist decolorisation, appearing violet/purple.

Gram negative bacteria are those that are decolorised completely and take up saffranine counter-stain, appearing red/pink (Fig. 3.3).

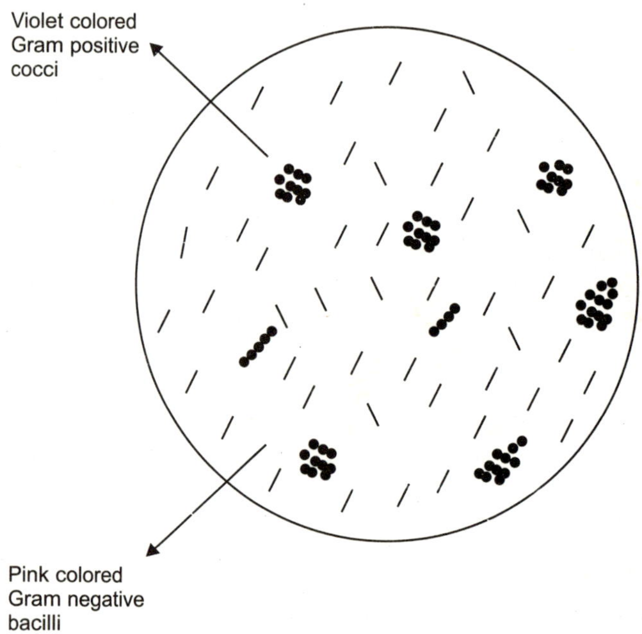

Fig. 3.3 Gram's stain.

Mechanism of Gram's reaction. Many theories have been postulated to explain the mechanism of Gram's reaction. They are as follows:

1. Gram positive bacteria have a more acidic protoplasm (pH 2-3) and retain basic dye (crystal violet) more strongly than Gram negative bacteria (pH 4-5).

2. When iodine is added to crystal violet, a dye-iodine complex is formed. Gram's reaction may be related to the chemical composition of cell walls and permeability differences in the two groups of bacteria, towards dye-iodine complex.

In Gram positive bacteria, the cell walls are thicker, have numerous teichoic acid cross-linkages and less lipids. They get dehydrated causing decreased porosity in the cell walls, trapping dye-iodine complex, during treatment with acetone/alcohol; appearing violet (Gram positive).

Gram negative bacterial cell walls are thinner, have a smaller amount of peptidoglycan, less extensively cross-linked and contain a high percentage of lipids. They dissolve during treatment with acetone/alcohol, forming larger pores in the cell wall, causing out-flow of dye-iodine complex and take up counter stain, thus appearing red/pink (Gram negative).

3. It has been found that Gram positivity depends on the integrity of cell wall and presence of specific Magnesium-ribonucleate-protein complex.

Thus, Gram positive bacteria may become Gram negative, if the cell is ageing, mechanically ruptured or by the action of ribonuclease.

Table 3.2 Gram positive and gram negative bacteria

Gram positive bacteria		***Gram negative bacteria***	
COCCI	– *Staphylococcus*	COCCI	– *Neisseria*
	– *Streptococcus*		
BACILLI	– *Corynebacterium*	BACILLI	
	– *Lactobacillus*		(*a*) Enterobacteria
	– *Bacillus*		– *Escherichia coli*
	– *Clostridium*		– *Klebsiella*
	– *Mycobacterium*		– *Salmonella*
			– *Shigella*
			– *Proteus*
			– *Yersinia*
(Some, Mycobacteria, including *Mycobacterium tuberculosis* are stained only faintly or not at all by Gram's method)			(*b*) *Pseudomonas*
			(*c*) *Vibrio*
			(*d*) Parvobacteria
			– *Hemophilus*
			– *Bordetella*
			– *Brucella*
			(*e*) *Bacteroides*

Differential qualities of Gram positive and Gram negative bacteria. Gram reaction is one manifestation of fundamental differences in the properties of Gram positive and Gram negative bacteria.

1. Composition of their cell well is different.
2. Gram positive bacteria have less synthetic ability and so more complex nutritional requirements.

3. Exotoxins are produced mainly by Gram positive bacteria. A few Gram negative bacilli may produce exotoxins e.g., *Vibrio cholera*, ETEC (Enterotoxigenic *E. coli*), *Shigella shiga*. In contrast, endotoxins are produced by Gram negative bacteria.

4. Gram positive organisms are more resistant to mechanical damage.

5. The two groups show different spectra of susceptibility to chemotherapeutic agents, disinfectants, dyes, simple chemicals and enzymes.

Relationship between Gram's reaction of bacteria and their antibiotic susceptibility.

1. Gram positive bacterial possess "penicillin-binding proteins (PBP)", some of which are transpeptidation enzymes. Penicillins can bind to this and inhibit cell wall formation. Gram negative bacteria do not possess these PBPs.

2. Bacterial possess a rigid cell wall, which protects the bacterium against high internal osmotic pressure. This internal osmotic pressure is 3 to 5 times greater in Gram positive than in Gram negative bacteria.

3. Polymyxins act only on Gram negative cells by binding to cell membrane and altering their permeability, so that macromolecules and ions escape from the cell leading to the death of the cell.

Antibiotics active against Gram positive bacteria are: Penicillin, methicillin, cloxacillin, erythromycin, vancomycin, clindamycin, lincomycin, bacitracin etc.

Antibiotics active against Gram negative bacteria are: Aminoglycosides, fluoroquinolenes (ciprofloxacin, norfloxacin, nalidixic acid).

Antibiotics active against Gram positive and Gram negative bacteria are: Tetracycline, chloramphenicol, ampicillin, cephalosporins.

Acid-fast staining/Ziehl-Neelsen's (ZN) staining

Acid-fast staining was first developed by Paul Ehrlich (1882) and later modified by Ziehl and Neelsen (1885).

***Principle*:** Some bacteria, such as mycobacteria are resistant to aniline dyes and the dye cannot penetrate into bacilli, because their surface is coated with a unsaponifiable wax. However, by using a strong solution of carbol fuchsin, that contains phenol (acts as a mordant), and by application of heat, the dye can be made to penetrate the bacillus. Once stained, they cannot be decolorised even with strong mineral acids. Hence, they are called **Acid-fast Bacilli (AFB)**. Some of them are also not decolorised by alcohol. Therefore, they are called as "**Alcohol-fast**".

Acid fastness is due to the presence of fatty acids, lipids and higher alcohols. A saponifiable wax, called mycolic acid (long chain fatty acid) is present in all Acid-fast bacilli. Acid-fastness is lost when the tubercle bacilli are exposed to Isoniazid (INH), but not by other drugs.

***Procedure*:** 1. Flood the smear with strong carbol fuchsin solution and heat the slide from below, intermittently, gently, until steam rises for 3 to 5 minutes. Care should be taken to see that the stain neither boils nor evaporates; then wash well with water.

2. Decolorize with:

(*a*) 20% sulphuric acid for about 1 minute, wash the slide and pour on fresh acid. Repeat this procedure several times (5 to 6 times atleast), each time for 1 minute, till the red color is changed to yellowish brown. 20% H_2SO_4 is used, when it is desired to stain all AFB.

(*b*) 3% Hydrochloric acid in 95% ethanol, if only tubercle bacilli is to be shown. Other mycobacteria are only acid-fast, whereas *Mycobacterium tuberculosis* is both acid and alcohol-fast.

(*c*) 5% sulphuric acid, to show the leprae bacilli (*Mycobacterium leprae*) in skin clippings or smears or sections.

3. Counterstain with Loeffler's methylene blue or malachite green or picric acid for 15 to 20 seconds.

Wash and blot dry, using blotting paper and examine under oil immersion lens of microscope (Fig. 3.4).

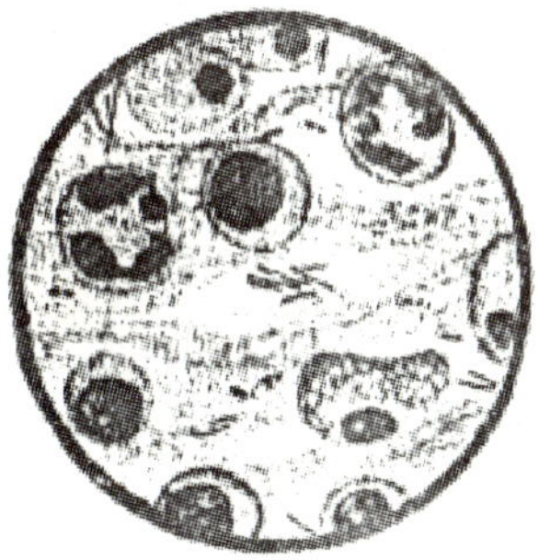

Pink coloured tubercle bacilli in sputum
smear against a blue back ground

Fig. 3.4 Ziehl-Neelsen's Staining (Pink colored tubercle bacilli in sputum).

Acid-fast bacilli appear bright pink, while other organisms, tissue cells and debris are stained blue (methylene blue) or green (malachite green) or yellow (picric acid) according to the counterstain used.

Acid-fast organisms **:**

1. All mycobacteria are acid-fast *e.g., Mycobacterium tuberculosis, Mycobacterium bovis, Mycobacterium leprae,* atypical mycobacteria.

2. *Nocardia asteroides, Nocardia braziliensis.*

3. *Cryptosporidium*-a protozoan coccidian parasite, which causes opportunistic infections in AIDS, is acid-fast.

4. Bacterial spores are weakly acid-fast.

Kinyoun's modification of acid-fast staining. Kinyoun's modification uses higher concentration of phenol in carbol fuchsin (primary stain) stain, hence heating is not required for the staining of AFB.

Gabbet's stain/cold acid-fast staining. Smears are flooded with carbol fuchsin-phenol stain, and allowed to stand at room temperature for 10 minutes. Longer exposure favours uniform penetration of the dye through the cell wall. Then washed in running water and counterstained with Gabbet's methylene blue for 2 minutes, and subsequently washed in tap water and air dried.

Gabbet's method differs from ZN method in that decolorisation and counterstaining are done in a single step using a mixure of H_2SO_4 and 2% methylene blue.

Cold acid-fast staining for Cryptosporidium. *Cryptosporidium* an acid-fast protozoan coccidian parasite causes diarrhoea, as an opportunist infection, paraticularly in AIDS cases. The oocysts of *Cryptosporidium* in feces smears are demonstrated by cold acid-fast staining.

Fecal smears are stained with carbol fuchsin for 5-10 minutes, Wash with water. For decolorisation 1% HCl-ethanol is used until color faded. Wash with water and counter stain with 0.25% methylene blue or malachite green for 30 seconds and wash with water.

Cryptosporidium oocysts appear as bright pink spherules against a blue or green background.

Fluorochrome staining for tubercle bacilli. Auramine 'O' dye can be substituted for carbol fuchsin in the Ziehl-Neelsen method, so that tubercle bacilli fluoresce and become easier to detect. Heating is unnecessary.

1. Stain a thin heat-fixed sputum smear with the Auramine solution for 15 minutes at room temperature.
2. Wash off with tap water.
3. Cover the slide with acid-alcohol decolorizing solution for 5 minutes.
4. Wash off with tap water and rinse well.
5. Cover the slide with potassium permanganate solution for 30 seconds.
6. Wash well with tap water. Dry in air, do not use blotting paper.
7. Examine the slide by fluorescence microscope. Tubercle bacilli are seen as yellow luminous rods in a dark field.

Silver impregnation method

Impregnation is done by precipitating a solution of metallic salts, such as silver salts, on the surface of organisms.

Impregnation methods are used to demonstrate very slender bacteria such as spirochetes and bacterial flagellae that are too thin to be seen under ordinary microscope. These slender organisms and thin flagellae are made thicker by coating or impregnating silver salts on their surface, so that they become visible under ordinary microscope.

Negative staining/background staining

Negative stains act by coloring the background and leaving the bacteria as clear objects. Negative staining is used to demonstrate bacterial capsules and very slender bacteria such as spirochetes.

In negative staining, bacteria are mixed with India Ink or Nigrosin and spread on a glass slide and examined under microscope. Bacterial capsules are seen unstained, as bright halos against a uniformly blackstained background (Fig. 3.5).

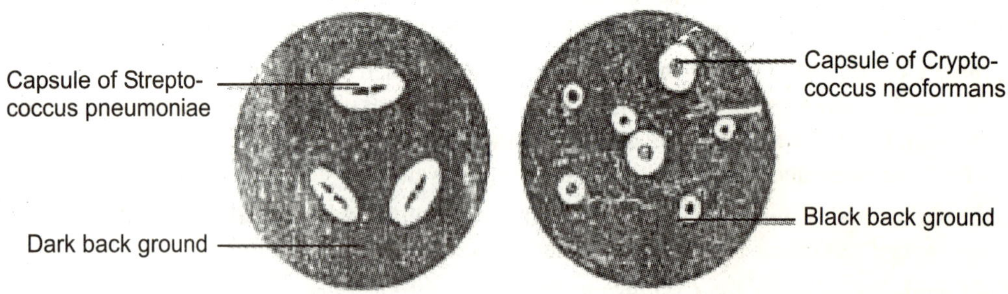

Fig. 3.5. Negative staining (Indian ink/Nigrosin preparation)

In negative staining, either wet films or dry films can be prepared. Dry film method is used for permanent preparations.

Special stains for Corynebacterium diphtheriae, stains to demonstrate metachromatic granules

Certain bacilli possess volutin granules in the protoplasm which aid in the identification of diphtheria bacilli. Several special and differential stains are used to stain diphtheria bacilli and to demonstrate their metachromatic granules.

1. Albert's stain
2. Neisser's stain
3. Ponder's stain
4. Pugh's stain.

1. Albert's stain

1. Prepare a thin smear of throat swab from a patient or culture, dry it.
2. Stain with Albert's stain (Albert's solution A) for 3 to 5 minutes.
3. Wash with a few drops of Albert's iodine.
4. Stain with Albert's iodine (Albert's solution B) for 1 to 2 minutes.

Wash with water and blot dry. Observe under the oil-immersion objective.

The metachromatic (volutin) granules of *Corynebacterium diphtheriae* stain bluish-black and the bacterial protoplasm green.

2. Neisser's stain

1. Stain the smear with Neisser's methylene blue for 3 minutes.
2. Wash off with dilute iodine and leave some of this solution on the slide for 1 minute.
3. Wash in water.
4. Counterstain with neutral red solution for 3 minutes.

Wash in water and dry. Observe under oil immersion lens. By this method the bacilli exhibit deep blue granules and the bacterial protoplasm takes pink color.

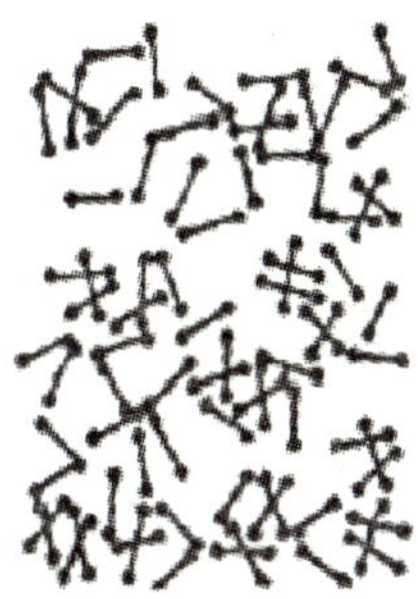

Fig. 3.6. Albert's stain.

3. Ponder's stain

1. Stain the smear with Ponder's stain for 1-2 minutes.
2. Wash with water and blot dry. Examine under oil immersion objective.

The volutin granules stain dark blue, whereas the bacillus pale blue.

4. Pugh's stain.

1. Stain the smear with Pugh's stain (toluidine blue) for 2 to 3 minutes.
2. Wash with water and blot dry. Examine under oil immersion objective. The volutin granules stain reddish purple and the remainder of the organism light blue.

Staining (or demonstration) of spores.

Spores can be demonstrated by several methods.

1. In unstained wet films, spores may be seen as dark refractile bodies.

2. If spore-bearing organisms are stained with ordinary dyes or simple stains or by Gram's stain, the body of the bacillus is deeply colored, whereas the spore is unstained and appears as a clear area in the organism.

Modified acid-fast stain.

1. Prepare thin smears of spore-bearing organisms dry and fix with minimum heating.

2. Stain with strong carbol fuchsin (Ziehl-Neelsen's) solution for 3-5 minutes, with intermittent heating till fumes arise and wash with water.

3. Decolorise with 0.25% or 0.5% sulphuric acid for one to several minutes (decolorisation can also be done by 2% solution of nitric acid in absolute alcohol; the slide is dipped once rapidly in the solution and immediately washed in water).

4. Wash with water.

5. Counterstain with 1% aqueous methylene blue for 3 minutes.

6. Wash in water, blot and dry. Examine under the oil immersion lens.

The spores are stained bright red and the protoplasm of the bacilli blue.

(**Note:** Bacteria are decolorised more readily than those of others and lipid inclusion granules may stain dark red, appearing like spherical spores).

Malachite green stain (schaeffer and fulton method)

1. Prepare the smears of spore bearing organisms dry and fix with minimum heating.

2. Place the slide over a beaker of boiling water, resting it on the rim with the bacterial film upper most.

3. When large droplets have condensed on the underside of the slide, flood it with 5% aqueous solution of malachite green and leave to act for 1 minute, while the water continues to boil.

4. Wash in water.

5. Treat with 0.5% saffranine or 0.05% basic fuchsin for 30 seconds.

6. Wash with water, dry and examine under oil immersion lens.

The spores take up green color and the vegetative bacilli red color. Lipid granules are unstained.

Demonstration of capsules

1. *Negative staining (Background staining)* :

Wet-Film India ink method. The best method for staining capsules is the wet-film India Ink method. It is the simplest, most informative and generally applicable method of demonstrating capsules. The dyes used for negative staining are India Ink, Nigrosin, eosin or colloidal silver.

1. Clean and wipe the slide free from particles, dust, grit. Place a large loopful of India Ink or Nigrosin on the slide.

2. Emulsify one or two colonies from solid culture or a small loopful of liquid culture in the ink.

3. Place a clean coverslip on the ink drop and press it with a blotting paper so that the film becomes very thin and pale.

Under phase contrast microscope, the bacteria appear dark and are surrounded by bright zones of capsules.

Under oil immersion objective, a clear space surrounding the refractile outline of the bacterium is seen. Non-capsulated bacteria do not show this clear space.

Positive staining by dryfilm method. Dry film methods in which positive staining of capsules is attempted are less reliable, because – (*i*) capsules may be shrunken so they become visible (*ii*) shrinkage spaces give the appearance of capsules so that non-capsulated bacteria look like capsulated.

Therefore, dry-film methods are used, if permanent preparations are required.

1. Place a loopful of India ink or nigrosin at one end of a clean glass slide. Add a small amount of bacterial culture to this and mix to form an even suspension.

2. Spread it over the slide in a thin film with the edge of a second glass slide, and air-dried.

3. Fix the film by pouring methyl alcohol over it; drain off excess and dry by warming over a flame.

4. Drop on methyl violet (or crystal violet) and stain for one or two minutes.

5. Wash in water. Blot and dry over a flame. Examine under oil immersion objective.

The bacteria appear violet and any capsule present appears as a clear zone between the stained bacterium and the black ink background.

3. Hiss stain. 1. Prepare a thin film on the capsulated bacterial suspension, dry and fix by warming.

2. Pour saturated alcoholic solution of gention violet on slide and heat gently until steam rises; allow the stain to act for 30 seconds.

3. Wash off with 20% copper sulphate and blot dry (copper sulphate acts as a mordant).

The capsules are stained pale violet and the bacteria deep violet.

Capsule swelling reaction/quellung reaction. Capsular material is antigenic and can be demonstrated by serological methods. When a suspension of capsulated bacteria are mixed with its specific anticapsular serum and a loopful of methylene blue solution, the capsule becomes swollen, refractile and prominent. Hence, known as capsule swelling (quellung) reaction. It was first described by Neufeld and widely employed for the demonstration of capsules and typing of pneumococci.

DEMONSTRATION OF FLAGELLAE

1. Flagellae are best demonstrated under electron microscope in metal-shadowed films or by negative staining with phosphotungstic acid.

2. Flagellae can also be demonstrated by the light microscope, using special staining techniques such as silver impregnation methods or Leifson method.

Leifson method. 1. Clean the glass slides with absolute alcohol, rubbing with a fine cotton cloth. Then immerse them in conc. H_2SO_4 saturated with potassium dichromate for several days at room temperature or for an hour at 90°C.

2. Using forceps, transfer the slides for rinsing, drying and storing (in coplin jars).

3. Rinse the slides with tap water thoroughly and finally with distilled water. Allow to dry in air. Before use, flame the slide for few seconds.

4. The smears are stained with stain solution of following composition:

Tannic acid	10 g
Sodium chloride	5 g
Basic fuchsin	4 g

Several smears should be prepared and stained for different times *e.g.,* for 6, 8, 10 and 12 minutes so that the best may be chosen.

The thickness of the flagellae increases with the duration of staining.

5. Rinse off the stain under a slowly running water tap.

6. Counterstain with methylene blue for 30 minutes to color the bacterial protoplast.

7. Wash with water, rinse with distilled water, drain, dry in air and examine by oil immersion lens.

The stain and tannic acid is deposited on the flagellae and appear pink, whereas bacterial protoplast blue.

Vital staining

Microorganisms may be stained in the living state. Many dyes are toxic and kill the cells on staining. Non-toxic staining, during which the cells retain their viability, is known as vital or intravital staining *e.g.,* Methylene blue dye test for *Toxoplasma.*

Supervital staining

The staining of living cells after their removal from the host has been referred to as supervital or supravital staining, where the cells remain viable during the staining process.

Staining of fungi

Lactophenol cotton blue wet mount. Tease out a fragment of fungal culture on a clean glass slide either in a drop of stain with a needle or straight wire. When it is spread satisfactorily, add a few drops of lactophenol cotton blue stain, apply a coverslip, avoiding air bubbles.

Excess stain, if any can be removed by blotting paper.

For permanent preparations, the edges of coverslips may be sealed with nail polish. Lactic acid is a preservative, phenol is a disinfectant and cotton blue provides blue color to fungal filaments.

Staining solutions

Loeffler's methylene blue

Saturated solution of methylene blue in alcohol	30 ml,
KOH (0.01%)	100 ml

Dilute carbol fuchsin

It is 10-15 times diluted Ziehl-Neelsen's strong carbol fuchsin.

Gention violet solution

Gention violet	1 gm
Distilled water	100 ml

It is one percent aqueous solution.

Gram's iodine

Iodine –	1 gm
Potassium iodide	2 gm
Distilled water	300 ml

Safranine solution

Safranine	1 gm
Distilled water	100 ml

Neutral red solution

Neutral red	1 gm
Glacial acetic acid (1%)	2 ml
Distilled water	100 ml

Crystal violet solution

Crystal violet	0.5 gm (or 1 gm)
Distilled water	100 ml

Strong carbol fuchsin (Ziehl-Neelsen's)

Basic fuchsin	1 gm
Absolute alcohol	10 ml
5% phenol in distilled water	10 ml

Auramine 'O' solution

Auramine 'O' 3 g	
Phenol	30 g
Distilled water	1 lit.

Acid-alcohol solution

Ethanol (75%, v/v) in distilled water containing 0.5% NaCl and 0.5% HCl.

Potassium permanganate solution

$KMnO_4$	1 gm
Distilled water	1 lit.

Albert's stain (Albert's solution-A)

Toluidine blue	1.5 gm
Malachite green	2 gm
Glacial acetic acid	10 ml
Alcohol (95% ethanol)	10 ml
Distilled water	1 lit.

Albert's iodine (Albert's solution-B)

Iodine	6 g
Potassium iodide	9 g
Distilled water	900 ml

Neisser's methylene blue stain

Methylene blue	1 gm
Ethanol (95%)	50 ml
Glacial acetic acid	50 ml
Distilled water	1 lit.

Pugh's stain

Toluidine blue	1 gm
Glacial acetic acid	25 ml
Alcohol (absolute)	10 ml
Distilled water	500 ml

Ponder's stain

Toluidine blue	0.02 gm
Glacial acetic acid	1 ml
Absolute alcohol	2 ml
Distilled water	100 ml

Lactophenol cotton blue stain

Phenol crystals	20 gm
Lactic acid	20 ml
Glycerol	40 ml
Distilled water	20 ml
Cotton blue (or methyl blue)	0.075 gm

Dissolve the phenol crystals in the liquids by gentle warming and then add the dye.

QUESTIONS

Essay Type Questions

1. Describe in detail the Gram's staining, its mechanism and the relationship between Gram's reaction of bacteria and their antibiotic susceptibility.
2. Give an account of differential stains.

Short Notes

1. Simple staining.
2. Gram's staining.
3. Mention reasons behind Gram positivity of bacteria (or) What is Gram positivity due to ?
4. Acid-fast stain or Ziehl-Neelsen's stain.
5. What is acid-fastness due to ?
6. Kinyoun's acid-fast staining.
7. Cold acid-fast staining.
8. Differential stains.
9. Negative staining.
10. Impregnation methods.
11. Capsule swelling reaction or quellung reaction.
12. Albert's stain.
13. Mention stains to demonstrate volutin granules of diphtheria bacilli.
14. What is the broad relationship between the Gram's reaction of bacteria and their antibiotic susceptibility ?
15. Lactophenol cotton blue stain.

4

Morphology of Bacteria

SIZE OF BACTERIA

Micron. The unit of measurement used in Bacteriology is the micron or micrometer. Most of the cocci have a diameter of 1 micron (μ) and bacilli measure 2-5 microns in length and 0.5-1 micron in width.

1 Micron (μ) or 1 micrometer (μm) = One thousandth of a millimetre

The unit micron is also used to measure the size of protozoan parasites, parasitic eggs and larvae.

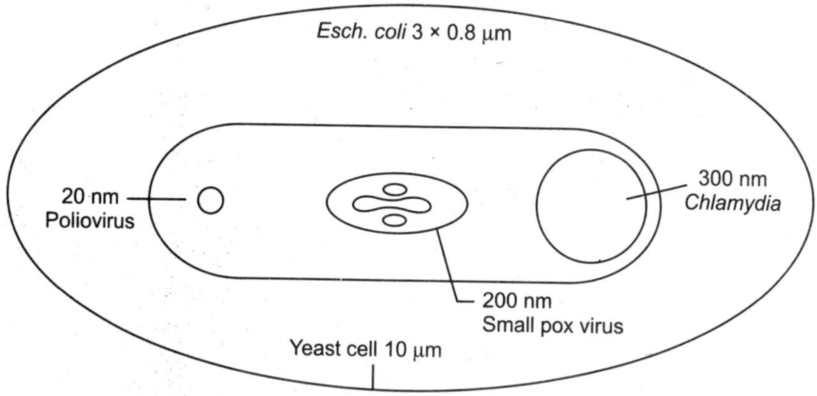

Fig. 4.1 Relative sizes of microorganisms.

Microscopic measurements

Micrometer (μm)	–	One millionth (10^{-6}) of a meter	or	one thousandth of a mm
Nanometer (nm)	–	One billionth of a meter (10^{-9})	or	one millionth of a mm
Angstrom (Å)	–	1/10 th of nm (one ten billionth of a meter (10^{-10})		

NANOMETER (nm) AND ANGSTROM UNIT (Å)

These units are used to measure the size of viruses and various cell organelles.

1 Millimicron (mμ)	–	one thousandth of a micron
or		or
1 Nanometer (nm)	–	one millionth of a millimetre
1 Angstrom unit (Å)	–	one tenth of a nanometre

MORPHOLOGY (SHAPES) OF BACTERIA

Bacteria can be classified into various groups, based on their shape.

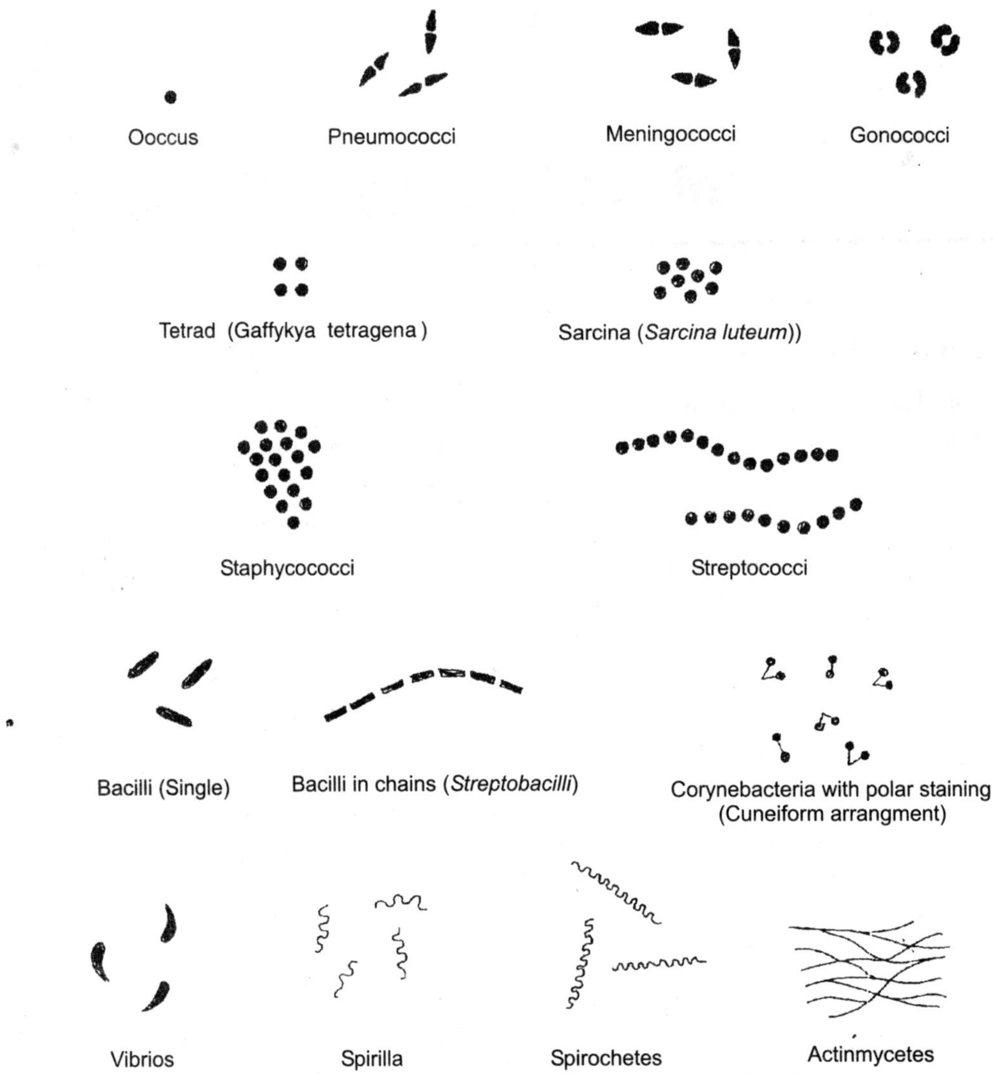

Fig. 4.2 Some morphological forms of bacteria.

I. Cocci (Kokkos-berry). They are spherical or oval shaped cells. The cocci can be arranged in different ways and different names are given according to their arrangement.

1. Micrococci. Cocci may exist as single isolated cell.

1. ***Diplococci.*** Cocci may be present in pairs

e.g, Pneumococci	– cells are lanceolate or flame shaped, Gram positive diplococci
Meningococci	– cells are oval shaped, Gram negative diplococci.
Gonococci	– cells are kidney or bean seed shaped, Gram negative diplococci.

2. ***Tetrads.*** Cocci are present in groups of four *e.g., Gaffykya* tetragena.

3. ***Sarcina.*** Cocci are present in groups of eight *e.g., Sarcina luteum.*

4. ***Staphylococci.*** Cocci are present in grape like bunches.

5. ***Streptococci.*** Cocci are arranged in chains.

II. Bacilli (Baculus-rod). They are rod shaped organisms. *e.g., E.coli, Clostridium, Mycobacterium*

Based on their arrangement, bacilli can be further named.

1. ***Streptobacilli.*** Bacilli are arranged in chains *e.g., Streptobacillus moniliformis, Bacillus anthracis.*

2. ***Chinese letter pattern or cuneiform arrangement.*** The bacilli are arranged at right angles to each other, resembling letters V or L, similar to chinese letter pattern or cuneiform arrangement *e.g., Corynebacterium diphtheriae.*

III. Coccobacilli. Short rod shaped organisms or small ovoid organisms are called coccobacilli *e.g., Brucella, Bordetella*

IV. Vibrios. They are comma shaped organisms. They can be described as curved bacilli. The name vibrio is derived from their vibratory motility. *e.g., Vibrio cholerae, Campylobacter, Helicobacter.*

V. Spirilla. They are rigid spiral forms *e.g., Spirillum minus.*

VI. Spirochetes (Speira = spiral; chaite = hair like). They are flexuous spiral shaped organisms having several coils. These coils may be arranged in two ways:

1. Relaxed coils – *Borrelia, Leptospira.*
2. Tight coils – *Treponema.*

VII. Actinomycetes (actis = ray; mykes = fungus). They are branching filamentous forms, having superficial resemblance to fungi. They are called as actinomycetes, because they look like radiating sun rays in tissue lesions. *e.g., Actinomyces, Nocardia.*

VIII. *Mycoplasma.* They are cell wall deficient and hence do not possess a stable morphology. They occur as spherical, oval, bacillary and filamentous forms. Bacteria lose their cell wall either spontaneously or in the presence of salts, penicillin like agents. Such cells are called L-forms, protoplasts or spheroplasts. *e.g., Mycoplasma pneumoniae, M.hominis, Ureaplasma urealyticum.*

QUESTIONS

Short Notes

1. Morphology of bacteria/shapes of bacteria.
2. Cocci
3. Morphological classification of bacteria.
4. Micron.
5. Nanometer.
6. Angstrom unit.
7. Size of bacteria.

5

Bacterial Anatomy/ Ultrastructure of Bacterial Cells

- *Introduction*
- *Cell envelope*
- *Cell wall*
  - *Chemical composition*
  - *Gram positive bacterial cell walls*
  - *Differences between Gram positive and Gram negative bacterial cell walls*
  - *Demonstration*
  - *Functions*
- *Cytoplasmic membrane*
- *Mesosomes*
- *Cytoplasm*
- *Cytoplasmic inclusions*
  - *Ribosomes*
  - *Volutin/metachromatic granules*
  - *Lipid granules*
  - *Polysaccharide granules*
  - *Vacuoles*
- *Bacterial nucleus (Nucleoid)*
- *Plasmids and episomes*
- *Glycocalyx, capsule, slime layer*
  - *Chemical composition*
  - *Demonstration*
    - *Negative staianing*
    - *Quellung reaction*
  - *Functions*
- *Flagellae*
  - *Parts of flagellum*
  - *Arrangement*
  - *Motility*
  - *Demonstration*
  - *Functions*
- *Fimbriae*
- *Bacterial spores (Endospores)*
  - *Sporulation*
  - *Structure*
  - *Germination*
  - *Shape and position*
  - *Demonstration*
  - *Uses*
- *Pleomorphism and Involution forms*
- *Protoplasts*
- *L-phase organisms*

INTRODUCTION

Bacteria are prokaryotic unicellular microorganisms, enclosed by a thin, elastic membrane known as plasma membrane. Outside, and closely covering this, there is cell wall; these two together are called "cell envelope". The cell envelope encloses protoplasm, that is differentiated into cytoplasm and nuclear material. The cytoplasm contains ribosomes, mesosomes, vacuoles and inclusion granules. Some bacteria may be enclosed by a viscous material known as capsule. Some bacteria carry filamentous appendages protruding from the cell membrane – the flagellae which are organelles of locomotion, and the pili or fimbriae which are organelles of adhesion (Fig. 5.1).

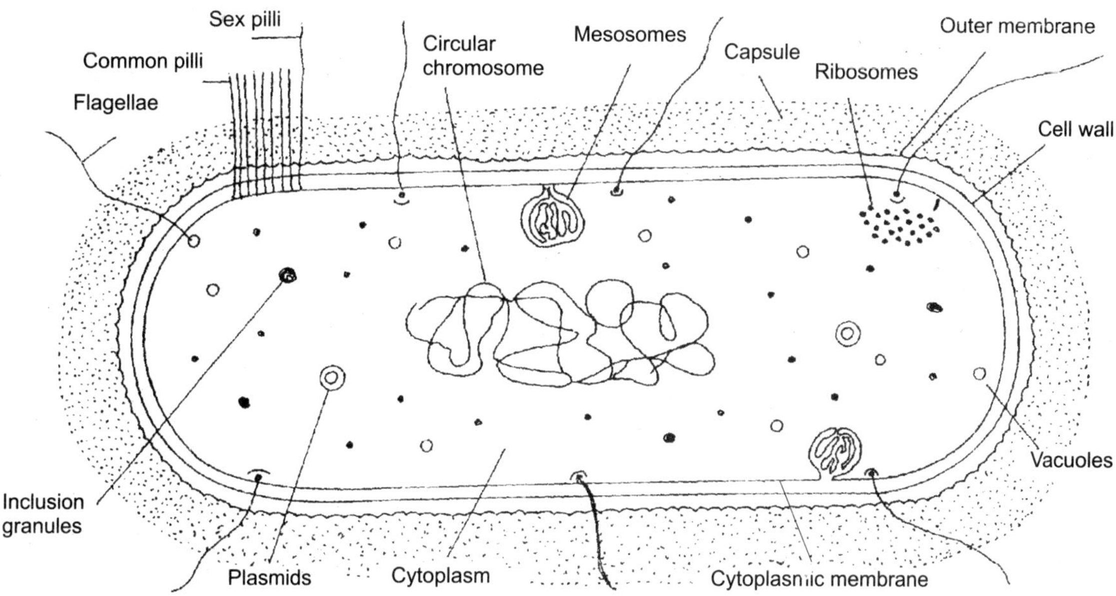

Fig. 5.1 The structure of bacterial cell.

CELL ENVELOPE

Various layers that surround the bacterial cell are collectively referred to as "cell envelope". The structure and organization of cell envelope differ in Gram positive and Gram negative bacteria.

The cell envelope in Gram positive bacteria consists of plasma membrane and cell wall and in some bacteria an outer layer called the capsule.

The cell envelope in Gram negative bacteria contains plasma membrane, cell wall, outer membrane and in some capsule. The plasma membrane in Gram negative bacteria is sometimes called "inner membrane" and the space between inner membrane and outer membrance is called the "periplasmic space."

CELL WALL

Cell wall encloses the protoplast and lies immediately external to the cytoplasmic membrane. It accounts for about 20-30% dry weight of the cell. It measures 10-25 nm in thickness. The cell walls of Gram negative bacteria are thinner (10-15 nm) and those of Gram positive bacteria are thicker (20-25 nm) (Fig. 5.2).

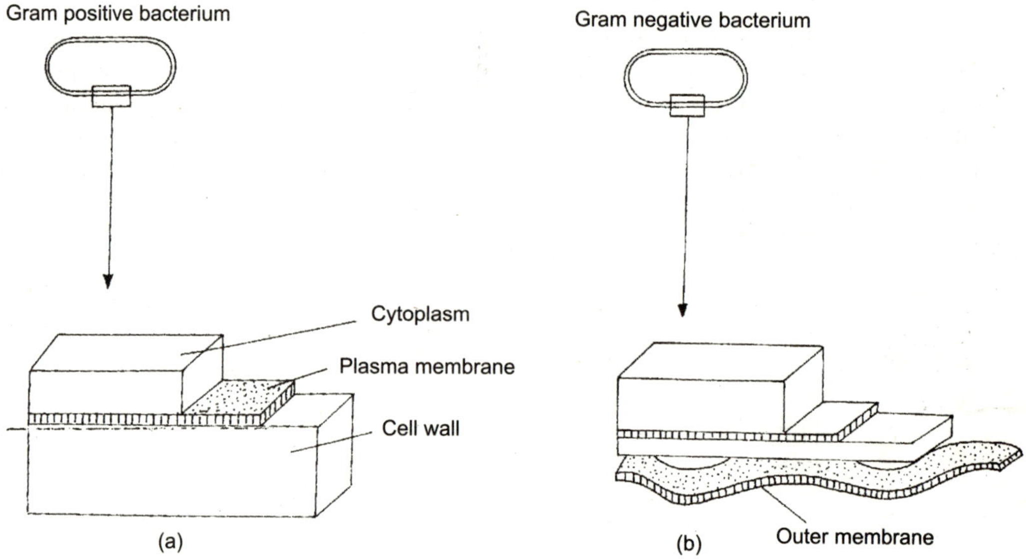

Fig. 5.2 Cell envelope.

Chemical composition

Chemically, the cell wall is made up of peptidoglycan (or mucopeptide or glycopeptide or murein) network, which is a polymer of glycan strands. Peptidoglycan is a single gigantic molecule of great strength and rigidity that surrounds the cell as a network. It consists of two hexose sugars N-acetyl glycosamine (NAG) and N-acetyl muramic acid (NAM) in alternating chains, interconnected by tri-, tetra- or penta-peptide chains containing D- and L-alanine, D-glutamic acid and either L-lysine, diaminopimelic acid, diaminobutyric acid or ornithine. These peptide chains are the target for penicillins, cephalosporins and other antimicrobial agents which kill microorganisms by inhibiting cell wall synthesis.

Bacteria themselves possess enzymes, called 'autolysins', able to hydrolyse their own cell wall, so that new polymer can be added and the cell can grow and divide (Fig. 5.3).

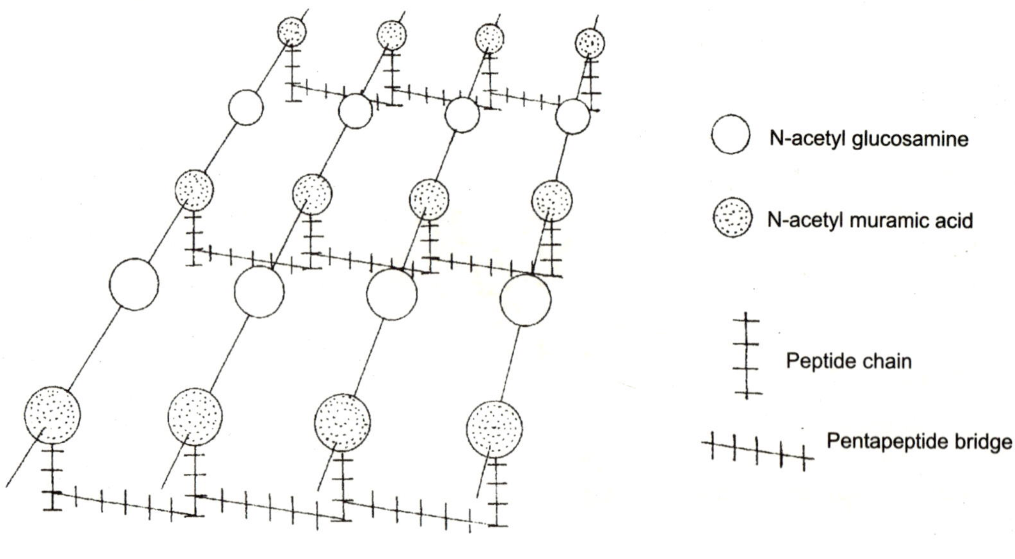

Fig. 5.3 The structure of bacterial cell wall.

Lysozyme, an enzyme normally present in tissue fluids, lyses susceptible bacteria, by splitting the cell wall mucopeptide linkages between NGA and NAM. It can completely destroy the cell wall of Gram positive bacterium, producing a "protoplast"; while the cell walls of Gram negative bacteria are more resistant to lysozyme and lose less of their cell wall producing a "spheroplast".

Gram positive bacterial cell walls

Gram positive bacterial cell walls contain large amount of peptidoglycan, account for 50 per cent or more of the dry weight of the cell wall and are thicker. Many Gram positve bacterial cell walls also contain polysaccharides called "**Teichoic acids**", which are polymers of glycerol and ribitol phosphates.

Teichoic acids are negatively charged, and aid in the transport of positive ions into and out of the cell and in the storage of phosphorous.

Some Gram positive bacterial cell walls contain lipids called mycolic acids *e.g.*, Mycobacteria; and miscellaneous components such as protein A in staphylococcal cell walls and M proteins in *Streptococcus pyogenes* cell wall.

Gram negative bacterial cell walls

Gram negative bacterial cell walls contain less amount of peptidoglycan, account for only 5 to 10 per cent of the dry weight of the cell wall and are thinner. These cell walls have an additional "outer membrane" that surrounds the peptidoglycan layer. The outer membrane is anchored to peptidoglycan by a lipoprotein layer, also called Braun's lipoprotein. The outer layer of the outer membrane is a bilayered structure consisting of phospholipids, proteins and lipopolysaccharides (LPS). The phospholipids of the outer membrane are similar to those in the cytoplasmic membrane.

Lipopolysaccharides are characteristic to Gram negative bacteria and found on the outer surface of outer membrane. It comprises three parts, which are covalently linked (Fig. 5.4).

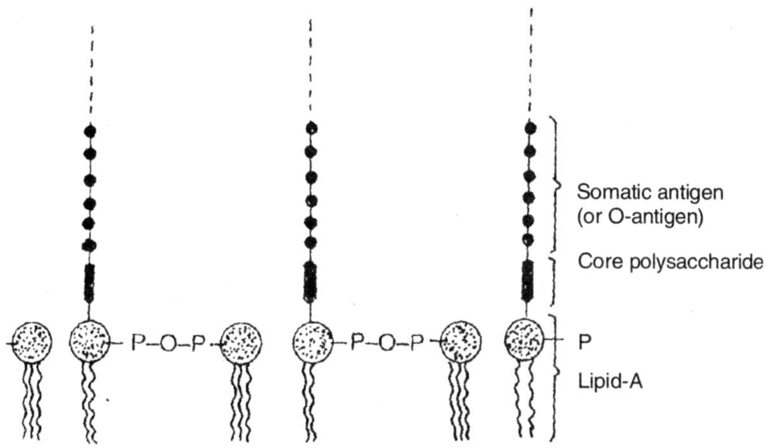

Fig. 5.4 Lipopolysaccharide.

1. Region I is a polysaccharide. It extends like whiskers (hair like) from the membrane surface into the surrounding medium. It is also called somatic antigen or O-antigen. It was first extracted by Boivin, hence known as Boivin antigen.O-antigens are important in serological tests such as widal test. They also serve as sites for bacteriophage attachment to bacterial cells.

2. Region II is core polysaccharide located at the membrane surface.

3. Region III is lipid A firmly embedded in the outer membrane. It is also known as endotoxin and can act as a poison – causing fever, diarrhea, lysis of RBC, and fatal shock.

Outer membrane contains various proteins, known as outer membrane proteins (OMP), which include porins and receptors.

Porins are special proteins that form diffusion channels; that are selectively permeable allow smaller molecules and act as a barrier for larger molecules. Various porins are specific for different kinds of small molecules, and some can allow passage of larger, essential molecules such as vitamin B_{12}. Porins allow secretion of extracellular enzymes. Porins facilitate signal transdusion. Some outer membrane proteins act as receptor sites for attachment of bacteriophages and bacteriocins. The region between outer membrane and plasma membrane is called **"periplasmic space".** It contains hydrolytic enzymes, binding proteins and oligosaccharides, that play an important role in osmotic regulation.

Demonstration of cell wall. Cell wall can be demonstrated by:

1. Microdissection.
2. Mechanical rupture of cell.
3. Electron microscope.
4. Differential staining procedures.
5. Plasmolysis–when bacterial cells are placed in hypertonic solution, cytoplasm loses water by osmosis and shrinks, while cell wall retains the original shape and size and appears like a bacterial ghost under the microscope.

Functions of cell wall:

1. accounts for the characteristic shape of the cell.
2. confers rigidity and ductility on the cell and gives mechanical support to the cell.
3. plays an important role in cell division by forming cross walls to separate the daughter cells.
4. supports weak cytoplasmic membrane against high internal osmotic pressure of the protoplasm.
5. carries antigens that are important in virulence and immunity.

Table 5.1 Differences between gram positive and gram negative bacterial cell walls

Character	*Gram positive cell walls*	*Gram negative cell walls*
1. Thickness	Thicker	Thinner
2. Peptidoglycan content	Larger, 50 per cent or more of the dry weight of the cell wall	Less, 5–10 per cent of the dry weight of the cell wall
3. Outer membrane	Absent	Present
4. LPS	Absent	Present
5. Teichoic acids	Present	Absent
6. Variety of amino-acids	Few	Several
7. Aromatic and sulphur containing amino-acids	Absent	Present
8. Lipids	Absent, Mycolic acids present in mycobacteria	Present, possess endotoxic activity
9. Lipoproteins	Absent	Present

CYTOPLASMIC MEMBRANE

Immediately beneath the cell wall is the cytoplasmic membrane; also called plasma membrane or cell membrane.It is thin, elastic and semipermeable, composed of phospholipids (20 to 30 per cent) and proteins (50 to 70 per cent). The phospholipids form a bilayer in which proteins are firmly held. These proteins are called the integral proteins (intrinsic protein) and may be removed by disruption of the membrane by treatment with detergents. There are other proteins that are loosely attached to the surface of the phospholipid bilayer, which are called peripheral proteins (extrinsic proteins). They can be removed by osmotic shock.

The lipids found in the phospholipid bilayer are phosphatidylethanolamine and phosphatidylcholine. Each phospholipid molecule contains a charged, polar head (the phosphate end) and an uncharged, nonpolar tail (the hydrocarbon end). In the phospholipid bilayer water-soluble, polar ends are lined on the outside, while the water-insoluble, non-polar ends are on the inside (Fig. 5.5).

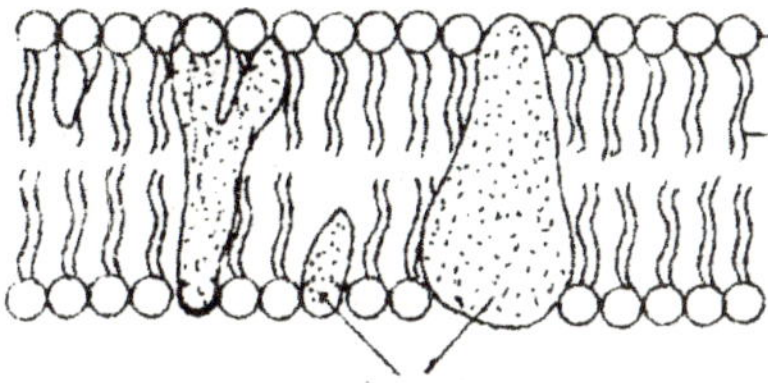

Fig. 5.5 Plasma membrane phospholipid bilayer.

According to fluid-mosaic model of Singer and Nicolson (1972), the phospholipids in the membrane make it fluid, allowing protein molecules to move around, which is essential for the various functions of the membrane.

Functions:

1. Plasma membrane carries specific enzymes called permeases, that transport small molecules into the cell by active transport.
2. Cell membrane also contains various enzymes, some of which are involved in energy production and cell wall synthesis.
3. The bacterial electron transport system is located in the cytoplasmic membrane.
4. The plasma membrane is selectively semi-permeable for the penetration of water soluble molecules. It allows the entry and exit of small molecules such as nutrients and waste products by simple diffusion.
5. Being semipermeable, the cell membrane regulates the osmotic concentration of cytoplasm.
6. The cell membrane is also a centre for the control of flagellar motility.
7. It contains several enzymes, including enzymes of Kreb's cycle and enzymes necessary for synthesis of cell wall.

MESOSOMES

Mesosomes are sites of respiratory enzymes and are analogous to mitochondira. They are vesicular, convoluted or multilaminated membranous bodies, formed by invagination or infolding of plasma membrane into the cytoplasm. They consist of convoluted tubules and vesicles. They are especially prominent in Gram positive bacateria.

Mesosomes are also known as "chondroids". Mesosomes may lie near the cytoplasmic membrane or deeper inside the cytoplasm. The deeper central mesosomes penetrate deeply into the cytoplasm and are located near the middle of the cell and seem to be attached to the cell's nuclear material. They are involved in DNA replication and cell division. The peripheral mesosomes barely penetrate the cytoplasm and are not centrally located, and are not associated with nuclear material. They are involved in the secretion of some extracelluar enzymes such as penicillinases (Fig. 5.6).

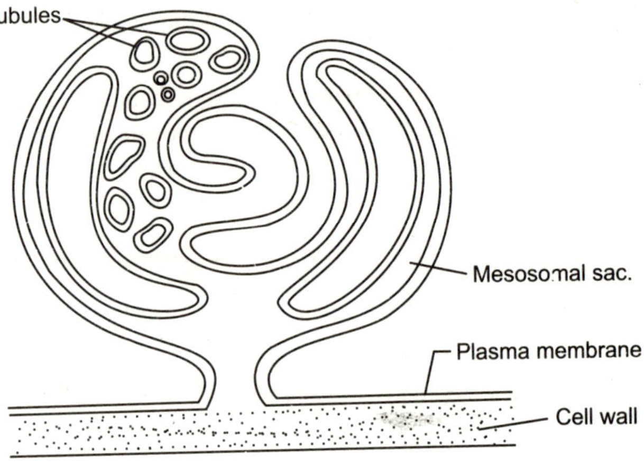

Fig. 5.6 Mesosome

CYTOPLASM

Cytoplasm is a colloidal system of viscous watery solution or soft gel, containing a variety of organic and inorganic solutes. It does not exhibit cytoplasmic streaming. Cell organelles such as ER, Golgi bodies, mitochondria, microsomes and plastids are absent.

The cytoplasm is largely consists a high percentage of water, along with nucleic acids, proteins, carbohydrates, lipids, inorganic ions and several low molecular weight compounds.

Cytoplasm stains uniformly in young cultures, but becomes granular with age and shows barred or beaded appearance in old cells.

CYTOPLASMIC INCLUSIONS

Cytoplasm contains ribosomes, several inclusion storage granules, nucleoid and vacuoles.

Ribosomes. They are present in the cytoplasm freely and are centres of protein synthesis. They may be found together on mRNA strand to form polysomes. Ribosomes in bacteria consists of two subunits – the larger 50S subunit and the smaller 30S subunit, together they form the 70S bacterial risbosome (the 'S' refers to the "svedberg unit", a measure of rate of sedimentation when centrifuged at high speed. Since both shape and size determine the rate of sedimentation, the 'S' units do not add up arithmetically).

Volutin granules or Metachromatic granules or Babes-Ernst granules. They are characteristically present in diphtheria bacilli (*Corynebacterium diphtheriae*) as round, dark bipolar bodies. The name 'volutin' refers to the bacterium *Spirillum volutans* in which these granules were first found. They take up reddish purple color when stained with Loeffler's methylene blue (stain red with blue dye) and therefore called metachromatic granules.

They are composed of polymetaphosphate and considered to be reserve sources of energy. They can to demonstrated by special stains;

1. Albert's stain—Volutin granules appear bluish black and diphtheria bacilli light green.
2. Neisser's stain—The granules appear deep blue colored and the bacilli pink color.
3. Ponder's stain—The granules appear dark blue and the organism pale blue color.
4. Pugh's stain—The volutin granules take up reddish-purple color and the diphtheria bacilli light blue color.

Poly β-hydroxy butyrate (PHB). They are reserve sources of carbon and energy and are clear, round areas and chloroform-soluble lipid materials. PHB granules can be stained with lipid soluble dyes such as Nile blue or sudan black.

Polysaccharide. Polysaccharide granules such as starch and glycogen, that stain brown with iodine may be found and may act as source of carbon and energy.

Vacuoles. Vacuoles are fluid containing cavities may be found in some bacterial cells.

BACTERIAL NUCLEUS or NUCLEOID

Bacteria possess a prokaryotic nucleus. They have no nuclear membrane or nucleolus and DNA is not associated with any protein. The DNA material is located or concentrated near the centre of the cell called the "nucleoid".

The nucleoid consists of a single circular chromosome, made up of a single molecule of double-stranded DNA, arranged in the form of a circle. It is haploid and replicates by simple fission. Mitosis is absent. It carries hereditary genetic information.

The nuclear material can be demonstrated by acid or ribonuclease hydrolysis and subsequent staining by fuelgen technique.

PLASMIDS AND EPISOMES

Plasmids are small circular, covalently closed, double-stranded DNA molecules found in cytoplasm. They are self-replicating extrachromosomal genetic elements that reproduce themselves and are thus conserved, apart from chromosome, through successive cell divisions and segregate into daughter cells.

Plasmids that may also become integrated into the chromosome are sometimes called episomes.

Plasmids may be transmitted from one bacterium to another bacterium either through conjugation or through the agency of bacteriophages by transduction. They are not essential for the life of the cell, they inhabit, but may confer on it certain properties like toxin production, drug resistance or resistance to heavy metals which may constitute a survival advantage.

Some plasmids, such as F factor endow the host cell with maleness or ability to conjugate with other cells. Following conjugation, the recipient acquires the plasmid, becoming male or donor cell in the process. The basis of maleness is the ability to form sex pili which are coded for by the plasmid (F factor).

Penicillinase plasmids which induces resistance in Staphylococci are transmitted from cell to cell through transduction.

R-plasmids confer drug resistance and readily transmitted from cell to cell by mechanisms of gene transfer. It is known as transferable or infectious drug resistance.

GLYCOCALYX, CAPSULE, SLIME LAYER

Many bacteria secrete a viscous, jelly-like, gelatinous material, that surrounds the cell wall is called "Glycocalyx". When glycocalyx is organized into a sharply defined structure and is attached firmly to the cell wall, it is a "capsule" *e.g., Streptococcus pneumoniae, Streptococcus pyogenes, Bacillius anthracis, Clostridium welchii, Klebsiella pneumoniae, Hemophilus influenzae, Niesseria meningitidis.*

When a capsule is too thin to be seen under light microscope, and detectable only by ındirect, serological means or by electron microscope, it may be termed "Microcapsule". When glycocalyx is disorganized without any definite shape, and seen as a loose undemarcated secretion and surrounds bacterial cells, as "matrix", in which several bacterial cells may be embedded; then it is termed "Slime layer" *e.g., Leuconostoc*. Some bacteria may have both capsules and slime layer *e.g., Streptococcus salivarius*.

Capsular gel consists largely of water and has only a small content (2 per cent) of solids. Bacteria producing large amount of capsular material, produce mucoid growth on agar medium, with a stingy consistency when touched with the wire loop. Capsulated strains from smooth (S) colonies whereas noncapsulated strains form rough (R) colonies. Capsule may be lost either spontaneously or due to mutations and is associated with loss of virulence.

Capsular material is soluble in water and may diffuse into liquid culture medium or infective exudates and tissues, and therefore called "Specific soluble substance (SSS)".

Under electron microscope, capsules are seen as a mesh or network of fine strands. Capsule may be chemically composed of polysaccharide *e.g., Streptococcus pneumoniae*; or polypeptide *e.g., Bacillus anthracis*; or hyaluronic acid *e.g., Streptococcus pyogenes*.

Polysaccharide capsules may be composed of a single kind of sugar and are termed "homopoly saccharide capsules". When polysaccharide capsules contain more than one kind of sugar, it is termed "heteropolysaccharide capsule". For example, the capsule of *Streptococcus pneumoniae,* type VI, consists of galactose, glucose and rhamnose.

In *Bacillus anthracis* capsule is made up of polypeptide, a polymer of D-glutamic acid. This polymer is unusual, because glutamic acid is usually found as L-isomer in nature.

Demonstration of Capsules. Capsule have no affinity for basic aniline dyes and cannot be stained by ordinary methods such as Gram's and Leishman stains.

Capsules can be demonstrated by 1. Negative staining, 2. Capsule swelling reaction (quellung reaction), 3. Special staining methods such as Hiss stain, in which copper salts are used as mordants.

Negative staining. When capsulated bacteria are mixed with Indian ink or nigrosin, and spread on a glass slide and examined under microscope; capsules can be seen as unstained bright halos against black dark background.

Capsule swelling reaction or quellung reaction. Capsular material is antigenic, and therefore may be demonstrated by serological methods. When a suspension of capsulated bacteria is mixed on a slide with a drop of type specific anticapsular serum and a loopful of methylene blue solution, and examined under the microscope, the capsule becomes swollen, refractile and prominent.

Quellung (= swelling) reaction was first described by Neufeld (1902). It was widely employed for typing of pneumococci when lobar pneumonia used to be treated with specific anticapsular serum, before sulphonamides were discovered.

Functions of Capsules:

1. Capsules protect pathogenic bacteria from being engulfed by phagocytes *i.e.,* inhibit phagocytosis and confer or promote virulence or greater infective ability.
2. Capsule protect bacteria by preventing adsorption and lysis by bacteriophages and from lytic enzymes and drugs.
3. Capsule may serve as reservoir of stored food.
4. Capsules can protect cells against temporary drying by binding to water molecules.
5. Capsule help in adherence, enabling the bacterium to attach to various surfaces.
6. Capsular vaccines may be used for immunization against diseases caused by capsulated bacteria.
7. Capsules give stability to bacterial suspension by preventing aggregation of cells as they carry a net negative charge due to which cells will repel each other.

FLAGELLAE

All motile bacteria, except spirochetes possess one or more long, unbranched hair like or thread like filamentous appendages, called flagellae, which are organelles of locomotion. They originate in the cytoplasm, extend through cytoplasmic membrane and extruded out through the cell wall. Each flagellum is a long, thin filament, twisted spirally (helical shape) in an open, regular wave form, which effect cork-screw like propulsive movements. Flagellae are usually several times longer than the cell, measuring 15 to 20 μ in length, with a diameter of 0.01 to 0.02 μ.

Parts of flagellum

Each flagellum has three distinct parts – basal body, hook and filament or shaft.

Basal body. It is embedded in cell envelope and consists of a small central rod surrounded by a series of rings. Gram negative bacteria have two pairs of rings, with the outer rings anchored to the cell wall and the inner rings attached to the cytoplasmic membrane. These rings are called sequentially as follows:

M ring – attached to plasma membrane

S ring – located in the periplasmic space above the plasma membrane

P ring – attached to the peptidoglycan

L ring – attached to lipopolysaccharide.

In Gram positive bacteria, only one pair of rings is present, the out set of rings (P ring and L ring) are absent. One ring, called M ring is embedded in the plasma membrane and the other S ring is attached to the inside of the peptidoglycan (cell wall) layer (Fig. 5.7).

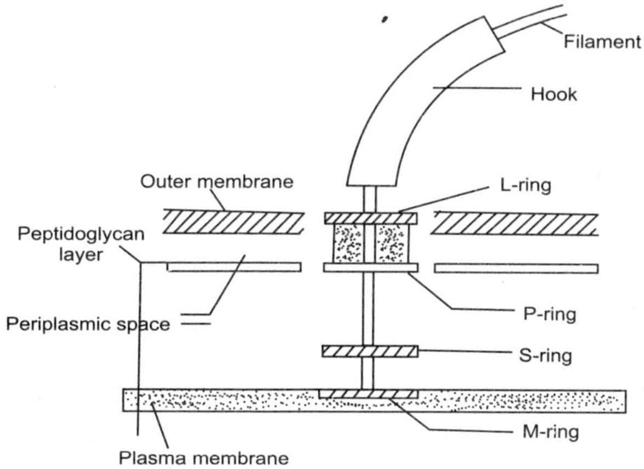

Fig. 5.7 The ultrastructure of bacterial flagellae.

Hook. Hook connects the basal body with the filament. The hook of Gram positive bacterial flagellum is longer than that of the Gram negative bacterial flagellum. Hook arises from basal body and positions the filament along its long aixs during motility.

Filament or shaft. It is external to the cell surface twisted helically and connected to the hook at the cell surface. The filament is composed of protein molecules called "flagellin" similar to keratin or myosin. These flagellin molecules are made within the cell and then passed along the hollow core of the flagellum to be added to the distal end of the filament. Thus, a flagellum grown at its tip rather than at its base.

Arrangement. Based on number and arrangement of flagellae, bacteria can be classified into different groups. The bacteria which do not possess flagellae may be termed "Atrichous". When bacteria contain flagellae at one or both ends. They are termed "Polar" flagellae (Fig. 5.8).

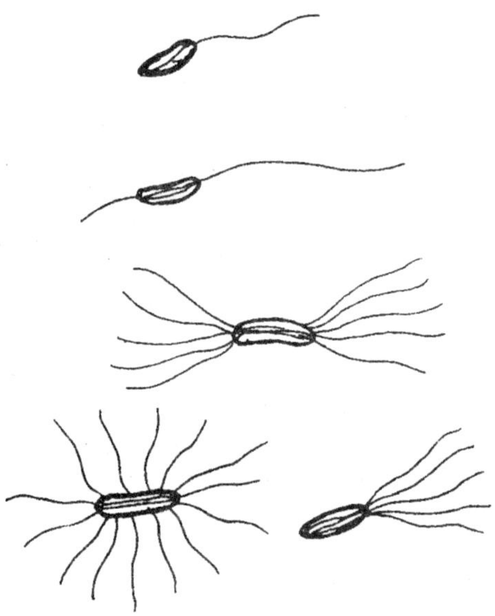

Monotrichous
e.g., Vibrio cholerae, Pseudomonas aeruginosa, Campylobacter sp.

Amphitrichous
e.g., Campylobacter, Alcaligenes fecalis

Amphitrichous
e.g., Aquaspirillus serpens

Lophotrichous
e.g., Spirillum minus, Pseudomonas fluorescens

Peritrichous
e.g., Salmonella typhi, E.Coli, Proteus, Clostridium tetani

Fig. 5.8 Number and arrangement of flagellae

1. ***Monotrichous*** (Greak monos = single; trichos = hair) – consists of a single polar flagellum ***e.g.,*** *Vibrio cholerae, Campylobacter* sp. *Pseudomonas aeruginosa.*

2. ***Amphitrichous*** – when bacteria has flagellae at both the ends. It could be a single flagellum at either end *e.g., Campylobacter* sp., *Alcaligenes fecalis*; or a tuft of flagellae at both the ends ***e.g.,*** *Aquaspirillum serpens.*

3. ***Lophotrichous*** – when a bacterial cell possesses a tuft of flagellae at one end, it is known as lophotrichous *e.g., Spirillum minus, pseudomonas fluorescenes.*

4. ***Peritrichous*** – when flagellae are present all around the bacterial cell surface, it is called peritrichous. *e.g., E.coli, Salmonella typhi, Proteus* sp., *Clostridium tetani.*

Cocci rarely have flagellae. But some cocci such as *Rhodococcus* are flagellated. Spirochetes are actively motile but do not contain external filaments instead they possess special flagellae called "axial filaments or periplasmic flagellae or endoflagellae", that arise at cell poles and wind around the cell body beneath the outer membrane of cell wall in the periplasmic space. They are responsible for cork-screw like rotatory movement of spirochetes.

Locomotion or Motility.

Bacteria having polar flagellae move or swim in back-and-forth fashion. Bacteria having peritrichous flagellae swim in a more complicated manner in a three dimensional random movement. Their flagellae form a bundle that extends behind the cell, so that cell moves/swims along a straight track. When the flagellar motors reverse, the bundle separates and the cell tumbles wildly. But soon the flagellar motors resume their bundle form and the cell moves in a different direction. Swimming bacteria exhibit chemotaxis, which is movement in response to chemicals in environment. Arginine stimulates motility (Fig. 5.9).

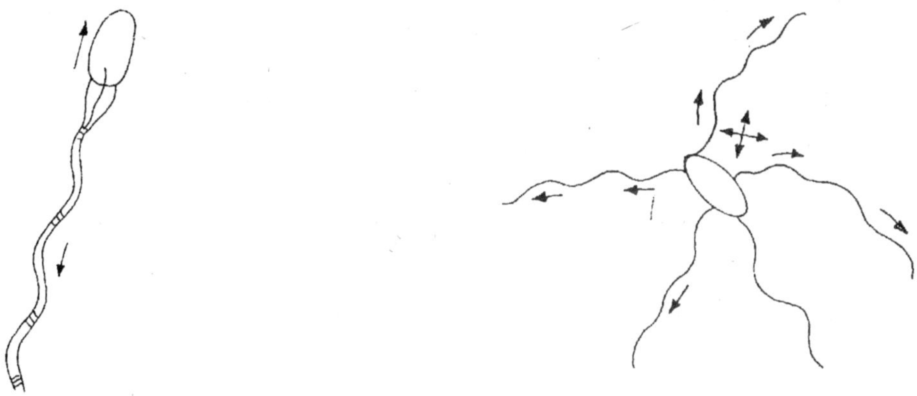

(*a*) While swimming the flagellae form a bundle twisted helicly counter clock-wise. Arrow on top indicates direction of swimming.

(*b*) During tumbling the flagellae reverse their rotation and the bundle flies apart.

Fig. 5.9 The arrangement of flagellae during motility.

It is essential to differentiate true motility from false motility under the microscope. True motility is directional where the organism changes its position in the field (displacement of position). *e.g.*,

1. *Salmonella typhi* exhibits serpentine motility
2. *Vibrio cholerae* moves by darting motility
3. *Bacillus* species exhibit slow stately motion
4. *Listeria monocytogenes* exhibits tumbling motility.

False motility, also called brownian movement is defined as an oscillatory movement exhibited by living as well as nonliving bodies, due to water convection currents or bombardment of water molecules.

Demonstration of flagellae

Flagellae can be demonstrated by several methods:

1. in electron microscope either by shadow-casting or by negative staining with phosphotungstic acid.

2. by silver impregnation methods, where the flagellae are made thick by impregnating or depositing silver salts on their surface so that they become visible under the microscope.

3. by dark field microscopy.

4. by special staining methods such as Leifson's staining.

5. the presence of flagellae can be inferred by demonstrating motility. The motility can be demonstrated (*a*) by hanging drop experiment or (*b*) by noting spreading or swarming growth on a semisolid agar medium.

Functions: Flagellae are organelles of locomotion. Motility helps bacteria to move towards favourable regions where there is a higher concentration of nutrients. Aerobic bacteria tend to move towards a region, where there is enough oxygen, while anaerobic bacteria move away. The active motility by pathogens, enable them to penetrate tissues and body fluids.

FIMBRIAE (or) PILI (Latin; fimbriae = fringes; pili = hair)

Many Gram negative bacilli possess very fine, shorter, straighter, thinner, non-helical hair like surface appendages called pili (singular pilus). Thay are not related to motility and may be found on both motile as well as nonmotile cells. They originate in the plasma membrane and protrude out through the cell envelope. They are more numerous than flagellae. They differ from flagellae in being thinner, (diameter 3-10 nm), shorter, straighter and nonhelical.

Fimbriae (singular fimbria) are widely found in Gram negative bacteria. They are also noticed in *Corynebacterium renale*, a Gram positive bacillus. Among the enterobacteria fimbriae are usually peritrichously arranged and cells may possess from a few to 1000 of pili. In some pseudomonads, fimbriae may be polar or bipolar.

Their length vary from 0.1 μ to 2 μ. They are chemically made up of a protein called "pilin". arranged in a spiral fashion around a central space to form pilus structure. The pili are genetically coded by plasmid DNA which can also integrate with chromosomal DNA. They cannot be seen under ordinary microscope, but can be seen under electron microscope in preparations that have been metal-shadowed or negatively stained with phosphotungstic acid.

Fimbriae are best developed and form surface pellicles in liquid culture media.Fimbriate strains may undergo a reversible variation between a fimbriate phase and a non-fimbriate phase. When grown in liquid media or due to subcultures in liquid media the fimbriate phase becomes predominant, whereas on solid media or due to subcultures on solid media, bacteria tend to lose pili.

Fimbriae are antigenic. But fimbrial antibodies are not useful in sero-diagnosis, because different genera may possess the same fimbrial antigen. Hence bacterial antigens employed for serological tests and preparation of antisera must be devoid of fimbriae.

Many fimbriated cells can agglutinate red blood cells of Guinea pigs, fowl, horses, pigs very strongly, human RBC moderately, sheep RBC weakly and ox RBC scarcely at all. This phenomenon is called "**Hemagglutination**". If a drop of fimbriated bacterial suspension is mixed with a drop of RBC suspension for a few minutes, clumps are formed, that is visible to the naked eye. This simple hemagglutination test can be used to determine the presence or absence of fimbriae. This hemagglutination is specifically inhibited by D-mannose or methyl-α-D-mannoside.

Several functions have been attributed to different types of fimbriae and they have been classified into the following major groups:

I. Based on function, pili are classified into 2 groups:

1. *Common pili or ordinary pili.* Help in adhesion to host cells or nutritionally favourable environments.

2. ***Sex pili.*** They are special type of fimbriae, which are longer and fewer in number than other fimbriae. They are found on male or donor or '+' strains and help in the attachment to female or recipient or '–' strains through hollow conjugation tubes and aid in gene transfer. The formation of sex pili or maleness is determined by F-plasmid or fertility factor.

II. Based on susceptibility to specific bacteriophages, pili are classified into different types *e.g.,* F, I.

III. Based on morphology, pili are classified into six morphological types or groups (Types 1 to 6).

BACTERIAL SPORES *OR* ENDOSPORES

Bacterial spores are highly resistant resting dormant forms, which are thick walled and highly refractile. They are commonly found in *Bacillus* and *Clostridium* species.

Bacterial spores are formed inside the cell, hence called as endospores. Each bacterium forms one spore, which on germination forms a single vegetative cell. Sporulation in bacteria, therefore, is not a method of reproduction.

Spores are dormant bacterial forms. They are non-metabolizing and non-reproducing. Spore DNA is not replicated, mRNA is not produced and the spore protein synthesizing system is defective. The spores are highly resistant to heat, UV radiation, mechanical disruption, chemical disinfectants and desiccation and can remain viable for many centuries. The extremely high resistance of spores is due to

1. low content of water
2. absence of metabolism and enzyme activity
3. high content of calcium and dipicolinic acid
4. impermeability of spore layers (spore cortex and spore coat).

The spores can be killed by moist heat at 100-120°C for a period of 10 min or preferably by autoclaving.

Spore Formation of Sporulation.

Spore formation occur to tide over the adverse or unfavourable conditions and is a mechanism for the safety of the propagation of species. Sporulation occurs during stationary phase when exponential or active growth terminates. During sporulation dehydration occurs.

The first stage in the formation of the spore is condensation of chromatin, in an area at one end of the bacterium known as "Spore field", which is separated by a transverse septum formed by invagination of cytoplasmic membrane and divides the developing spore, now known as "forespore", from the rest of the bacillus, known as the "sporangium". The transverse septum completely encircles the forespore as a double-layered membrane; the inner layer becomes the "spore wall". The "spore cortex" is then laid down between the inner and outer layers and the outer layer is transformed into "spore coat" and "exosporium" (Fig. 5.10).

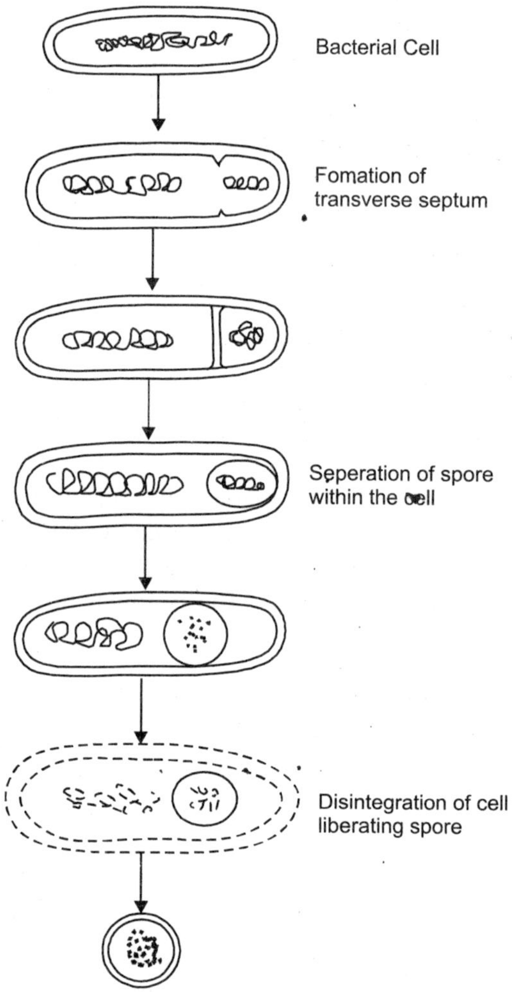

Fig. 5.10. Sporulation.

When the spore is fully formed, the body of the organism degenerates and the spore is set free. Sporulation process completes within 4 to 8 hours.

Spore structure. Spores exhibit marked differences from vegetative cells in morphology, chemical composition and antigenic structure (Fig. 5.11). The core of a fully developed spore has homogenous protoplasm, containing chromosome, enzymes of glycolysis and protein synthesis. The protoplast is surrounded by a membrane called "**spore wall**". It contains normal peptidoglycan, from which the cell wall of future vegetative bacterium develops. Outside the spore wall is a thick "spore cortex" consisting of dipicolinic acid, calcium and an unusual type of peptidoglycan. Spore cortex is surrounded by "spore coats", usually two or upto three may be present.Spore coat is composed of Keratin like protein consisting of sulfur containing aminoacids with intramolecular disulfide bonds. Spore coat is highly impermeable and responsible for the resistance of spores. Outside the spore coats, there is a wrinkled outerlayer with ridges and folds, known as "**exsoporium**", containing mainly lipoprotein and some carbohydrate.

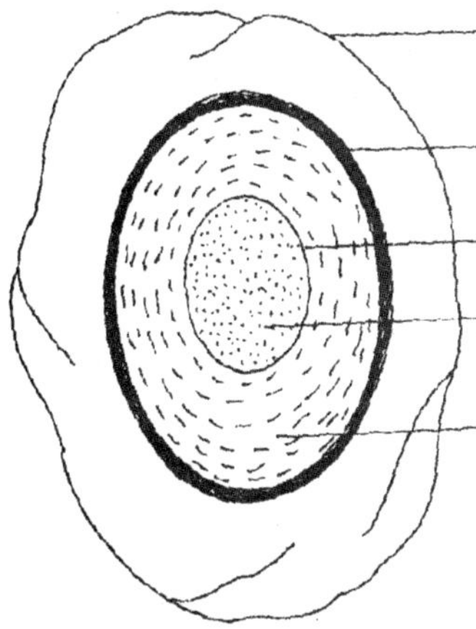

Fig. 5.11 Structure of a bacterial spore.

Germination

The process by which a spore is converted into a vegetative cell is called germination. The process of germination occurs in 3 stages-activation, initiation and outgrowth.

1. ***Activation.*** Spores may be activated from dormancy by trigger nutrients like sugars (glucose), aminoacids (L-alanine), ribosides (adenosine, inosine) or agents like heat, acidity, abrasion, surface active agents and compounds containing free sulfhydryl groups.

2. ***Initiation.*** The initiation of germination takes place under favourable conditions. Initiation is triggered by L-alanine in some and adenosine in some others. Binding of these effectors activate autolysin, which degrades cortex peptidoglycan water is taken up so that spore swells; calcium dipicolinate is released, and spore constituents are degraded by hyrolytic enzymes.

3. ***Outgrowth.*** Vegetative cell consisting of spore protoplast with surrounding wall emerges breaking open spore coat. This outgrowth requires a supply of all nutrients essential for cell growth. After a period of biosynthesis, cell division follows.

Shapes and Position of Spores. The spores may be spherical, oval or elongated in shape. The spores may be narrower than the cell or broader causing bulging of parent cell. Spores may occupy terminal, subterminal or central (equatorial) position. In Clostridium species the spores are broader than bacillary body and gives a swollen appearance, resembling a spindle. Bacteria may be classified based on the shape and position of spores.

1. Spores are spherical in shape and terminal in position and broader than vegetative cell giving the bacillus a drum-stick appearance, *e.g., Clostridium tetani.*

2. Spores are oval in shape and terminal in position and broader than parent cell, giving the bacillus a tennis racket appearance, *e.g., Clostridium tertium.*

3. Spores are oval and subterminal in position between the center and one of the poles of the bacillus and broader than parent cell casuing bulging, *e.g., Clostridium welchii* (*perfringens*), *Clostridium septicum, Clostridium sporogenes.*

4. Spores are spherical and equatorial in position; narrower than parent cell and do not bulge cell, *e.g., Bacillus anthracis* (Fig. 5.12).

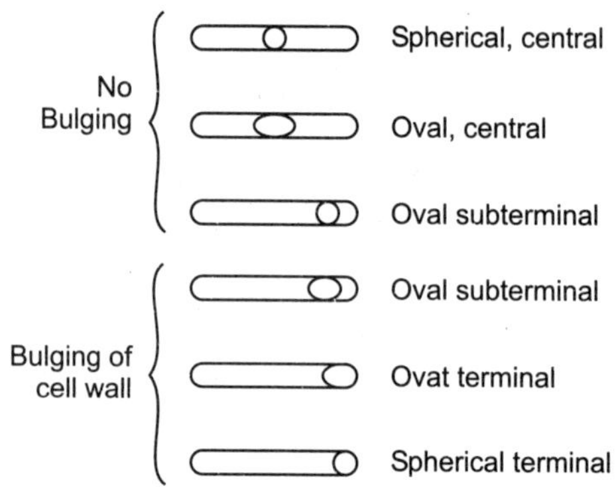

Fig. 5.12 Shape and position of spore in the bacterial cell.

Demonstration of Spores. The spores can be demonstrated by several methods.

1. Spores are seen as refractile bodies within parent cell in unstained preparations, under phase-contrast microscope.

2. Spores can be seen as unstained haloes (clear space) in stained cell protoplasm in simple stains and Gram's staining, since spores resist coloration.

3. Spores are slightly acid-fast and may be stained differentially by a modificaiton of Ziehl-Neelsen's staining.

4. Spores can be demonstrated by special staining methods –

Schaeffer-Fulton method: The spores stain green (malachite green) and the cells red (saffranine).

Dorner's method: The spores stain pink (carbol fuchsin) and the cell colorless. Nigrosine or Indian ink may be used to provide a dark background (negative staining) for contrast.

Uses of Spores :

1. Spores are used to define sterilisation process.

2. The spores of *Bacillus stearothermophilus* are used as sterilisation controls to determine the efficiency of moist heat sterilisation by biological testing. Its spores are killed at 121°C for 12 minutes by moist heat.

3. *Bacillus thuringiensis* forms paracrystalloid proteinaceous spores which are toxic to insect larvae and used as biopesticides to control pests in agriculture.

PLEOMORPHISM AND INVOLUTION FORMS

During the course of growth, bacteria of a single strain may exhibit variation in size and shape, a phenomenon known as pleomorphism. The cells may become swollen, spherical, pear-shaped, elongated filaments and filaments with localized swellings. These abnormal cells are called "involution forms". This phenomenon is commonly seen in *Streptobacillus moniliformis, Yersinia pestis, Neisseria gonorrhoeae* and *Corynebacterium diphtheriae.*

Pleomorphism occurs in ageing cultures on artificial media, particularly in the presence of antagonistic substances such as penicillin, sodium chloride, glycine, lithium chloride in high concentrations and organic acids at low pH. These involution forms are non-viable; some of them may grow and revert back to normal form when transferred to a suitable medium.

PROTOPLAST

A protoplast is a cell wall deficient microbial form, bounded by cytoplasmic membrane and do not contain any cell wall material; produced by enzymatic degestion of peptidoglycan of Gram positive bacteria such as *Bacclus*, Enterococci, Micrococci.

Protoplasts are readily produced from Gram positive bacteria by treatment with lysozyme enzyme or egg-white which lyses mucopeptide linkages. Protoplasts are osmotically sensitive or fragile and undergo rapid lysis in hypotonic or isotonic solutions. Because of this protoplasts can be maintained in intact form only in hypertonic solutions. Protoplasts when maintained in osmotically protective medium, they remain viable, metabolize and grow. They do not divide or multiply. They cannot form cell wall and cannot revert back to their parent form.

SPHEROPLASTS

Spheroplast is a cell wall deficient microbial form produced from Gram negative becilli such as *E.coli*. Spheroptast differs from protoplast in that it contains outer membrane and some amount of cell wall material.

Spheroplasts are readily produced from Gram negative bacilli in the presence of penicillin and other antibiotics, which inhibit the synthesis of peptidoglycan; or by culturing on media lacking nutrients such as diaminopimelic acid, lysine or a hexosamine derivative, which are required for cell wall synthesis.

Spheroplasts are not as osmotically sensitive as protoplasts, since they contain residual cell wall material. Spheroplasts may reproduce and multiply and are capable of growing on ordinary agar medium. They can synthesize their cell wall and revert back to their original parent form when transferred to a medium lacking cell wall inhibitor.

L-FORMS (L-PHASE) OF BACTERIA

L-forms were discovered by Klieneberger-Nobel (1935, 1942) in *Streptobacillus moniliformis*, at Lister Institute, London; hence the name.

L-forms are cell wall deficient, capable of multiplication and develop either spontaneously, or in the presence of antibiotics which inhibit cell walls synthesis such as penicillin or chemical agents such as salt (NaCl). In other words, protoplasts and spheroplasts that are capable of multiplicaiton are called L-forms. L-forms are usually unstable, and their morphological abnormality is maintained only in the presence of inducing agents and may revert back to their normal parent form, when inducing agent is absent. Some times L-forms may be stable, and become permanent feature of the organism and cannot revert back to their parent form, even in the absence of inducing agent. For example, Mycoplasmas represent stable L-forms derived from an unknown parent form.

L-forms do not possess definite shape and size, because of the absence of cell wall. They vary in size from minute bodies of 0.1 μ to 10 – 20 μ in diameter. The smallest forms can pass through bacteria-stopping filters. Their shape varies, may occur as granules and filaments of various sizes. The granules may be coccoid, balloon, disc, ring or star shaped. The filaments are slender of varying lengths.

The colonies of L-phase organisms are typically biphasic and exhibit fried-egg appearance with a central, opaque, dark, thick centre extending deep into the medium surrounded by a lace like textured flat, translucent peripheral zone. Since the colonies are highly fragile, L-forms are best examined in situ in an agar block bearing the growth under microscope. L-forms can be maintained by culturing in a soft agar medium containing 20% horse serum.

QUESTIONS

Long Essay

1. Describe briefly the anatomy of bacterial cell.

Short Notes

1. Cell envelope.
2. Bacterial cell wall.
3. Periplasmic space.
4. Porins.
5. Lysozyme.
6. Draw a neat diagram of bacterial cell and label its parts.
7. Mesosomes.
8. Volutin granules or Metachromatic granules or Babes-Ernst granules.
9. Bacterial nucleus.
10. Capsule or bacterial capsule.
11. Negative staining.
12. Capsule swelling reaction or quellung reaction.
13. Plasmids or episomes.
14. Filamentous appendages of bacteria.
15. Bacterial flagellae.
16. Fimbriae or pili.
17. Sex pili.
18. Bacterial motility.
19. Bacterial spores or endospores.
20. Pleomorphism and involution forms.
21. Protoplasts.
22. Spheroplasts.
23. What are the similarities and differences between protoplasts and spheroplasts ?
24. L-forms.

6

Bacterial Nutrition

- *Nutritional classification*
- *Autotrophs or Lithotrophs*
  - *– Photoautotrophs or photolithotrophs*
  - *– Chemoautotrophs or chemolithotrophs*
- *Heterotrophs or organotrophs*
  - *– Photoheterotrophs or photoorganotrophs*
  - *– Chemoheterotrophs or chemoorganotrophs*
- *Mixotrophs*
- *Nutritional requirements of bacteria*
  - *– Water*
  - *– Source of energy*
  - *– Source of carbon*
  - *– Source of nitrogen*
  - *– Hydrogen, oxygen, sulfur and phosphorous*
  - *– Macronutrients/Inorganic salts/minerals*
  - *– Micronutrients/Trace elements*
  - *– Growth factors/bacterial vitamins*
- *Physical (Environmental) growth requirements of bacteria*
  - *– Oxygen requirement*
  - *– Carbondtoxide requirement-capnophiles*
  - *– O-R potential (Eh)*
  - *– pH*
  - *– Temperature*
  - *– Light*
  - *– Effect of moisture and desiccation*
  - *– Effect of osmotic pressure*
  - *– Effect of mechanical and sonic stress*

NUTRITIONAL CLASSIFICATION

Bacteria may be classified nutritionally into various nutritional forms.

I. Based on energy requirements, bacteria are classified into two types.

1. Phototrophs – derive energy from sunlight
2. Chemotrophs – derive energy from oxidation of chemical compounds.

II. Based on the ability to synthesize essential metabolites, bacteria are classified into two types.

1. Autofrophs (Lithotrophs) – can synthesize their own metabolites.

2. Heterotrophs (organotrophs) – cannot synthesize their own metabolites, hence, depend upon preformed readymade organic compounds.

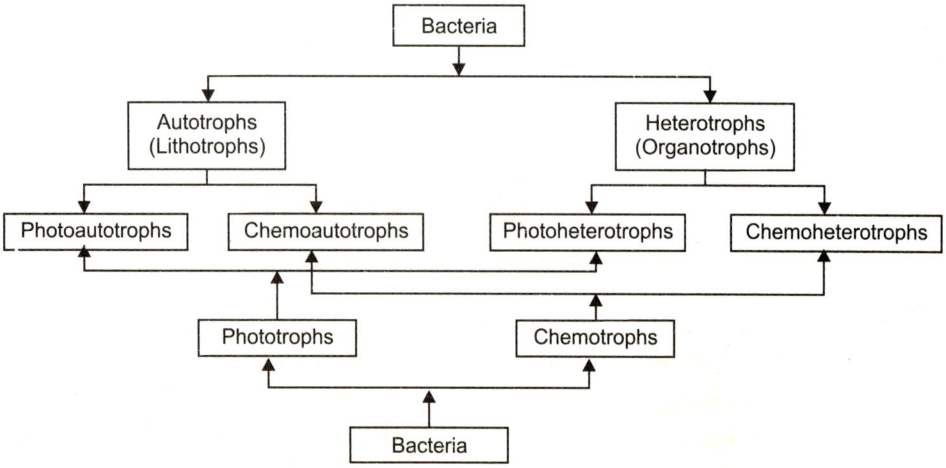

Fig. 6.1

AUTOTROPHS (OR) LITHOTROPHS

They can utilise atmospheric CO_2 and are capable of independent existence in soil and water. They are vitally important in agriculture and maintenance of soil fertility; they are of no medical importance.

Autotrophs can be further subdivided into two groups.

Photoautotrophs/photolithotrophs/photosynthetic autotrophs. They utilise sunlight as a primary source of energy and carry out photosynthesis to synthesize organic compounds from CO_2, *e.g., Chlorobium, Chromatium, Cyanobacteria.*

Chemoautotrophs/chemolithotrophs. They derive their energy by oxidation of inorganic compounds. Chemoautotrophs can be further subclassified into groups based on the type of inorganic compound used as a source of energy. *e.g.,* Nitrifying bacteria, sulphur bacteria, iron bacteria, hydrogen bacteria.

HETEROTROPHS (ORGANOTROPHS)

They cannot synthesize their own metabolites and depend upon preformed readymade organic compounds such as amino-acids, nucleotides, lipids, carbohydrates and growth factors or co-enzymes.

Heterotrophs are further subclassified into two groups.

Photoheterotrophs/photoorganotrophs. They utilise sunlight as a source of energy and organic compounds such as alcohols, fatty acids and amino-acids as a source of carbon. *e.g., Rhodospirillum.*

Chemoheterotrophs/chemoorganotrophs. Majority of heterotrophs are chemoheterotrophs. They utilise organic compounds as a source of energy as well as directly as a source of carbon. They constitute medically important bacteria, that can be grouped into commensals and parasites. Parasitic bacteria may be pathogens or non-pathogens. *e.g., Salmonella typhi, Mycobacterium tuberculosis.*

MIXOTROPHS

Some bacteria are capable of living as chemoautotrophs and as well as chemoheterotrophs. They obtain their energy from inorganic compounds but carbon from organic compounds e.g., *Desulfovilerio.*

NUTRITIONAL REQUIREMENTS OF BACTERIA

Microorganisms need a variety of chemical compounds as nutrients for their growth and multiplication and also to maintain the structure and organization of the cell.

The minimum nutritional requirements are

1. water
2. a source energy
3. a source of carbon (for the majority of bacteria, the same nutrient may serve both the purposes of energy and carbon).
4. a source of nitrogen
5. hydrogen, oxygen, sulphur and phosphorous
6. macronutrients/inorganic salts/minerals
7. micronutrients/trace elements
8. growth factors/bacterial vitamins.

Water

Water is the major constituent of bacterial cell and an integral part of the protoplasm. It is a prime nutritional requirement. Water participates in the metabolic reactions and acts as a medium for the entry of nutrients and for the excretion of waste products. Thus, water acts as a life supporting medium.

Source of Energy

Bacteria which derive their energy from sunlight are called phototrophs and those that obtain energy from chemical reactions are called chemotrophs. Usually carbohydrates are the sources of energy; amino acids and nucleotides may also serve as energy source. For the majority of bacteria the same nutrient may serve both the purposes of energy and carbon.

Source of Carbon

Carbon is one of the most important chemical required as building block for microbial growth. All microorganisms require carbon in some or other form.

The microorganisms that use organic compounds such as carbohydrates, lipids, aminoacids, nucleotides as their major carbon source are called heterotrophs; and those that use CO_2 as sole source of carbon are called autotrophs.

Source of Nitrogen

Nitrogen is the essential part of aminoacids, that together form proteins. Nitrogen serves mainly as a source of structural unit. Bacteria are particularly versatile in the utilization of nitrogen. Some bacteria use atmospheric gaseous nitrogen for cell synthesis through a process called nitrogen fixation, which is vital for the maintenance of soil fertility in agriculture. Others use inorganic nitrogen compounds such as nitrates, nitrites or ammonium salts, while some require organic nitrogen compounds such as amino acids or peptides.

Hydrogen, Oxygen, Sulfur and Phosphorous

Hydrogen and oxygen form part of many organic compounds. Water also serves as the source of hydrogen and oxygen. Hydrogen serves as the main electron donor and oxygen as the chief electron acceptor. Sulphur and phosphorous, the constituents of certain aminoacids and nucleotides are also required in smaller amounts. Phosphorous is essential for the synthesis of ATP and nucleic acids. ATP is a compound that is extremely important for energy storage and transfer. Sulphur is needed for the biosynthesis of the aminoacids cysteine, cystine and methionine.

Macronutrients/Inorganic Salts/Minerals

Bacteria require a supply of inorganic salts, particularly the anions-phosphates, sulphates and the cations-sodium, potassium, magnesium, iron, and calcium. These are normally present in the natural environments where bacteria live, but will have to be supplied in culture media.

Magnesium functins to stabilise ribosomes, cell membranes, nucleic acids and is required for the activity of many enzymes. Sodium is required by the permeases that transport nutrients into the cell. Potassium is required for the activity of many enzymes. Some essential elements are required as cofactors for enzymes for example, iron is required as a cofactor for enzymes like cytochromes, catalase etc.

Micronutrients/Trace Elements

Most microorganisms require manganese, zinc, copper, cobalt, molybdenum, selenium, boron and nickel in minute quantities. These trace elements are usually supplied in adequate amounts as impurities in major inorganic salts.

Manganese is an activator of enzymes and a part of superoxide dismutase. Zinc (Zn^{++}) and is required for the activity of enzymes like DNA and RNA polymerases, alcohol dehydrogenase and carbonic anhydrase. Copper (Cu^{2+}) is a prosthetic group of several enzymes, like cytochrome oxidase involved in respiration. Cobalt is a constituent of vitamin B_{12}. Molybdenum is present in molybdoflavoproteins. Nickel is present in hydrogenases. Selenium is an essential component of several enzymes such as glutathione peroxidase.

Growth Factors/Bacterial Vitamins

Some bacteria require certain organic compounds in minute quantities for growth. These are known as growth factors. In many cases, these growth factors are identical with the vitamins belonging to the B-complex group and hence known as "Bacterial vitamins". They include thiamine, riboflavine, nicotinic acid, pyridoxine, p-aminobenzoic acid, folic acid, biotin, vitamin B_{12} etc. Aminoacids, purines and pyrimidines also serve as growth factors.

e.g., Hemophilus influenzae requires X and V factors
Salmonella typhi requires tryptophan
Gonococci requires glutathione
Brucella abortus requires niacin
Clostridium tetani requires riboflavine
Bacillus anthracis requires thiamine (vitamin B_1)
Lactobacillus requires pyridoxine (vitamin B_6)

Growth factors may be of two types:

1. ***Essential growth factors.*** They are essential for the growth and the growth does not occur in their absence.

2. ***Accessory growth factors.*** They are not essential for the growth, but when present can enhance growth.

PHYSICAL/ENVIRONMENTAL GROWTH REQUIREMENTS

Bacteria require environmental factors for growth in optimum concentrations. They are as follows:

1. Oxygen
2. Carbon dioxide
3. Oxidation-reduction potential (Eh)
4. pH
5. Temperature
6. Light
7. Moisture and drying
8. Osmotic effect
9. Mechanical and sonic stress.

Oxygen requirement

The proper oxygen tension is essential for balanced growth. The bacteria which require oxygen for growth are known as "**Aerobes**"and those that do not require oxygen are known as "**Anaerobes**".

Based on the influence of oxygen on growth and viability, bacteria may be classified into different groups.

1. ***Obligate aerobes.*** They grow only in the presence of oxygen. Oxygen is used as terminal electron acceptor. *e.g., Pseudomonas, Mycobacterium.*

2. ***Facultative anaerobes.*** They can grow in the presence or absence of oxygen. *e.g.*, Staphylococci, *Salmonella, E.coli.*

3. ***Microaerophiles.*** They are aerobes which grow best with less oxygen than found in air *e.g., Campylobacter.*

4. ***Obligate anaerobes.*** They can grow only in the absence of oxygen, presence of small amounts of oxygen may be toxic and kills the bacterium. They do not use oxygen as an electron acceptor. Anaerobic bacteria use nitrates and sulphates (inorganic compounds) as terminal electron acceptors. In the absence of oxygen, energy is produced by fermentation. *e.g., Clostridium, Bacteroides.*

5. ***Aerotolerant anaerobes.*** They are anaerobes which are not readily killed by oxygen. *e.g.,* most Streptococci, Lactobacilli.

In the presence of oxygen, hydrogen peroxide, super oxide radicals and other toxic peroxides accumulate. The enzymes superoxide dismutase and catalase, which splits superoxide radicals and hydrogen peroxide is present only in aerobic bacteria but absent in anaerobes. Moreover, obligate anaerobes may possess enzymes that are active only in the reduced state.

Carbondioxide requirement

All bacteria require small amounts of carbondioxide for their growth. This is provided by the atmospheric air or endogenously by the metabolic reactions within the cell.

Capnophiles. Some bacteria grow best at a high CO_2 tension than those found in atmosphere. Several bacteria are stimulated by partial pressures that are greater than those normally found in air. These bacteria, which have high CO_2 requirement are called capnophilic bacteria. *e.g., Brucella,* gonococci, meningococci etc. require 3–10% CO_2 for their primary isolation from clinical specimens. Hence, these cultures are incubated in a CO_2 incubator (capnoeic incubator) or candle jar, that provides a 3–10% CO_2.

Oxidation-Reduction Potential (Eh) Requirement

The growth of the aerobic and anaerobic bacteria is greatly dependent upon the oxidised or reduced state of the environment than the presence or absence of oxygen.

The oxidising or reducing condition of a system or medium is indicated by the net readiness of all the components in that system to accept or donate electrons. This is known as oxidation-reduction potential (redox potential) of the system.

The redox potential of a medium is estimated by measuring the electrical potential difference set up between the mediumn and an unattackable electrode immersed in it. This electrode potential (Eh) can be measured in millivolts (mV). A simple method of measuring the redox potential is the use of oxidation-reduction indicators such as methylene blue, and noting the color change. The more oxidised the system, the higher is potential.

For most bacteria, the optimum Eh is about + 0.2 to + 0.4 millivolts at pH 7. Obligate anaerobes are unable to grow, unless the Eh is atleast as low as – 0.2 millivolts.

During the growth of both aerobic and anaerobic bacteria, there is a progressive decrease in the Eh of the environment.

pH requirement

Bacteria are very sensitive to variations in pH. Each microorganism has a "**pH range**" and the growth does not occur above the maximum or below the minimum of this range. Every microorganism has a well-defined pH optimum, at which it grows best. Majority of bacteria grow best at neutral or very slightly alkaline reaction *i.e.,* 7.2 to 7.6. These are called **neutrophiles**, since they grow at and around neutral pH. But some microorganisms grow best at acidic pH, known as "**acidophiles**". *e.g., Lactobacilli.* Fungi and yeasts grow best at acidic pH. Some bacteria are very sensitive to acid, but tolerant of alkali and grow at alkaline pH. They are known as "**alkaliphiles** or **basophiles**". *e.g., Vibrio cholerae* grows at a pH of 8.5 to 9.

Strong acid or alkali (*e.g.*, 5% HCl or NaOH) can rapidly kill bacteria, but mycobacteria are exceptionally resistant to them.

The pH of a culture medium is adjusted by adding NaOH (alkali) if the pH is acidic or HCl (acid) if the pH is alkaline.

Temperature requirement

Bacteria differ in their requirements of temperature for growth. For each species, there is a "temperature range", and growth does not occur above the maximum or below the minimum of the range. The temperature at which growth occurs best is known as the "**optimum temperature**". Most pathogenic bacteria grow best at an optimum temperature of 37°C. In the laboratory, bacteria are grown at this optimum temperature in a thermostatically controlled incubator.

Based on temperature requirement, microorganisms can be broadly classified into five groups:

1. Psychrophiles
2. Mesophiles
3. Thermodurics
4. Thermophiles
5. Hyperthermophiles

Psychrophilic bacteria are those which grow best at temperatures below 20°C, usually quite well at 0°C and in some cases even at – 7°C. These microorganisms grow in refrigerated and frozen foods and cause spoilage.

Mesophilic bacteria are those which grow at a temperature range of 25 to 40°C. Some mesophiles have a wide growth temperature range *e.g.,* 5 to 43°C for *Pseudomonas aeruginosa*; whereas some others have a more restricted range of temperature *e.g.,* 30 to 39°C for gonococci. A few mesophiles can grow at temperatures below 5°C, as in a domestic refrigerator or at temperatures above 45°C.

Many saprophytes of soil and water are mesophilic. Parasites of humans and warm-blooded animals are also mesophilic.

Thermoduric bacteria are those mesophiles that are capable of surviving pasteurisation, although they do not necessarily grow at such temperatures.

Thermophilic bacteria are those which grow at high temperatures between 55 and 80°C. They are usually non-parasitic. They may cause spoilage of under processed canned foods. Some bacteria such as *Bacillus stearothermophilus* and *Clostridium botulinum* form spores that are extremely heat resistant.

Hyperthermophilic bacteria are those which grow at temperature of above 80°C, some of them grow even at 250°C.

Thermophiles are found in hot springs, geysers and industrial heated wastes.

Thermophiles offer advantages in biotechnology microbial processes carried out at high temperatures. Enzymes from thermophiles are capable of catalyzing biochemical reactions at high temperatures and are more stable than enzymes from mesophiles.

Light requirement. Many bacteria, except phototrophic organisms require darkness for growth and viability. Sunlight, UV light and ionizing radiations can kill microorganisms. Hence, cultures are incubated in an incubator under dark to protect them from sunlight, clinical specimens containing meningococci. *e.g.,* CSF, should not be exposed to sunlight. Exposure to sunlight may influence pigment production. e.g., photochromogenic mycobacteria form pigment only on exposure to light.

Effect of Moisture and Desiccation

There is a wide variation in the ability of bacteria to survive drying. Bacterial spores (*e.g.,* anthrax spores, tetanus spores) are extremely resistant to desiccation and can survive many years in a moisture free environment.

Vegetative bacteria are much less resistant to drying and require moisture. It is for this reason culture media should be fresh and contain water of condensation. Otherwise delicate organisms like Streptococci, gonococci and meningococci cannot grow well.

Treponema pallidum and gonococci cannot withstand drying and die quickly whereas *Staphylococcus aureus*, tubercle bacillus can withstand drying for weeks.

Delicate, nonsporing organisms can survive drying for many years, if they are desiccated rapidly, completely while frozen and maintained in vacuum in the dark. This is the basis of preservation of cultures by "**Freeze-drying** or **Lyophilisaiton**".

Effect of Osmotic Pressure

Bacteria are more tolerant to osmotic variation than most other cells due to the mechanical strength of their cell walls.

When bacteria are placed in hypertonic solution (*e.g.*, 20% NaCl), water (solvent) passes out, from the interior of the cell through semipermeable cell membranes, into the solution surrounding the cell (by osmosis), so that cells become dehydrated, resulting in shrinkage of cell. This phenomenon is called "Plasmolysis". Here, the cell wall retains the original shape and size, appearing as bacterial ghost. Plasmolysis occurs more readily in Gram negative than in Gram positive bacteria.

Some bacteria can grow and tolerate high salt concentrations. They are known as halophilic organisms, usually found in sea water.

Some pathogenic bacteria such as *Staphylococcus aureus* can grow in the presence of 8–10% NaCl and *Enterococcus* at a concentration of 6.5% NaCl.

When bacteria are placed in hypotonic solution (*e.g.*, distilled water, 0.01% NaCl), the water enters the cell from the surroundings causing swelling and may even burst the cell. This phenomenon is called "**Plasmoptysis**" or "**Imbibition**".

Effect of mechanical and sonic stress. Though bacteria have tough cell walls, they may be ruptured by mechanical stresses, such as grinding or vigorous shaking with glass beads. They may also be disintegrated by exposure to ultrasonic vibrations.

QUESTIONS

Essay Type Questions:

1. What are the heterotrophic bacteria ? Discuss the nutritional and physical requirements for the growth of the bacteria.

Short Notes:

1. Heterotrophs.
2. Growth factors/bacterial vitamins.
3. Oxygen requirement of bacteria.
4. Capnophilies.
5. Psychrophiles.
6. Thermophiles.
7. Mesophiles.
8. Lyophilisation/freeze drying.
9. Plasmolysis.
10. Plasmoptysis.

7

Growth and Multiplication of Bacteria

- *Reproduction in bacteria*
- *Generation time/population doubling time*
- *Batch cultures*
- *Bacterial counts*
  - *Total count*
  - *Viable count*
- *Bacterial growth curve*
- *Continuous cultures*
- *Synchronous cultures*

REPRODUCTION IN BACTERIA

Bacteria reproduce asexually by transverse binary fission. When a bacterium size increases and reaches its critical stage, it divides and produces two daughter cells. Bacterial cell division consists of following stages :

1. DNA replication. The two strands of DNA separate and each strand replicates to form a new complementary strand. Nucleus replicates by simple fission. Mitosis is absent.

2. The replicated double stranded DNA molecules are distributed into two daughter cells equally.

3. The cell divides into two by an inward growth of cytoplasmic membrane across the cell, known as transverse septum or cross wall. Mesosome (chondroid) attached to the cytoplasmic membrane plays an important role in the formation of transverse septum. This is followed by the formation of cell wall material, and finally the two daughter cells separate. Sometimes, the daughter cells may remain together, even after cell division.

GENERATION TIME/POPULATION DOUBLING TIME

The time required for a cell to divide to form two daughter cells or the interval of time between two cell divisions is known as generation time or population doubling time.

Bacteria multiply by binary fission, in which each cell produces two daughter cells. Thus, if we start with a single bacterium, the increase in population is by geometric progression :

$$1 \rightarrow 2 \rightarrow 2^2 \rightarrow 2^3 \rightarrow 2^4 \rightarrow 2^5 \text{ -------}\rightarrow 2^n$$

Therefore, a single bacterial cell can theoretically give rise to 10^{21} progeny in 24 hours.

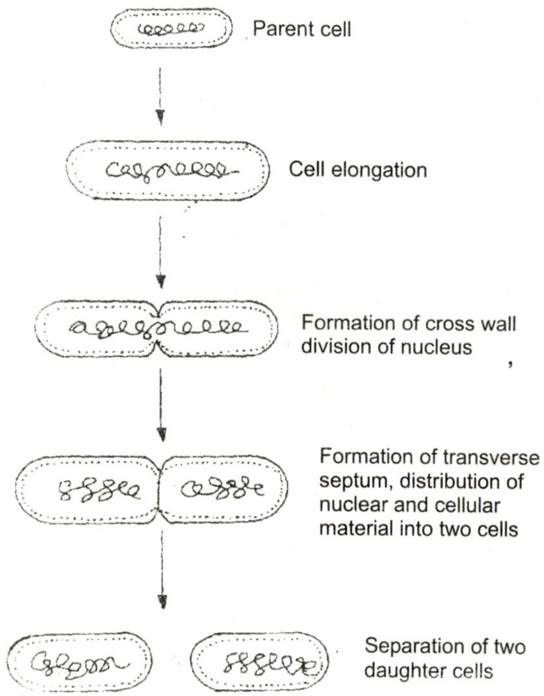

Fig. 7.1 Reproduction/multiplication of bacteria by transverse binary fission.

Generation time can be calculated by examination of culture under phase contrast microscope with photography, by recording the sequence of events, automatically and at a predetermined time intervals; or by analyzing the growth with some simple mathematical expressions.

$$G = \frac{t}{n}$$

G = generation time

t = time interval (the time elapsed between final and initial population)

n = number of generations

Table 7.1 Generation times of some bacteria

Microorganism	*Generation time*
Escherichia coli	20 minutes
Staphylococcus aureus	30 minutes
Mycobacterium tuberculosis	20–24 hours
Mycobacterium leprae	20–30 days

The generation time of most of the medically important bacteria is about 20 minutes. It varies with the species and environmental conditions. Generation times in nature are usually much longer than in culture media.

BATCH CULTURE

When microorganisms are cultivated in a liquid medium, in a closed system such as in a conical flask or a large fermentor vessel; that is when they are incubated and grown in a single batch of medium, the multiplication of bacteria, after some time, comes to a halt, due to depletion of nutrients and accumulation of toxic waste metabolites; because no fresh medium is provided during incubation. Such culture is known as "Batch culture" and grown each time by inculating into fresh medium, in batches. Such a closed system culture is very useful in studying the growth characters of microorganisms.

If the number of cells present at different time intervals after inoculation, in a limited volume of liquid medium is measured and plotted, a growth curve (batch growth curve) is obtained (Fig. 7.2).

BACTERIAL COUNTS

Bacterial growth in numbers can be studied by bacterial counts. Two types of bacterial counts can be made, total count and viable count.

Total count is the total number of cells present in a sample, irrespective of whether they are living or not. Total counts can be obtained by

1. Direct counting under the microscope using counting chambers such as Neubauer chamber and Petroff-Hausser chamber.
2. Counting in an electronic device such as coulter counter.
3. Direct microscopic count (DMC) by Breed's method employs direct counting using stained smears prepared by spreading a known volume (0.01 ml) of the sample over a measured area (one square cm) of a slide.
4. Proportional count method employs counting bacteria by comparing the number of cells in smears in proportion (or in relation) to the known number of particles such as tiny plastic beads.
5. Turbidity measurements using photoelectric colorimeter or spectrophotometer or nephalometer.
6. Separating the cells by centrifugation or filtration and measuring their wet or dry weight.
7. Chemical assay of cell components such as nitrogen.

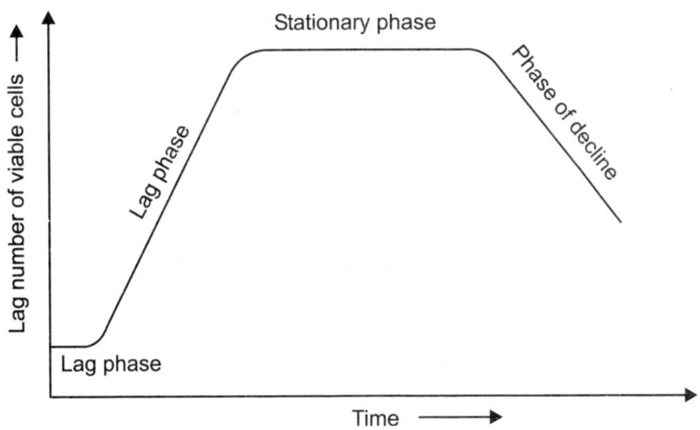

Fig. 7.2 (*a*) Growth curve for viable count.

Viable count measures only those cells capable of growing and producing a colony on a suitable nutrient medium. In other words, it measures the number of living cells, that is, cells capable of multiplication.

Viable counts are obtained by

1. Standard plate count (SPC) by pour plate method,

2. Membrane filter method, and

3. Mean probable number (MPN) or presumptive coliform count used in the bacteriological analysis of water.

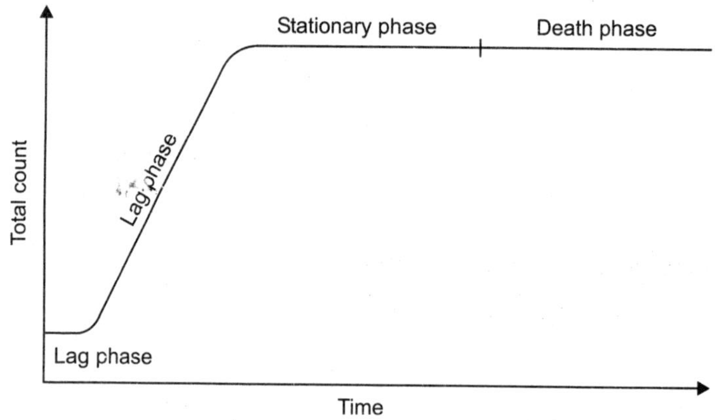

Fig. 7.2 (*b*) Growth curve for total count.

BACTERIAL GROWTH CURVE

Growth curve is a graphic representation of rate of multiplication (or number) of cells plotted against time. For all organisms including microbes the growth curve is sigmoid.

When bacteria are cultivated in a liquid medium, in a closed system and bacterial counts are made at regular time intervals and plotted in relation to time; a growth curve is obtained. The growth curve shows four distinct phases Fig.7.2.

1. Lag phase.

2. Log phase/Logarithmic phase/Exponential phase.

3. Stationary phase

4. Death phase/phase of decline.

1. Lag phase. When a microorganism is inoculated into a fresh culture medium, usually no immediate increase in cell numbers or mass occurs because no cell division occurs. Therefore, this period is called the lag phase. It is the time taken by the organism to adjust physiologically to the given conditions and build up an internal supply of metabolites, ribosomes, ATP, enzymes and co-enzymes.

The duration of the lag phase varies with the species, amount of inoculum, nature of culture medium and environmental factors such as pH, temperature etc. The bacteria will have maximum size towards the end of lag phase.

Log phase/Logrithmic phase/Exponential phase. Following the lag phase, the cells grow at constant rate, start dividing by binary fission and their numbers increase exponentially or by geometric progression with time. There is a linear relationship (strength line on the graph) between the time and logarithm of the number of cells. That is why, sometimes infection overtakes body defences and gets out of control.

During log phase the cells are smaller in size, young, actively multiplying, the metabolic activity is at its peak, and the population is most uniform in terms of chemical and physiological properties, and stain uniformly. Therefore, log phase is most suitable for studying biochemical and physiological properties of cells.

Stationary phase. During this period, the nutrients begin to disappear, and there is a balance between cell growth and division and cell death; the growth curve becomes horizontal or plateau.

The stationary phase is due to the depletion of nutrients, and the accumulation of toxic metabolic wastes such as organic acids in the culture medium.

In the stationary phase, the cells are Gram variable and show irregular staining due to the presence of intracellular storage granules such as polysaccharides, lipids. In spore forming bacteria, sporulation occurs in this phase. In this phase, some bacteria produce secondary metabolites such as exotoxins and antibiotics.

Death phase/Decline phase. Due to nutrient deprivation and accumulation of toxic metabolites such as organic acids leads to the death of cells logarithmically. Bacteria die at different rates. Some species such as gonococci die rapidly due to autolysis. It leads to a decline phase, the reverse of log phase. Involution forms are common in phase of decline.

CONTINUOUS CULTURES

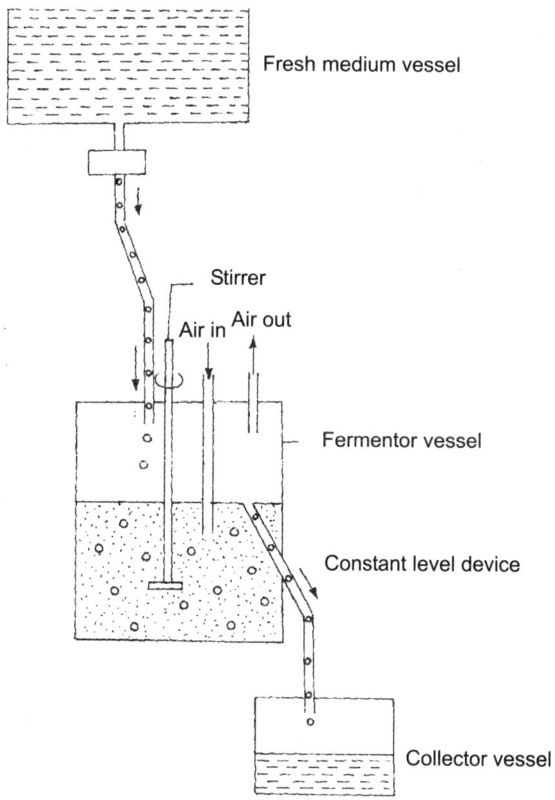

Fig. 7.3. Chemostat for continuous cultures.

Batch culture is the usual method of growing bacteria. However, it is possible to grow microorganisms in an open system, through continuous provision of nutrients and removal of wastes, so that cells continuously multiply and remain in logarithmic phase and at a constant biomass concentration. This method is called continuous culture, may be similar to a situation occurring in human and animal disease.

Continuous cultures are useful, 1. for the production of industrially important fermentation products, 2. in selective isolation of certain rare microorganisms and, 3. for research studies, to obtain population at logarithmic phase, which can grow continuously in limiting concentrations of nutrients.

There are several devices to maintain continuous cultures.

Chemostat. It is a continuous system cultivator in which the sterile nutrient medium is continuously fed into the culture vessel at the same rate as media containing waste products, old and dead cells of microorganisms is removed. The level of growth is controlled by maintaining in fixed, limiting concentration of an essential nutrient (*e.g.*, Amino acid).

Turbidostat. It has an optical sensing device or photocell that measures the absorbance or turbidity of the culture in the growth vessel. The flow rate of media through the culture vessel is automatically regulated to maintain a predetermined turbidity or cell density.

The turbidostat differs from chemostat in several ways. The culture medium in turbidostat lacks a limiting nutrient, and its dilution rate varies rather than remaining constant. The turbidostat operates best at high dilution rates; whereas the chemostat is most stable and effective at low dilution rates.

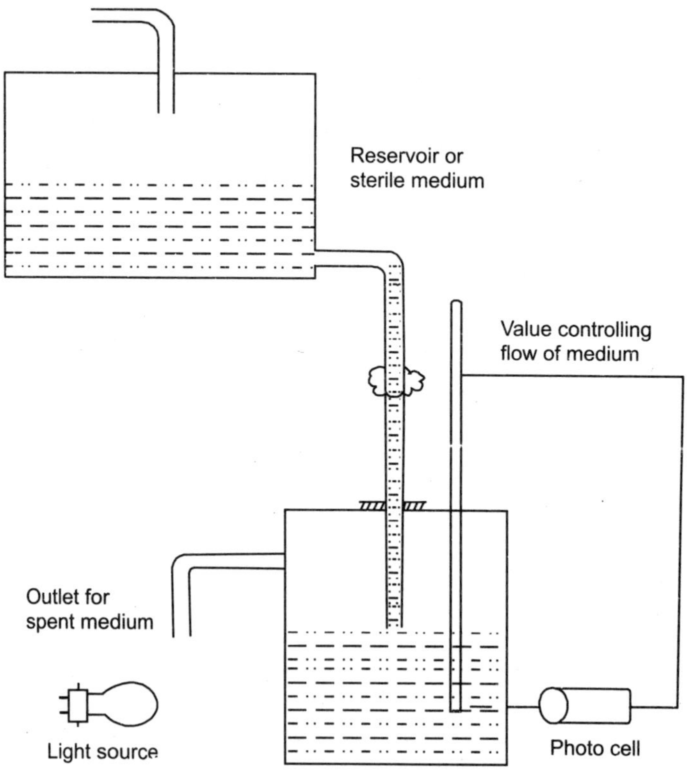

Fig. 7.4. The turbidostat.

Dialysis technique is another method which maintains the culture in the logarithmic phase for a slightly longer periods.

SYNCHRONOUS CULTURES

In normal bacterial cultures, different cells divide at different times. But synchronous cultures are composed of populations of cells that are at the same stage of their life cycle. All the cells in the culture will divide at the same time, will grow for a generation time, and all will divide again at the same time. Thus, the entire population is kept uniform with respect to growth and division. In microbiology, it is not possible to analyze a single bacterial cell and synchronous cultures provide the entire cell crop in the same stage of growth. Measurements made on such synchronous cultures are equivalent to the measurement made on individual cells, which is essential for critical biochemical, physiological and genetic experiments.

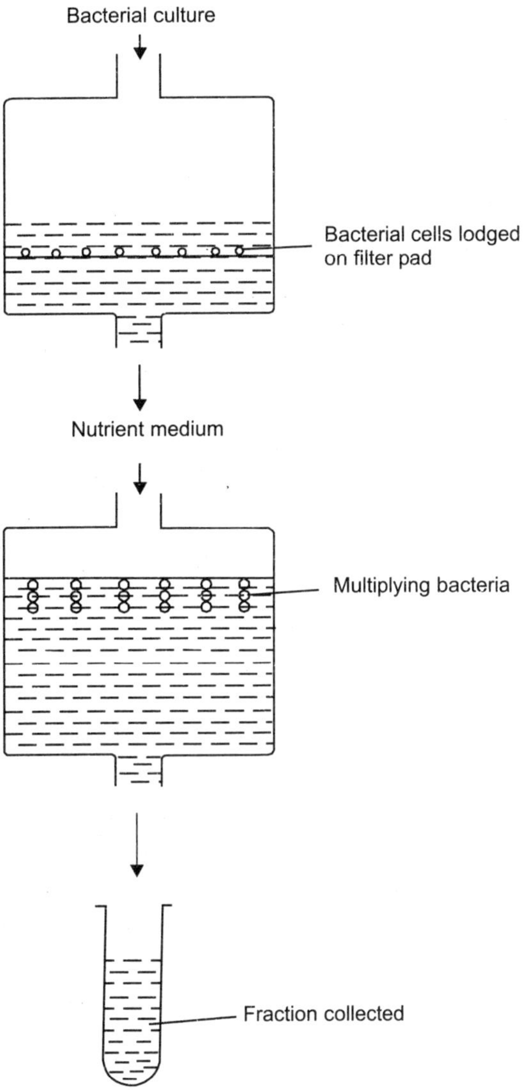

Fig. 7.5. The Helmstetler-Cummings apparatus for obtaining synchronous cultures.

Synchronous cultures of bacteria may be obtained by several methods.

1. A synchronous population of cells can be selected or sorted out according to size and age by physical separation of cells, such as filtration, centrifugation and density gradient methods. Usually Helmstetler-Cummings filter pad technique is employed.

2. A culture is induced by manipulating the physical environment or the chemical composition of the medium to obtain a synchronously dividing population.

The techniques based on selection are preferable to those based on induction, since induction is likely to introduce distortions in the physiologic state of the cells.

QUESTIONS

Short Notes

1. Reproduction in bacteria/binary fission.
2. Generation time/population doubling time.
3. Batch culture.
4. Bacterial counts.
5. Total count.
6. Viable count.
7. Bacterial growth curve/growth phases of bacteria.
8. Continuous cultures.
9. Chemostat.
10. Turbidostat.
11. Synchronous cultures.

8

Sterilization

- *Introduction*
- *Definition*
- *Factors influencing destruction of micro-organisms*
- *Sterilization methods*
  - *– Physical methods*
  - *– Chemical methods*
  - *– Mechanical methods*
- *Heat sterilization*
  - *– Dry heat sterilization*
    - *– Red heat*
    - *– Flaming*
    - *– Incineration or burning*
    - *– Hot air oven*
    - *– Infrared conveyor sterilizer*
    - *– Sterilization controls*
  - *– Moist heat sterilization*
    - *– Mode of action of steam*
    - *– Thermal death point*
    - *– Thermal death time*
    - *– Decimal reduction time (D-value)*
    - *– Physical characteristics of steam*
    - *– Advantages of steam (moist heat) over dry heat*
    - *– Moist heat below 100°C*
    - *– Inspissation*
  - *– Moist heat at 100°C*
    - *– Tyndallization*
  - *– Moist heat at above 100°C*
    - *– Autoclaving*
  - *– Sterilization controls*
- *Ionizing radiation/cold sterilization*
  - *– Gamma rays*
  - *– High energy electrons (cathode rays)*
- *Gaseous chemosterilizers*
  - *– Low Temperature Steam with formaldehyde (LTSF)*
  - *– Ethylene oxide*
  - *– Formaldehyde gas/fumigation*
  - *– Beta propiolactone*
  - *– Gas plasma*
- *Liquid chemosterilizers*
  - *– Formalin solution*
  - *– Glutaraldehyde (cidex)*
  - *– Iodine*
- *Filtration*
  - *– Applications*
  - *– Types of bacterial filters*
  - *– Diatomaceous earthenware candle filters*
  - *– Unglazed porcelain/ceramic filters*
  - *– Asbestos disk (seitz) filters*
  - *– Sintered glass filters*
  - *– Membrane filters*
  - *– Polypore filters*
  - *– HEPA filters*
  - *– Sterilization controls*

INTRODUCTION

The sterilization procedures are important particularly in the microbiological laboratories and in hospital practice. In microbiological work the sterilization of culture media, glass ware, containers and instruments is essential for the isolation and maintenance of pure cultures. In hospital practice, the sterilization of instruments, dressings, drugs and other supplies is important for the prevention of infection.

Sterilization procedures are also important and widely practiced in food, drug and pharmaceutical industries.

DEFINITION

Sterilization can be defined as a process by which any article, objects, surface, culture medium, specimen or material is freed from all living microorganisms including vegetative bacteria and their spores, viruses, vegetative fungi and their spores, both pathogenic and nonpathogenic.

"**Sterility**" is an absolute state. "**Sterile**" is an absolute term-an item/article is either sterile or nonsterile. It can never be "partly sterile" or "almost sterile" or "semisterile".

METHODS OF STERILIZATION

Sterilization may be accomplished by physical, chemical and mechanical methods.

Physical Methods

I. Heat

A. ***Dry heat***

1. Red heat
2. Flaming
3. Incineration or burning
4. Hot air oven
5. Microwave ovens.

B. ***Moist heat*** **(*steaming*)**

1. Steaming below 100°C or below atmospheric pressure
   - Inspissation
2. Steaming at 100°C or at atmospheric pressure
   - Tyndallization
   - Single exposure for 90 minutes
3. Steaming under pressure, above 100°C or above atmospheric pressures
   - Autoclaving

II. Ionizing radiation (cold sterilization)

- Gamma rays
- Particulate high energy electrons.

Chemical methods/chemcsterilants/chemical sporicidal agents

III. Gaseous chemosterilizers

1. Low temperature steam and formaldehyde (LTSF)

2. Ethylene oxide gas
3. Formaldehyde gas
4. Betapropiolactone

IV. Liquid chemosterilizers

6. Formalin (formaldehyde solution)
7. Glutaraldehyde solution

Mechanical methods

V. Filtration

1. Diatomaceous earthenware candle filters *e.g.,* Berkefeld filters, Mandler filters.
2. Unglazed, porcelain filters *e.g.,* Chamberland filters, Doulton filters, Jenkins filters.
3. Asbestos disk filters *e.g.,* Seitz filters.
4. Sintered glass filters (fritted glass filters/Morton filters).
5. Membrane filters (ultra filters).
6. HEPA (High efficiency particulate air) filters.

HEAT STERILIZATION

Heat is the simplest and reliable means of sterilization. Practical procedures by which heat is employed are divided into 2 categories – dry heat and moist heat.

A. Dry Heat Sterilization

The lethal effect of dry heat is due to:

– oxidative damage to cell constituents
– protein denaturation
– increased levels of electrolytes.

1. Red heat. Inoculation wires, wire loops, points of forceps and spatulas are held in Bunsen flame till they become red hot, to sterilize them.

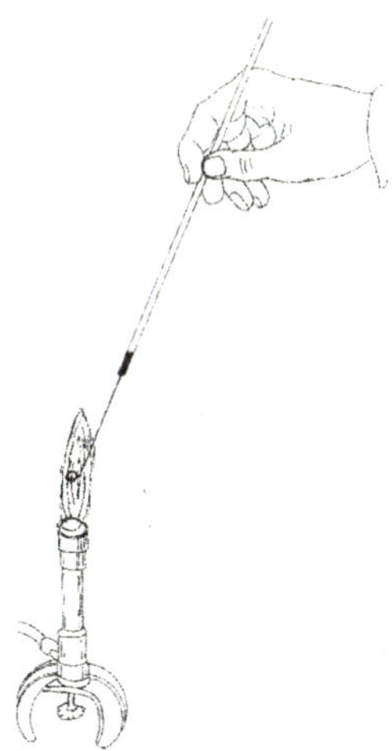

Fig. 8.1 Method of sterilization by red heat (dry heat). Inoculation loop heated to redness before and after inoculation. Aseptic technique to prevent contamination.

If inoculation loops contain infectious proteinaceous material, it should be washed in chemical disinfectant before heating to avoid the spread of infected particles by spattering.

2. Flaming. Scalpels, needles, necks of flasks, mouths of culture tubes, glass slides, coverslips etc. could be passed a few times through the bunsen flame without allowing them to become red hot.

Needles, scalpels, basins, inoculation loops are sometimes treated by immersing in methylated spirit and burning off the alcohol

3. Incineration or burning. It is an efficient method for the sterilization and disposal of hazardous infectious hospital waste. Soiled dressings, pathological materials, animal carcasses, infected linen/ bedding, sharp needles and other clinical waste are literally burned to ashes at temperatures of 870°C to 980°C in incinerator by electricity.

Plastics such as disposable syringes, rubber catheters, culture plates, specimen containers made of polyvinyl chloride (PVC) and polyethylene may emit dense black smoke when incinerated. They can be autoclaved before disposal.

Toxic air emissions during incineration and heavy metals in ash may constitute health hazard.

4. Hot air oven/Hot air sterilizer. It is the most important, widely used and the best method of sterilization by dry heat.

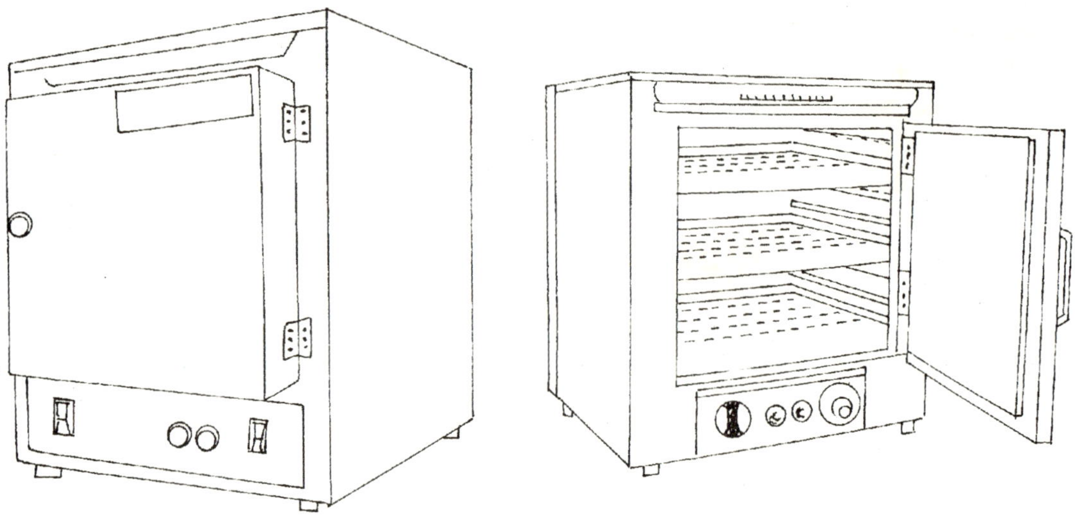

Fig. 8.2 Hot air oven.

Principle. Dry heat is transferred from source to load (article) by conduction or radiation. Since hot air is a bad conductor of heat with less penetrating power; high temperatures and long exposure times are required for dry heat sterilization than moist heat sterilization.

Uses. Hot air oven is used for the sterilization of following items:

1. Glass ware such as test tubes, conical flasks (or any other flasks), petri plates, pipettes, measuring cylinders, ampoules etc.

2. Glass syringes.

3. Surgical metal instruments like needles, fine cannulae, forceps, scissors, scalpels etc.

4. Materials such as oils, petroleum jelly, waxes, glycerol, fats, grease and liquid paraffin which are impervious to steam.

5. Sulphonamides.

6. Powders, talc, dusting powder that may form paste by steam can be sterilized by dry heat in hot air oven.

Cotton wool plugs, wrappings of kraft paper, aluminium tins, aluminium tubes, aluminium foils may be used to retain sterility after processing.

Hot air oven is not suitable for fabrics and dressings which are poor conductors of heat and ruined (charred) by excessive heating.

Rubber articles like washers, corks, plastics, gloves, tubing or catheters should not be sterilized in hot air oven. However, silicone rubber can withstand dry heat sterilization.

Structure of hot-air oven. Hot air oven consists of an insulated double walled cabinet made of aluminium or stainless steel and is constructed to withstand high temperatures. It is heated by electricity and has a thermostat, which regulates the temperature inside the chamber at a desired level, and a thermometer is fitted for recording the temperature. Large hot air ovens may have a motor and fan fitted either at the bottom or back of the oven to circulate hot air uniformly throughout the chamber. The shelves (partitions) within the oven are perforated to ensure proper air circulation.

Temperature and holding period used for sterilization. Sterilization in hot air oven is done by two methods:

(*i*) using a temperature of 160°C for one hour

(*ii*) using a temperature of 180°C for 30 minutes. Infact, the total heating cycle time is much longer, since it includes the time required to attain the desired temperature, prior to sterilization time, plus the time required to cool down after sterilization.

Heating at 150°C for two hours is used for sterilization of cutting instruments such as those used in opthalmic surgery.

Precautions. The following precautions have to be taken during sterilization by hot air oven.

1. The glassware must be thoroughly washed, cleaned and perfectly dry.
2. Test tubes and flasks must be stoppered with non-absorbent cotton wool plugs.
3. All glassware must be neatly wrapped in kraft paper.
4. Care must be taken to avoid overloading and the articles should be arranged in such a way as to ensure the uniform circulation of hot air between the individual items in the load.
5. After sterilization is over, the oven must be allowed to cool gradually before the door is opened. Otherwise, the sudden inrush of air into the chamber may result in cracking of glassware and wrappings may catch fire.
6. Rubber articles like washers, caps, gloves, plastics, rubber tubings, corks should not be sterilized by hot air oven as they get melted by dry heat. Similarly fabrics and dressings should not be sterilized as they get charred. Fluids and culture media should not be sterilized in hot air oven.

5. **Microwave ovens.** Microwave ovens can be used for dry heat sterilization of small items.

Sterility tests for dry heat sterilization or sterilization controls for hot air oven.

To determine the efficiency of dry heat sterilization, various sterilization controls are employed. They are as follows:

Physical methods. 1. By recording temperature with centigrade thermometers.

2. Thermocouple measurement. Thermocouples are temperature–sensitive, electronically operated sensors (probes) for measuring temperature and are more accurate than routine thermometers.

A thermocouple is inserted inside any article in the hot air oven chamber and its wire leads are carried out to a potentiometer which indicates the temperature inside the chamber during sterilization.

3. **Chemical methods – Browne's tube.** Browne's tube contains a red color indicator solution which turns green when adequate temperature is maintained for a fixed time by dry heat sterilization and is a convenient method for routine use.

A Browne's tube is included with the load to be sterilized in the hot air oven and immediately inspected at the end of the sterilization cycle for color change.

4. **Biological method/bacteriological test.** For determining efficiency of dry heat sterilization by microbiological testing, paper strips impregnated with 10^6 spores of a non-toxigenic strain of *Clostridium tetani* are placed in envelopes and inserted into hot air oven chamber. After sterilization is over, the strips are taken out and inoculated into RCM broth or thioglycollate broth and incubated for sterility test under strict anaerobic conditions at 37°C for 5 days.

MOIST HEAT STERILIZATION

Moist heat (steaming) under pressure is the only method of sterilization that is both reliable, widely applicable and efficient and always should be the method of choice, wherever applicable.

Moist heat kills bacteria by

- denaturation of enzymes and proteins
- coagulation of cytoplasm.

1. Moist heat below 100°C or steaming below atmospheric pressure.

Inspissation and serum inspissator. Inspissation is a process used to sterilize and solidify culture media containing substances like serum, egg and other coagulable proteins, which cannot withstand high temperatures, in an apparatus called inspissator.

Culture media such as Lowenstein-Jensen (LJ) media, Dorset's egg media and Loeffler's serum slope are rendered sterile and solid, simultaneously by inspissation.

Inspissator consists of a chamber made of copper plate with a water jacket around it and the chamber can be closed with a glass lid. The temperature is regulated automatically by a thermostat. There are small openings in the inner wall communicating with the top of the water chamber above the level of the water, so that water vapor (steam) can enter the interior of the inspissator, and the medium is exposed to moist heat.

The tubes or bottles containing media are kept in a slanting position inside the chamber and exposed to a temperature of 80–85°C for 30 minutes on three successive days, without disturbing their position. Hence, the sterilization takes place by the principle of tyndallization. The first day heating kills all vegetative bacteria; spores, if present, being in a favourable medium, will germinate and be killed on subsequent heatings.

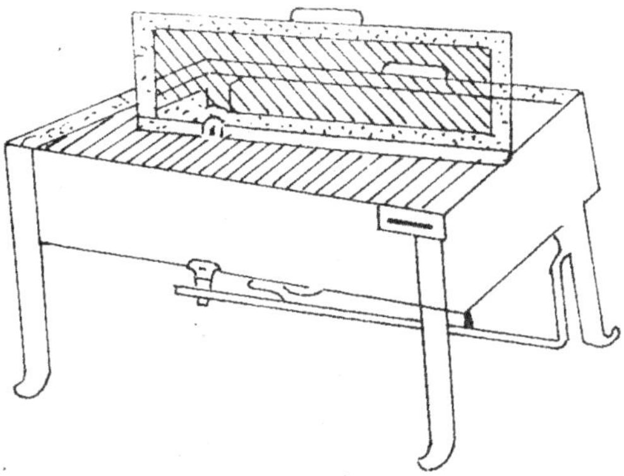

Fig. 8.3 Inspissator.

2. Moist heat at 100°C or steaming at atmospheric pressure –

Tyndallization/fractional sterilization/intermittent sterilization. This method was introduced by John Tyndall, hence known as Tyndallization.

This method is used to sterilize culture media which might damage at higher temperature, such as sugar media, media containing gelatin, milk etc., with a free-flowing steam at atmospheric pressure.

A Koch steamer or Arnold steamer is widely used for tyndallization. It is a vertical metal cylinder or rectangular vessel, with a removable conical lid, with an opening at the top for escaping of steam. At the bottom, there is a water reservoir, which can be heated either by using electricity or gas. A perforated tray situated above the water bears the articles to be sterilized. It is also possible to operate an autoclave with free-flowing steam for tyndallization.

The tubes and flasks plugged with cotton wool are arranged in wire baskets and covered with kraft paper to avoid damping of plugs with condensed steam.

The container and the medium are simultaneously sterilized. Tyndallization is done by heating to 100°C for 30 minutes (or 20 to 45 min.) on three successive days. The principle is that first exposure kills all vegetative bacteria, and between heatings, spores, if present, being in a favourable medium will germinate and be killed on second day and third day heatings. Since, sterilization is done by heating intermittently or in fractions, it is also called intermittent sterilization or fractional sterilization.

The advantages of tyndallization are that the apparatus is simple, cheap, easy to operate and no loss of volume of the medium due to evaporation.

This method may not kill spores of thermophilic organisms and anaerobic spore bearers, unless the incubation is carried out anaerobically.

Single exposure at 100°C for 90 minutes. Sterilization in a steamer can be done by a single exposure to heat at 100°C for 90 minutes (1½ hour). This steaming period of 90 minutes includes the time required for the articles to be heated up from room temperature to 100°C. The spores of some thermophiles may survive, but usually, sterilization is effective.

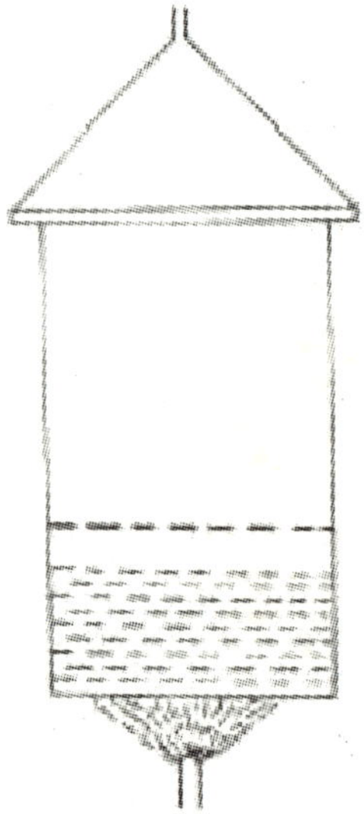

Fig. 8.4. Steam sterilizer.

3. Moist heat at a temperature above 100°C (or) steaming at a temperature above atmospheric pressure (or) saturated steam under increased pressure in an autoclave.

Autoclave (or) high pressure sterilizer. Autoclave (self-locking) was originally designed by Chamberland (1880) in Pasteur's laboratory. An autoclave is a strong boiler or cylinder with a lid which can be hermetically sealed and constructed strongly to withstand high pressures. Autoclave is an essential equipment required in microbiology laboratories.

Principle of autoclaving. Autoclave works on the principle of pressure cooker. Infact, a large pressure cooker can be used as an autoclave for sterilization of small articles in clinics and laboratories.

When the water is boiled within a closed vessel at increased pressures, the boiling point of water will rise above 100°C, depending on the pressure employed. Thus an increase in pressure yields an increase in effective temperature. This is the principle employed in the pressure cooker and autoclave.

Table 8.1 Temperatures attained at different pressures

Steam pressure	*Temperature attained*
0 lb/in^2 (atmospheric pressure)	100°C
5 lb/in^2	108°C
10 lb/in^2	115.5°C
15 lb/in^2	121°C
20 lb/in^2	127°C
25 lb/in^2	135.5°C
30 lb/in^2	133.5°C

The sterilization by steam under pressure depends upon four properties of dry, saturated steam:

– high temperature

– ability to form water by condensation

– liberation of latent heat when steam condenses on a cooler surface

– instantaneous contraction in volume that sucks more steam during condensation.

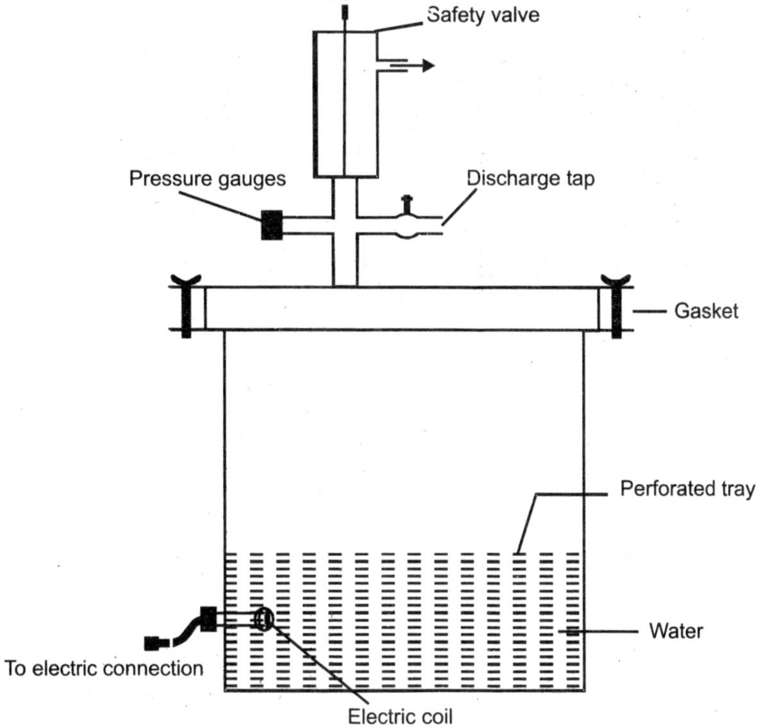

Fig. 8.5 A simple non-jacketed autoclave.

Holding period. In autoclave, sterilization is done by steaming under 15 lb/in^2 (1.05 kg/cm^2) pressure for 15 min, where the temperature is attained to 121°C. Some laboratories employ a holding period of 20–30 min.

A pressure of 30 lb/in^2 (2.1 kg/cm^2) equivalent to 134°C for 3 minutes can be used rarely.

Articles to be sterilized in an autoclave : Autoclave is generally used for the sterilization of following articles :

– surgical dressings

– surgical instruments

– culture media

– liquids which can withstand high temperatures

– dilution blanks (measured quantities of normal saline or distilled water in test tubes or bottles)

– rubber articles like tubing, washers, caps etc.

– rubber gloves

– discarded media with growth.

Substances that are immiscible in water, such as greases, waxes, fats and oils cannot be sterilized by autoclaving, as steam cannot penetrate into them.

Types of autoclaves : Several types of autoclaves are available.

1. A simple non-jacketed laboratory autoclave.
2. Downward displacement autoclaves or steam jacketed autoclave with automatic air and condensate discharge (Fig. 8.6).
3. Automatic high pre-vacuum autoclaves.

Simple laboratory autoclave. It consists of a vertical or horizontal cylinder made up of strong gun metal or stainless steel. It may be single chambered or double chambered. The articles/items to be sterilized are placed in a perforated vessel or tray above the water level. The lid is fastened by screw clamps, rendered air-tight by an asbestos gasket/washer. On the lid, there is a pressure gauge (indicates the steam pressure built up inside), a discharge tap (for discharge of air and steam mixture) and a safety valve (that can be set to release steam at the chosen pressure). The cylinder contains water upto a certain level and is heated by electric heater.

Autoclaving. Sufficient water is poured into the cylinder and the articles to be sterilized are placed on a perforated tray above the water level. The discharge tap is opened and the lid is tightened with screw clamps. The water in the chamber is heated by electricity. When water begins to boil the air-steam mixture escapes through discharge tap and it is closed when the chamber is filled with steam. When the steam pressure rises to 15 lb/in^2 inside the chamber, a temperature of 121°C is attained and should be maintained for 15–20 minutes. It is the temperature that kills the organisms and spores.

Then the heater is switched off and autoclave is allowed to cool down slowly so that the pressure comes down to atmospheric pressure. The discharge tap is opened and air allowed to enter the chamber and the lid can be opened. Autoclave should not be opened under positive pressure as it may cause explosion, scalding and the liquids may boil and spill over.

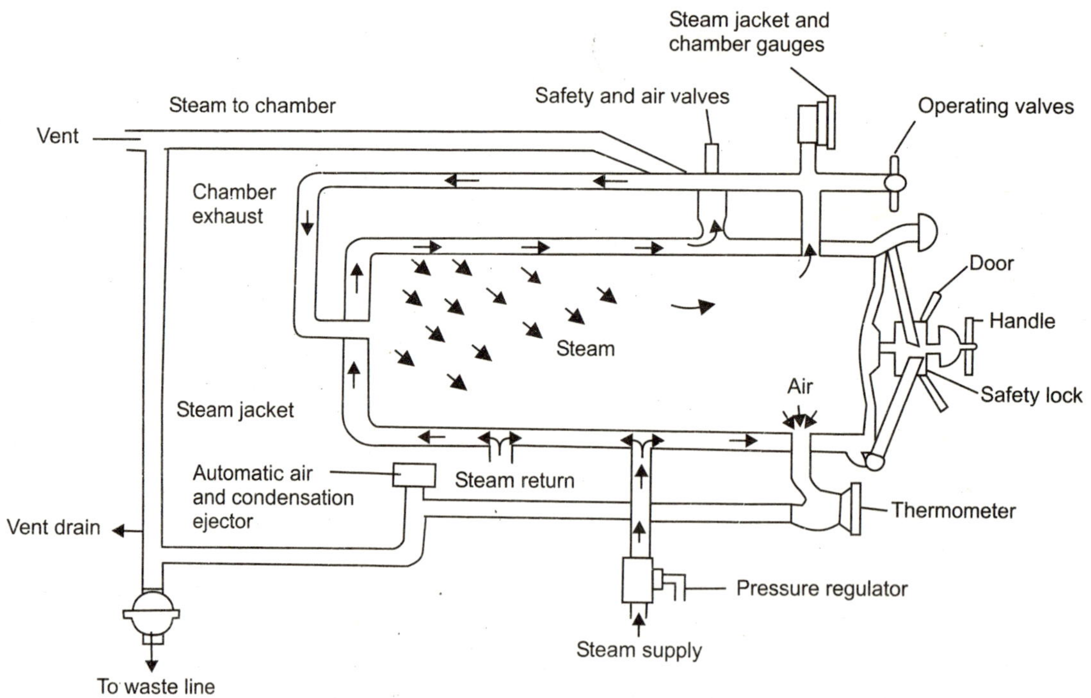

Fig. 8.6 Steam-jacketed autoclave with automatic gravity discharge of air condensate and system for drying by vacuum and intake of filtered air.

This simple laboratory autoclave is efficient but has some disadvantages.

1. The method of air discharge is inefficient. Air trapped in the chamber lowers the working temperature which may go undetected, because these simple autoclaves are not furnished with thermometers.

2. Articles become wet/moistened during sterilization due to condensation of steam. These autoclaves lack the facility for drying articles after sterilization.

Sterilization controls for moist-heat sterilization or sterility tests for autoclaving

To determine the efficiency of moist heat sterilization or autoclaving various sterilization controls are employed.

Physical methods:

1. Centigrade thermometers in the outlet drain records temperature inside the autoclave chamber, which is displayed on dial.

2. Thermocouple measurement. Thermocouples are temperature-sensitive and electronically operated sensors (fine probes consisting of two different metals *e.g.,* copper and constantan) for measuring temperature and are more accurate than routine thermometers. A thermocouple is inserted inside a test article in the autoclave chamber and its wire leads are carried out through valves in the autoclave wall and linked to a galvanometer, the dial of which gives a reading of the temperature.

Chemical methods:

(1) Autoclave tapes – Bowie-Dick test. The test consists of placing autoclave tapes into the center of the load and examining the tape after the sterilizing cycle. If the diagonal lines in the tape are evenly changed and become dark colored, it indicates that the sterilization was effective. If there is no dark color in the diagonal lines, it indicates the sterilization was not effective.

(2) Adhesive indicator tapes (steritapes). These are impregnated with a dye that show a color change from colorless (or white) to various shades-brown to grey to black on completion of sterilization.

3. Browne's tube. It contains a red color indicator solution which turns green when adequate temperature is maintained for a fixed time by moist heat sterilization. A Browne's tube is included with the load to be sterilized in tha autoclave chamber and immediately inspected at the end of the sterilization cycle for a color change.

Biological or bacteriological test. To determine the efficiency of moist heat sterilization, *Bacillus stearothermophilus* is used as indicator for microbiological testing. *Bacillus stearothermophilus* is a thermophile, grows optimally at 55-60°C. Its spores are killed at 121°C in about 12 min.

Paper strips impregnated with 10^6 spores of *Bacillus stearothermophilus* are placed in envelopes and inserted into different parts of load in the autoclave chamber; and after sterilization, the strips are inoculated into a suitable medium and incubated for sterility test at 55°C for 5 days.

An autoclaved spore strip is cultured as a positive control and an uninoculated medium as negative control.

IONIZING RADIATION (COLD STERILIZATION)

Electromagnetic radiations such as gamma rays, X-rays and high speed electron beams which have energies of more than about 10 eV, are called ionizing radiations, because they have enough energy to pull electrons away from molecules and ionize them.

Two sources of ionizing radiations are used:

1. Gamma rays from radioactive isotopes cobalt-60 and cesium-137.
2. Particulate high energy electrons from a linear electron accelerator or Van de Graaf generator.

The application of ionizing radiation, particularly gamma radiation to sterilize biological materials and heat sensitive materials is called **"cold sterilisation",** because ionizing radiations produce no heat in the material being irradiated. Thus, cold sterilization finds application in food and pharmaceutical industries and in medical field to sterilize heat-sensitive materials.

Ionizing radiations have a high penetrating power and when pass through cells, pull electrons away from molecules and creates free hydrogen, hydroxyl radicals and peroxides which in turn can cause different kinds of intracellular damage. Since this damage is produced in a wide variety of materials, ionizing radiations are rather non-specific in their effects.

1. Gamma Radiations

Gamma rays are high energy radiations emitted from certain radioactive isotopes such as cobalt-60 and cesium-137. Gamma rays are similar to X-rays but are of shorter wavelength. They have very high penetrative power and lethal to all life including microorganisms by causing damage to DNA and other vital cell constituents. Because of this, they can be used for sterilization of materials of considerable thickness or volume *e.g.,* packaged items.

The items can be packed before sterilization in sealed aluminium foil or plastic packs contained in outer carton ready for despatch; can be sterilized by gamma rays, avoiding any handling and recontamination after sterilization. A dose of 2.5 M rad is usually used.

Gamma rays are used for sterilizing disposable items such as plastic syringes, needles, suture materials, scalpel, blades, rubber gloves, catherters, swabs culture, plates, animal feeds, cardboard, oils, greases, fabrics and metal foils.

Micrococcus radiodurans, a nonsporing organism is most resistant to gamma rays.

Sterilization controls. To determine the efficiency of sterilization be gamma radiation, various sterilization controls are employed.

Chemical method. The most commonly used chemical indicator is small, circular, adhesive disc (containing azo dye indicator) which changes color from yellow to red.

Biological method. Paper strips impregnated with 10^6 spores of *Bacillus pumilus* are placed between plunger and barrel of plastic syringe. After sterilization with gamma rays, the paper strips are taken out and inoculated into a suitable medium and incubated for sterility test at 37°C for 5 days.

2. High energy Electron or Cathode rays

Accelerated electron beams are used for the sterilization of surgical supplies, drugs and other materials. The material can be sterilized after packing (the electrons penetrate the wrappings) and at room temperature. Since the degree of penetration is low, usually single and small items are sterilized by electron beams.

Two types of equipment are used to produce high intensities (millions of volts) of accelerated electrons – Van de Graaf generator and linear electron accelerator.

Chemical sterilants may be gases or liquids.

GASEOUS CHEMOSTERILIZERS

1. Low Temperature Steam with Formaldehyde (LTSF)

Combination of steam at low temperature and formaldehyde vapor can be used for sterilization of heat-sensitive materials such as endoscopes, polythene tubing and blankets which cannot withstand steam at high temperatures.

A specially designed LTSF sterilizer or an autoclave is modified to admit steam at subatmospheric pressures, at a temperature of 73-80°C and formaldehyde gas for one hour (or 30 min. to 2 hrs). Materials should be packed in such a way that allows the vapor to penetrate.

The efficiency of sterilization by LTSF method can be determined by microbiological testing, by using *Bacillus stearothermophilus* spores as sterilization indicators.

2. Ethylene Oxide Gas

Ethylene oxide is a highly reactive colorless liquid with a boiling point of 10.8°C; above this temperature it is a gas and it is used in this gaseous state for sterilization of heat-sensitive materials. It is highly flammable and carries the risk of explosion even in low concentrations. This problem can be overcome by mixing ethylene oxide with inert diluents like CO_2, Freon and nitrogen. These mixtures are non-flammable and retain the microbicidal and sporicidal activity.

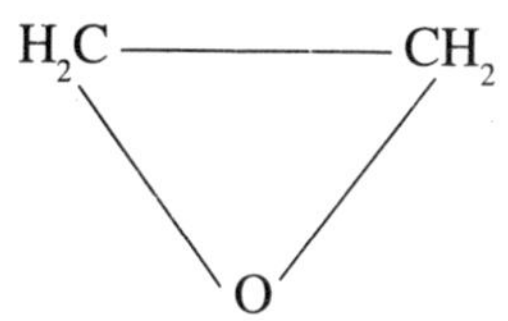

Molecular structure of ethylene oxide

The action of ethylene oxide depends upon temperature, concentration, time and presence of water vapor (humidity). Usually 10% ethylene oxide mixture (CO_2 or freon or nitrogen) and 30% humidity are used. The recommended gas concentration is between 450 and 900 mg/lit.

The gas can be used at low temperature, does not corrode or damage materials and used for sterilizing materials which would be ruined by both heat and ionizing radiation. It is used to sterilize plastic syringes, needles, transfusion sets, polythene tubing, respirators, heart-lung machines, cardiac catheters and pacers, sutures, surgical equipment, dental equipment, hospital bedding, blankets, books, ophthalmic and anesthetic equipment, endoscopes, electronic and medical equipment, biological materials, crude drugs, powders and culture media. Items such as syringes can be packed first and sterilized.

Ethylene oxide gas has been used for sterilization of space craft components.

Ethylene oxide vapors are toxic, irritating, mutagenic and carcinogenic. Controlled conditions are essential for load packing and sterilization.

Ethylene oxide acts by inactivating enzymes and other proteins by alkylating the amino, carboxyl, hydroxyl and sulphydryl groups.

Sterilization controls are used to determine the efficiency of ethylene oxide sterilization.

(*a*) Green gas sensitive tape turns deep to pale green after exposure to ethylene oxide gas.

(*b*) The spores of *Bacillus subtilis* (sub *species* – niger; var – *globigii*) are used as indicators for biological testing.

3. Formaldehyde Gas or Fumigation. Formaldehyde gas is used for the sterilization of instruments, heat-sensitive catheters, clothing, bedding, woolen blankets, furniture, foot wear etc. It is mainly used for the sterilization of enclosed areas such as operation theaters, wards, sick rooms, babies' incubators, respiratory ventilators and laboratories by fumigation. The temperature and humidity affects the action of formaldehyde. The temperature must be 22°C and the humidity between 60 and 80%.

Fumigation can be achieved by several ways

- formaldehyde gas can be sprayed
- formalin solution can be heated so that it liberates fumes
- paraformaldehyde solid can be heated so that it liberates gaseous vapors, as it is highly volatile
- formalin solution can be added to potassium permanganate to generate gas. Usually 150 gms of $KMnO_4$ to 280 ml formalin for every 1000 cu.ft (28.3 cu.mt) of room volume. The reaction produces considerable heat and so heat resistant vessels should be used.

After starting generation of formaldehyde vapor the doors, windows and other outlets should be sealed and left unopened for atleast 48 hrs.

The gas is irritant and toxic when inhaled and carcinogenic. Its irritant action can be neutralized by exposure to ammonia vapor.

4. Beta Propiolactone (BPL). It is a colorless liquid at room temperature, with a high boiling point of 155°C. It is more active for sterilization and more efficient for fumigation than formaldehyde. But it is not widely used due to its carcinogenicity and lack of penetrating power. Liquid BPL is used in the preparation of veterinary vaccines.

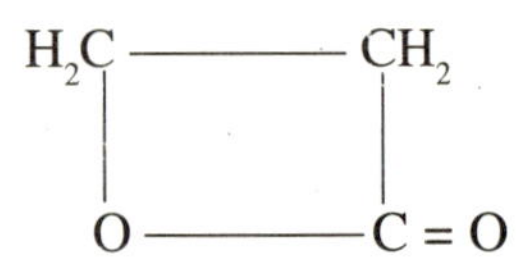

Molecular structure of BPL

LIQUID CHEMOSTERILIZERS

1. Formalin (Formaldehyde) Solution. It is marketed in aqueous solution as formalin, which contains 37 to 40% (w/v) formaldehyde. Methanol is added to (10 to 15%) to prevent polymerization of formaldehyde.

Formalin solution has several uses:

- for sterilization of clean instruments, furniture, fibres, leather etc.
- to preserve anatomical specimens
- 10% formalin solution is used for killing bacterial cultures and suspensions
- to destroy anthrax spores in hair, wool and hair brushes
- as a fixative for fixation of tissue specimens
- as a microbicidal agent in the preparation of killed vaccines
- to prepare toxoids from toxins
- as an antiseptic mouth wash
- for sterilization of membranes in dialysis equipment
- for sterilization of shoes and foot wear to prevent fungal infections such as athlete's foot.

2. Glutaraldehyde. It is usually employed as a 2% buffered solution "cidex". It has a broad spectrum of action against viruses, fungi, fungal spores, bacteria, bacterial spores and tubercle bacilli. Its antimicrobial action is due to cross-linking and precipitation of proteins.

It is used to sterilize urological instruments, instruments with lenses, rubber anaesthetic tubes, face maskes, plastic endotracheal tubes, bronchoscopes, metal instruments, polythene tubing, fibre-optic endoscopes, cystoscopes.

It does not corrode lenses, metal or rubber. It is less toxic and less irritant to the eyes and the skin than formaldehyde.

Glutaraldehyde is stable in acidic pH. But is most active in alkaline solution. It is unstable under alkaline pH due to gradual polymerization. Hence, the alkali has to be added to the glutaraldehyde, shortly before use. For example, cidex 25%, an aqueous solution of glutaraldehyde is diluted to 2% with an alkali (0.3 % Na_2CO_3) and can be used for sterilization of articles. These alkaline solutions of glutaraldehyde may be active for two weeks at 20°C.

Glutaraldehyde is also used as a fixative in leather tanning, in electron microscope and in biochemistry.

3. Iodine. It is sporicidal, bactericidal, fungicidal, virucidal and amoebicidal. Iodine kills microorganisms by denaturation of enzymes by oxidizing Sulphydryl groups and by binding to tyrosine.

FILTRATION

Filtration is used to sterilize heat labile liquids such as antibiotic solutions, sera, carbohydrate solutions, pharmaceutical fluids and certain laboratory media, which would be damaged by heat, ionizing radiation or chemicals.

Several types of filters are available. They render liquids bacteria-free but not virus-free or *Mycoplasma*-free.

Filtration is usually carried out under carefully controlled negative pressure, the fluid being sucked through the filter into receiving flask, which is connected to an exhaust pump.

Uses or Applications of Filtration

1. Used for sterilization of heat-labile liquids such as carbohydrate solutions, sera, antibiotic solutions, blood products and other parenteral and ophthalmic fluids.
2. Used to obtain bacteria-free filtrates of toxins, enzymes and bacteriophages.
3. To separate microorganisms which are scanty in fluids.
4. For clarification of water.
5. For microbiological analysis of water. The organisms from water or infected fluids may be recovered on the surface of the filter discs and placed on suitable culture media to obtain the viable count.
6. For sterilization of certain culture media.
7. For determination of viral particle size.
8. Cotton wool is an efficient air filter used to preserve the sterility of culture media in test tubes and flasks.

9. Filters of glass wool, slag wool, gauze, spun glass fibres are used for air filtration in hospitals particularly in operation theater, isolation units, ICU and dressing rooms to control cross-infections.

10. In food and drug industries, air filtration is employed to maintain aseptic condition.

11. Specially designed filters may be used in respirators to protect patients from respiratory pathogens.

Types of Filters

Several types of filters are used for filtration.

1. Diatomaceous earthenware candle filters, *e.g.,* Berkefeld filters, Mandler filters.
2. Unglazed porcelain filters, *e.g.,* Chamberland filters, Doulton filters, Jenkins filters.
3. Asbestos disk filters, *e.g.,* Seitz filters, Carlson filters, Sterimat filters.
4. Sintered glass filters (fritted glass filters/Morton filters).
5. Membrane filters (ultra filters).
6. HEPA (high efficiency particulate air) filters.

Diatomaceous Earthenware Candle Filters

These filters are usually made in the form of hollow candles open at one end. A metal nozzle is inserted and cemented in the open end.

Berkefeld German filters are made from kieselguhr (infusorial earth), a fossilised diatomaceous earth.

Mandler American filters are made from kieselguhr (60-80%), asbestos (10-30%) and plaster of paris (10-15%).

These filters are manufactured in different grades of porosity, They are mainly used for the clarification of water. They can be cleaned with sodium hypochlorite, but without scrubbing.

Unglazed Ceramic Filters or Porcelain Filters.

Filters of this type are hollow cylinders and unglazed except for a short distance at the open end. They are made up of hydrous aluminium silicate (kaolin) and sand. They are manufactured in different grades of porosity and used for large-scale clarification of water. They can be cleaned with sodium hypochlorite and by scrubbing.

e.g., Chamberland (French) filters, Doulton (English) filters, Jenkings filter–designed for the filtration of small quantities of liquid.

For use, the candle is mounted in a silicone rubber bung, which fits over the glazed portion and filtration is effected from within outwards.

Asbestos Disk Filters

These filters are made up of compressed filter sheet of asbestos fibres. They have high adsorbing capacities and tend to alkalinate solutions being filtered. Asbestos filters include – seitz filters, carlson filters, sterimat filters.

Seitz filters are made from chrysotile type of asbestos, chemically composed of magnesium silicate. They are available in different grades of porosity. Seitz filters have a pore size of between 0.5 µm and 0.75 µm.

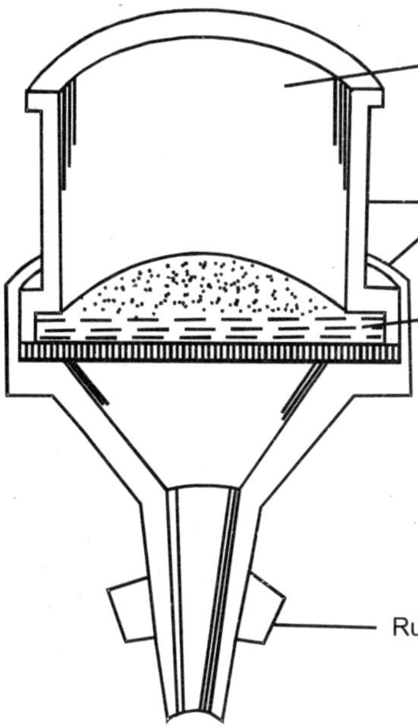

Fig. 8.7. Sietz filter.

They are particularly useful in the laboratory for removing bacteria from serum and fluid culture media. Seitz filters are also used to sterilize hydatid fluid.

The filter disc is fitted to a funnel like structure supported on a metal mount and is inserted rough side up ensuring that the metal support grid is in position. The filter is attached to a vacuum flask through a silicone rubber bung. The whole assembly can be sterilized by autoclaving. After use, the filter is discarded.

Sintered Glass Filters/Fritted Glass Filters/Morton Filters

They are prepared by molding finely pulverized glass in disk form. Glass for such a filter is ground into fine mesh powder of uniform size and then fused (fritted) in a furnace by heating sufficiently to leave small pores. This is then sealed into the body of the funnel and thoroughly cleaned by treating with H_2SO_4 containing sodium nitrate. The acid treatment quickly oxidizes and dissolves organic matter, if any. The acid is removed later by repeated washing with distilled water.

The funnel fitted with sintered glass filter disc is then attached to a collecting flask either by a rubber stopper or through a ground glass joint.

Fritted glass filters are available in various pore sizes – EC (extracoarse), C (coarse), M (medium), F (fine) and UF (ultrafine).

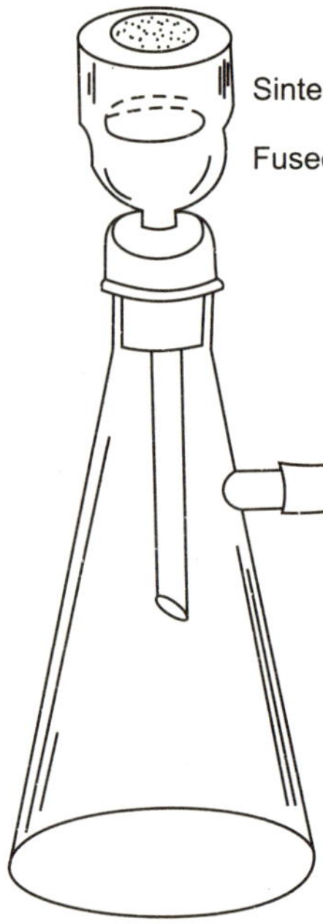

Fig. 8.8. Sintered glass filter.

Membrane Filters (Ultra Filters)

Membrane filters have the ability to filter out all forms of microorganisms and are the best and most useful when total elimination of microorganisms (absolute sterility) is required.

Membrane filters are composed of polymeric materials such as cellulose nitrate, cellulose diacetate, polycarbonate and polyester.

The older type membrane filters are composed of cellulose nitrate and are called Gradocol membrane filters, whereas the modern filters are made of cellulose acetate and are known as millipore filters (as they were originally manufactured by Millipore Corporation, USA). They are available in a range of pore sizes from 12 μm down to 0.015 μm.

The membrane filters have a highly uniform pore size and the pores occupy 80-85% of total filter volume and the cellulose matrix occupying only 15 to 20%, which facilitates high flow rate of liquids. Moreover, membrane filters are resistant to dilute acids, alkalies etc.; free of biological inhibitors, remain stable at high temperatures and high pressures and thus are superior to other filters. The membranes allow large volumes of liquid to pass through rapidly under suction.

Membrane filters are used for achieving absolute sterility and are used for

- sterilization of heat-labile liquids
- obtaining sterile solutions for parenteral use
- microbiological analysis of water
- sterility testing
- separating microorganisms and for collecting microbial samples

Specially designed equipment are available to hold membrane filters, while liquids pass through them

- membrane filters can be mounted on reusable holders and fitted to filtration vessels, the whole assembly being autoclaved as a single unit
- membrane filters may be supplied with plastic holder, presterilized, for single use (disposable, use and throw)
- to sterilize small volumes of fluids, syringe filters may be used, where small membrane filters are fitted in syringe holders.

High Efficiency Particulate Air (HEPA) Filters

Several laboratory procedures involve working with infectious microorganisms or diseased animals, and as a result microbial population of air is high in microbiology laboratories.

Special biological safety cabinets with laminar air flow system have been developed to filter and sterilize the air. It has an open front through which air is drawn in and away from the worker. The air then exits the cabinet through HEPA filters, which traps all particulate matter, including microorganisms. Thus, the laminar air flow system sucks the air in the room continuously and blows out the air through a pack of filters.

HEPA filters are made up of cellulose acetate, pleated around aluminium foil. Laminar air flow systems that employ HEPA filters have become an integral part of microbiological laboratories, dressing rooms, isolation rooms, operation theatres, intensive care units, pharmaceutical laboratories, food industries, electronic industries and computer rooms.

Sterilization Controls/Sterility Tests for Filtration

Filters used for sterilization should retain or hold back *Serratia marcescens*, a small Gram negative bacillus of 0.7 μm size.

The test is carried out by diluting 4 ml of *Serratia marcescens* culture to 100 ml with sterile nutrient broth. Then, the culture is filtered at a negative pressure through vacuum. Aseptically, around 50 ml filtrate is transferred to sterile nutrient broth and incubated for sterility at 37°C for 5 days.

QUESTIONS

Essay Types Questions

1. Define sterilization. Classify the methods of sterilization. Describe various methods of sterilization.
2. Define sterilization. Classify the methods of sterilization. Write briefly all about autoclave.
3. Define and classify the methods of sterilization. Describe moist heat sterilization.
4. Define sterilization. Classify the methods of sterilization be heat. Write in detail about dry heat sterilization.
5. Define and classify sterilization. Describe the various types of filters and their applications.

Short Notes

1. Define sterilization and mention two important uses of autoclave.
2. Explain how autoclave function. Specify the commonly used temperature, pressure and quality control measures.
3. Incineration.

4. Hot air oven.
5. Sterilization controls for dry heat sterilization/hot air oven.
6. Inspissation or serum inspissator.
7. Tyndallization or intermittent sterilization of fractional sterilization.
8. Articles sterilized in an autoclave.
9. Autoclave.
10. Sterilization controls for autoclave.
11. Cold sterilization.
12. Use of ionizing radiation in sterilization of lab. material.
13. Sterilization by radiation and its practical applications.
14. Filtration.
15. Bacterial filters.
16. Asbestos disc filters.
17. Seitz filters.
18. Membrane filters.
19. Gaseous sterilization.
20. Fumigation.
21. Chemical sporicidal agents.
22. Applications (uses) of filtration.
23. Applications (uses) of membrane filters.
24. HEPA filters.
25. Sterility tests for filtration.
26. Sintered glass filters (fritted glass filters).
27. Gamma radiation.

9

Disinfection

- *Definition*
- *Mode of action*
- *Methods of disinfection*

  Disinfection by moist heat

  – Pasteurisation

  – Boiling

  – low temperature (subatmospheric steam)

  Nonionizing radiation

  – UV radiation

  Chemical disinfectants

  – Aldehydes

  – Alcohols

  – Phenolics

  – Diguanides

  – Halogens

  – Surface active agents

  – Salts of heavy metals

  – Oxidising agents

  – Dyes

  – Acids

  – Alkalies
- *Testing of antimicrobial potency of disinfectants and antiseptics*

  – Tube dilution technique

  – Agar plate technique

  – Phenol coefficient technique

  – Rideal walker test

  – Chick Martin test

  – Kelsey-Sykes capacity tests

  – In-use tests

DEFINITION

Disinfection is defined as the destruction of many microorganisms, but not usually spores. The term "Disinfection" is usually applied to the treatment of inanimate objects.

Disinfection is not as effective as sterilization.

Disinfectants are chemical substances that are used for disinfection. Chemical disinfectants are strongly microbicidal and are generally used to eradicate microorganisms from inanimate materials. Disinfectants kill vegetative bacteria, fungi viruses but not usually spores.

Antisepsis refers to prevention of infection, usually by inhibiting the growth of bacteria.

Antiseptics are chemical disinfectants that can be safely applied to skin and mucus membrane surfaces.

Any given chemical can be used as disinfectant at a high concentration, and as an antiseptic at very low concentrations.

MODE OF ACTION

Chemical disinfectants and antiseptics kill microorganisms by various mechanisms

1. Coagulation of proteins
2. Disruption or damage to cell membrane which results in alteration of cell permeability
3. Removal of free sulphydryl groups from the active sites of enzymes, so that enzyme activity is destroyed, so that cell dies
4. Substrate competition – A chemical compound resembling the essential substrate misleads the enzyme by competing for substrate, so that metabolism is prevented causing cell death
5. Oxidation of protoplasm
6. Hydrolysis
7. Formation of salts

METHODS OF DISINFECTION

Disinfection by moist heat

1. Pasteurization
2. Boiling
3. Low temperature (Subatmospheric steam)

Non-ionizing radiation

1. UV radiation

Chemical disinfectants

1. Aldehydes – formaldehyde, Glutaraldehyde
2. Alcohols – Ethyl alcohol, Isopropyl alcohol
3. Phenolics – Phenols, Cresols, Hexyl resorcinol, Lysols, Hexachlorophene, Chloroxylenol (Dettol)
4. Diguanides – Chlorohexidine (Hibitane)
5. Halogens – Iodine compounds chlorine compounds
6. Surface active agents
   – anionic detergents–soap
   – cationic detergents (Quaternary ammonium compounds) – cetrimide, benzalkonium chloride
7. Salts of heavy metals – Mercury compounds, silver nitrate, copper sulphate, Zinc compounds
8. Oxidizing agents- hydrogen peroxide, potassium permanganate
9. Dyes – Aniline dyes, Acridine dyes
10. Acids
11. Alkalies.

These methods of disinfection should always be preceded by a thorough cleaning with a detergent and hot water, of the item to be disinfected, which will remove the majority of microorganisms present.

Disinfection by Moist Heat

1. Pasteurization. It was devised by Louis Pasteur to prevent spoilage of wine and beer. It is now widely used it kill majority of microorganisms in milk, cream, alcoholic beverages (wine and beer) and food industries. It is often used in conjunction with other methods of preservation such as cold storage, refrigeration or drying.

There are three methods of pasteurization

(*i*) Holder method (or) low temperature holding method (LTH) – milk is heated at 62.8°C (145°F) for 30 minutes, followed by cooling to 13°C.

(*ii*) Flash method (or) High temperature short time method (HTST) – Milk is heated to a temperature of 71.7°C (161°F) for 15 seconds, followed by sudden cooling to 13°C.

(*iii*) Ultra high temperature (UHT) method –The milk is heated to a very high temperature of 130°C for 1 or 2 seconds and then rapidly cooled.

In all the above processes, rapid cooling is important because

– It minimizes the multiplication of surviving nonpathogenic bacteria

– sudden variation in temperature may also kill microorganisms to certain extent.

Coxiella burnetti, the causative agent of Q fever may survive holder method but can be killed in other methods.

Pasteurization is not a method of sterilization, and it only reduces the microbial count.

Pasteurization of cystoscopes – Many cystoscopes would be damaged by high temperature and are disinfected, not sterilized, for this reason. The term "Pasteurization" should only be applied to the processing of milk; but it is colloquially used to describe the total immersion of instruments such as cystoscopes in a water bath at 75°C for 10 min. to destroy nonsporing organisms.

Pasteurization is recommended for decontamination of babies' milk bottles in hospitals and for anaesthetic apparatus, face masks and tubing.

2. Boiling. Total immersion of contaminated materials, objects and instruments in boiling water at 100°C for 5 min. can bring about disinfection. This required 5 min. time is measured from the time when the water actually boils again after the last instruments have been immersed. Sterile forceps may be used to remove instruments from boiler after processing.

3. Low-temperature steam disinfection (sub-atmospheric steam). Steam may be generated at 75°C for 20-30 min , by using sub-atmospheric pressure in a specially designed autoclave, which can be used for disinfection of heat-sensitive materials such as ventilator tubing .

For sterilization or a higher degree of disinfection, combination of low temperature steam and formaldehyde at subatmospheric pressure may be used. This low temperature formaldehyde process is used for disinfection of some endoscopes. However, some fibre-optic endoscopes may be damaged by heat.

Non-ionizing Radiation

UV RAYS. UV radiation can be produced artificially by mercury Vapor lamps. UV rays are effective against both Gram positive and Gram negative bacteria and Viruses. It has low penetrating power and its main application is to reduce the bacteria in air, water and on contaminated surfaces.

UV radiation is mainly used

– to disinfect drinking water and to obtain a Pyrogen-free water

–for air disinfection in hospital wards, operation rooms, laboratories, ventilated safety cabinets and enclosed areas such as entry ways and corridors.

UV radiation is absorbed by the proteins and nucleic acids and kills microorganisms by the chemical reactions it sets up in the bacterial cell.

Prolonged exposure to sunlight and fresh air is the most pleasant and perhaps an oldest anti-infection method.

The disadvantages of UV radiation:

- Causes damage to eyes, hence dark glasses must be worn or light source must be screened
- Excessive exposure to skin produces burns
- The energy of UV radiation is low, travels in straight lines and its penetrating ability into solids and liquids is poor. Hence, it has no effect on microorganisms present in the shadows or shielded from the incident beams.

Chemical Disinfectants

1. Aldehydes

Formaldehyde can be used in liquid form or gaseous form.

Formaldehyde gas is used for fumigation of operation theaters, sick rooms, wards, laboratories, post-mortem rooms, terminal room disinfection of premises occupied by TB, anthrax cases, safety cabinets, respiratory ventilators and babies incubators.

Formaldehyde gas can be liberated by spraying or by heating formalin solution or by heating solid paraformaldehyde. The atmosphere must have a humidity of over 60% (Preferably 80-90%) at a temperature of 18°C.

Formaldehyde is highly toxic and irritating. This effect can be neutralized by exposure to ammonia.

Small articles, instruments, blankets, surfaces of mattresses, shoes hair brushes are disinfected in a cabinet, by exposure to formaldehyde gas for atleast three hours, by boiling formalin.

Glutaraldehyde is an effective disinfectant against both Gram positive and Gram negative bacteria, including tubercle bacilli and sporicidal. It is used to treat heat sensitive articles such as respirators, fibre-optic endoscopes, corrugated rubber anaesthetic tubes, plastic endotracheal tubes, metal instruments, polythene tubing and lensed instruments such as bronchoscopes and cystoscopes. It has no deleterious effect on cements or lenses of these instruments and is an advantage over formaldehyde.

Glutaraldehyde is less corrosive than hypochlorites and therefore can be used to disinfect centrifuges and automated equipment.

2. Alcohols. Isopropyl alcohol, ethyl alcohol and methylated spirit (denatured alcohol) are bactericidal in aqueous solutions at a concentration of 70-75%. They are effective against Gram positive bacteria, Gram negative bacteria, Acid fast bacilli and viruses. They can kill vegetative cells, but are non-sporicidal and non-fungicidal. Since, alcohols are volatile they are used as rapidly drying antiseptics for skin, and disinfectants for inanimate surfaces.

Alcohols are used as skin antiseptics before and after venepuncture, cutaneous injections and hypodermic injections, for hand disinfection and applied as hand rubs on dry skin. 70% alcohols in combination with chlorhexidine (0.5%), Iodine (1 to 2%), laurolinium acetate (5%) are superior to alcohol alone .

The presence of organic matter delays the action of alcohols. Hence, they are used as disinfectants on physically clean surfaces; such as thermometers, instruments and equipment such as trolley tops, clean glass slides, mouths of culture bottles.

There is a gradual increase in the bactericidal action of alcohols, as their molecular weight increases. Thus, the bactericidal activity of isopropanol is greater than ethanol and being less volatile, widely used for the sterilization of thermometers. Whereas, alcohols with a molecular weight higher than that of propyl alcohol are not miscible in water, and are not used as disinfectants.

Methyl alcohol is less bactericidal than ethanol and it is highly poisonous. The fumes may produce permanent damage to eyes and not generally used.

Alcohols, being organic solvents can damage lipid membranes and also act by denaturation of cellular proteins. They are also dehydrating agents. That's why absolute alcohol is ineffective on dry cells, as very high concentrations of alcohol dehydrates cell so much that the alcohol is unable to penetrate. Thus, alcohols for their bactericidal action; require water and are more active at 70-75% aqueous solutions, than at 95% concentrations.

3. Phenolics. Phenols were the first antiseptics used in surgery by Joseph Lister (1865).

Phenols are widely used as disinfectants and antiseptics and used for decontamination of infective discharges, spillages, bathrooms, bed pans, environmental surfaces, walls, floors, furniture, instruments, bedding and as aerial disinfectants.

Phenols are also used as a preservative in sera and vaccines at a conc. of 0.5%.

Phenols are bactericidal to both Gram positive and Gram negative bacteria whereas spores are resistant. Phenols are active at acidic pH and their activity is reduced at alkaline pH. Presence of organic matter delays or inactivates the action of phenols. They may be bactericidal or bacteriostatic depending on the concentration used.

Phenol (carbolic acid) – at 2 to 5% aqueous solution used to disinfect materials such as sputum, urine, feces and contaminated instruments and utensils. Because phenol is toxic and has an unpleasant odor, it is replaced by several chemically related compounds.

Due to early recognition in the field of disinfection, phenol is used as the standard disinfectant against which the efficiency and activity of others is measured.

Cresols – ortho, Meta and para cresols are more bactericidal than phenol and employed as a mixture of tricresol. Their emulsions in liquid soaps and alkalies are used for practical applications.

Hexylresorcinol is used in a solution of glycerin and water. It is a strong surface-tension reductant, which accounts for its bactericidal action and used as general antiseptic.

Lysols are made of a soap solution containing phenolic compounds (o-phenyl phenol, o-benzyl-p-chlorophenol, xylenols) used to disinfect inanimate objects such as floors, walls, table surfaces, contaminated hospital items such as rectal thermometers, excreta and secretions from infected patients.

Hexachlorophene is a chlorinated phenolic bacteriostatic agent active against Gram positive bacteria such as Staphylococci and not active against Gram negative bacteria. It is used to reduce staphylococcal sepsis in maternity and neonatal units. In combination with soap it is used for hand washing and skin cleaning in operation theaters and clinical areas

It was formerly used at a conc. of 3% in soaps, shampoos, deodorants, tooth pastes, ointments and cosmetics.

It may be absorbed through intact skin and causes skin irritation and neurotoxicity.

Chloroxylenol (Dettol) is popularly used as disinfectant and antiseptic and active against both Gram positive and Gram negative bacteria.

Clear soluble phenolics-such as hycolin, clearsol, stericol and sudol are more efficient than phenol and more resistant to inactivation by organic matter.

Mode of action of phenols. 1. Alter the semipermeability of cell membrane causing leakage of vital intracellular constituents.

2. Causing denaturation and inactivation of proteins such as enzymes.

4. Diguanides or Biguanides

Chlorhexidine (Hibitane; 1, 6-di-4′-chloro phenyl guanido hexane) – It is the most widely used nontoxic, non-irritating skin antiseptic in medical dental and veterinary practice.

It is very active against Gram positive bacteria (*e.g.*, Staphylococci) and moderately active against Gram negative bacteria, but less active against *Pseudomonas* and *Proteus* sp.

It has no action against spores, tubercle bacilli fungi and viruses.

Its action is inactivated by organic matter, pus, serum, soaps, hard water, anionic compounds and some plastics.

It is available as a dihydrochloride, diacetate and gluconate. The most widely used one is chlorhexidine gluconate in 0.5%, 2%, 4% concentrations.

Uses – a general antiseptic for skin and mucus membrane surfaces

– used before operation, lumbar puncture or bone marrow aspiration

– 4% solution in a compatible detergent (Hibiscrub) is used as antiseptic for hand washing of hospital staff and preoperative scrub for surgeons.

– 0.5 to 1% solution in isopropyl alcohol (Hibisol) is used for rapid hand antisepsis in hospitals. The alcohol present results in a rapid antibacterial effect together with drying of the hands.

– chlorhexidine-cetrimide mixture (Savlon) is a useful antiseptic for wounds.

– Skin disinfection in urology and gynaecology.

5. Halogens – Halogens are strong oxidizing agents. Iodine (skin antiseptic) and chlorine (water disinfectant) are frequently used.

Iodine – It is one of the oldest and most effective disinfectant. It is sporicidal, bactericidal, fungicidal, virucidal and amoebicidal. Iodine kills microorganisms by denaturation of protein enzymes by oxidizing sulphydryl groups and by binding to tyrosine.

Iodine is used as skin antiseptic, to disinfect small quantities of water and food utensils. Iodine vapor is sometimes used to disinfect air. It is traditionally used as antiseptic in the form of "tincture of Iodine". The term "tincture" refers to an alcoholic solution of a medicinal substance. Several preparations of Iodine are used.

Aqueous solution of Iodine consists of 5% Iodine, 10% potassium Iodide in distilled water.

Alcoholic solution of Iodine consists of 7% Iodine, 5% potassium Iodide in 83% alcohol.

Tincture of Iodine consists of 2% Iodine, 2% sodium iodide diluted in 70% alcohol.

Iodophores are compounds of iodine with detergents *e.g.*, povidone-Iodine (Betadine, wescodyne) is a complex of lodine and polyvinyl pyrrolidone. Iodophores have the advantages of non-staining and non-irritating to the skin. Povidone Iodine is used for hand washing, surgical scrubbing, preparation of the skin prior to invasive procedures such as injection, aspiration and surgery and for prophylaxis against post-operative infections.

Chlorine. It is most widely used either in the form of gas or in certain chemical combinations.

Compressed and liquefied chlorine gas is the choice for disinfection of drinking water or municipal water supplies, swimming pools and for the treatment of effluents and used at a concentration of 0.5 to 1.0 ppm (mg/Lit). Many compounds of chlorine are more convenient to use than chlorine gas. *e.g.*, Inorganic chlorine compounds such as hypochlorites – *e.g.*, calcium hypochlorite ($Ca(OCl)_2$) and sodium hypochlorite (NaOCl). Calcium hypochlorite is used for sanitizing utensils in restaurants and equipment in food and dairy plants.

A solution of 1% sodium hypochlorite is used for personal hygiene and to disinfect baby-bottles. High concentrations, such as 5-12% are used as household bleaches, disinfectants and as sanitizers in dairy and food processing plants and for kitchen hygiene Sodium hypochlorite kills spores, bacteria, fungi, protozoa and viruses. It is particularly useful because of its activity against HIV and Hepatitis B virus .The disadvantages being corrosion of metals and its action can inactivated by the presence of organic matter.

It is efficient for disinfecting linen, clothing, spills, stainless steel instruments, syringes and needles before disposal/autoclaving.

Organic chloramines are used as antiseptics and for dressing wounds *e.g.*, mono-chloramine (NH_2Cl), chloramines-T and Azochloramide. The advantages of chloramines are stable and release chlorine over a long period of time than do hypochlorites.

Eusol is a chlorinated lime and boric acid compound used for wound dressings but too irritant for wound irrigation.

Dakin's solution (surgical chlorinated soda solution) and electrolytic sodium hypochlorite are used for wound irrigation and dressings.

Mode of action of chlorine. When added to water, hypochlorites and chloramines undergo hydrolysis giving rise to hypochlorous acid which changes to nascent oxygen, which is a powerful oxidizing agent that can severely damage vital cell constituents.

$$Cl_2 + H_2O \longrightarrow HCl + HClO \text{ (hypochlorous acid)}$$

$$HClO \longrightarrow HCl + O \text{ (nascent oxygen)}$$

6. *Surface active agents/surfactants/surface tension depressants/wetting agents/synthetic detergents.* Compounds that have the property of concentrating at interfaces and alter the energy relationships at interfaces producing a reduction of surface tension of interfacial tension causing disruption of cell membrane are called as surface active agents.

They possess wetting and cleansing properties and disinfectant activity. They are used in laundry, disk washing powders, shampoos, other washing preparations and for hand washing.

They arc of 4 types – anionic, cationic, non-ionic and Amphoteric (Tego) compounds. Among these anionic and cationic detergents are very useful for disinfection and cleaning purposes.

Anionic surface active agents – Detergents in which a long-chain hydrocarbon has a negative charge are called anionic *e.g,,* soaps, fatty acids and bile salts. They dissociate in aqueous solution to form a large, complex anion, which is responsible for lowering surface tension.

They are mainly effective against Gram positive bacteria, Acid fast bacilli and some viruses.

Soft soaps derived by combination of unsaturated fatty acids (*e.g.*, oleic acid) with NaOH or KOH are more efficient than hard soaps formed by combination of saturated fatty acids (*e.g.*, coconut oil) with NaOH or KOH.

Cationic surface active agents/quaternary ammonium compounds. Possess both bactericidal and detergent properties. They are active against Gram positive bacteria but less active against Gram negative bacteria. *Pseudomonas aeruginosa*, *Proteus* and tubercle bacilli are particularly resistant. Selective media for the cultivation of *Pseudomonas aeruginosa* contains cetrimide, and is known as **cetrimide agar**. They are sporistatic and funsistatic and are active against enveloped viruses but not against non-enveloped viruses.

They are most active at alkaline pH. Acid, organic matter, blood inactivates them. Their action is neutralized by anionic surface active agents, soaps, hard water and various chemicals.

Examples for Quaternary ammonium compounds are:

1. Cetyl trimethyl ammonium bromide (cetrimide or cetavlon)
2. Benzalkonium chloride (zephiran)
3. Cetyl pyridinium chloride
4. Laurolinium acetate (laurodin)
5. Dequalinium acetate
6. Triclobisonium chloride

They possess a peculiar adsorptive property which is of practical importance. When applied to skin they form an antibacterial surface film. They are readily adsorbed to glass ware and to fabrics. They are, therefore, widely used for the disinfection of food utensils in hotels and restaurants, milk containers in dairy industry, blankets in hospitals.

They are widely used for preoperative skin preparation of the skin and mucus membrane surfaces, as surgical scrub and as antiseptic for abrasions and wounds. They are also used for disinfection of bench-tops, floors and other surfaces in laboratories.

7. Salts of heavy metals. The term "heavy metals" refers to metals such as mercury, silver, copper, zinc and lead. They are protein coagulants and combine with free sulphydryl (–SH) groups of enzymes and thus kills the bacteria.

Mercuric chloride ($HgC1_2$) was widely used as a general disinfectant. Organic mercury compounds such as Merbromin (mercurochrome), thiomersal (merthiolate), nitromersol (metaphen) were used for treatment of minor cuts, wounds and infections. Merthiolate (1 in 10,000) is used for inactivation of vaccines and preservation of sera and antitoxins.

1% silver nitrate ($AgNO_3$) was widely used to disinfect the eyes of infants at birth to prevent ophthalmia neonatorum, a gonococcal infection. Currently, it is sometimes replaced either by antibiotics such as penicillin or erythromycin or by antiseptics such as chorohexidine. Sponges or layers of gauze impregnated with 0.5% silver nitrate has been used to prevent infections of burns.

Copper sulphate is an effective algicide in open bodies of water such as tanks, reservoirs and pools. It is also a fungicide and a constituent of Bordeaux mixture used to control fungal infections of plants.

8. Oxidizing agents. Hydrogen peroxide, potassium permanganate, ozone, chlorine dioxide, peracetic acid are some oxidizing agents find application in disinfection and antisepsis.

Hydrogen peroxide is active against both Gram positive and Gram negative bacteria and sporicidal at high concentrations. It is used as antiseptic for cleansing wounds, abscesses, for the removal of adhering dressings and for irrigation. It liberates oxygen when in contact with organic material. The effervescence helps mechanically to loosen slough and pus in a wound.

Potassium permanganate is used as mouth wash, gargle and for wound cleaning. It is also used to purify well water. Ozone (O_3) is bactericidal, sporicidal and virucidal and used to disinfect vegetables and fruits.

9. Dyes. Two groups of dyes, the aniline dyes and the acridines can be used as skin and wound antiseptics. Both are bacteriostatic at high dilution but are of low bactericidal activity.

Aniline dyes (Triphenyl methane dyes). Crystal violet, brilliant green, malachite green are included in this group. They are more active against Gram positive bacteria than Gram negative bacteria. Hence, selective media prepared by incorporating these dyes are used to grow coliform bacilli (Gram negative bacilli such as E.coli) in bacteriological analysis of water.

These dyes have no action on tubercle bacilli. Hence, malachite green is used as a selective agent in Lowenstein-Jensen (LJ) medium for the cultivation of tubercle bacilli.

Acridine dyes. Proflavine, acriflavine, euflavine and aminacrine are included in this group. Though they are more active against Gram positive bacteria than Gram negative bacteria, they are not as selective as the aniline dyes. Their action is usually not affected by the presence of organic matter. Presently, they have less application and are used to some extent for the treatment of burns, wounds, ophthalmic application and for bladder irrigation.

9. Acids. The antimicrobial action of acids is related to hydrogen ion concentration.

Several acids such as acetic, propionic, benzoic and sorbic acids are used as preservatives in the food industry, and to some extent in pharmaceutical and cosmetic products. Acids may be added to various foods as acidulants.

Citric acid is an effective disinfectant against foot-and-mouth virus.

Lactic acid has been used as an aerial disinfectant against non-sporing bacteria.

Formic and propionic acids are useful in controlling *Salmonellae* in feed stuffs.

Hydrochloric acid, at a concentration of 2.5%, used for disinfecting hides and skin contaminated with anthrax spores.

Sulphuric acid at a concentration of 5%, usually in combination with phenol is used for decontaminating floors, feed boxes etc.

10. Alkalies. The antimicrobial action of alkali is related to hydroxyl ion concentration.

Sodium hydroxide kills most common vegetative bacteria, and high concentrations are lethal to anthrax spores.

Calcium hydroxide is formed and heat liberated when calcium oxide is mixed with water. Calcium hydroxide is effective for white washing surfaces, which kills nonsporing bacteria.

Sodium carbonate is used as a cleaning agent for washing.

TESTING OF ANTIMICROBIAL POTENCY OF DISINFECTANTS AND ANTISEPTICS

There are several procedures available to evaluate antimicrobial potency of chemical agents

1. Tube dilution technique

2. Agar plate technique
3. Phenol, coefficient technique
   (*a*) Rideal-walker test
   (*b*) Chick-Martin test
4. Kelsey-Sykes capacity tests
5. In-use tests

Tube Dilution Technique

The disinfectant is made into several dilutions and an equal amount (*e.g.*, 5 ml) of each dilution is taken into sterile test tubes. Then a specific amount (*e.g.*, 0.1 ml) of the test organism is added to each tube and incubated. At regular intervals of time, subcultures are made and incubated and examined for growth.

"No growth" indicates the dilution at which the chemical agent has killed the test organism when exposed to a particular period of time.

Agar-Plate Technique

The test organism is inoculated on to nutrient agar and the chemical is placed in the center of the plate. If the chemical agent is in liquid form, an absorbent paper disk impregnated with the solution can be placed on the agar medium or a small volume of solution can be held in a hollow cylinder set upon the agar surface. After incubation, the plate is observed for a zone of inhibition.

Alternatively, the chemical can be incorporated into the nutrient agar and then poured into the plates. The medium is inoculated with the test organism, incubated and examined for microbial growth.

Phenol Coefficient Technique/Rideal-Walker Test

It is used extensively to test disinfectants. The Rideal-walker test compares the action of the antiseptic or disinfectant with that of phenol on *Salmonella typhi* in distilled water. It is expressed in terms of phenol coefficient.

$$\text{Phenol coefficient} = \frac{\text{Dilution of the disinfectant which kills the test organism in the given time}}{\text{Dilution of the phenol which kills the test organism in the same time}}$$

The disinfectant is made into several dilutions in one set and similarly phenol is taken in several dilutions in another set. To each of these tubes, the test organism (*Salmonella typhi*) is added and allowed to react over a definite time interval – 2.½, 5, 7 and 10 minutes at 37°C for two days and observe for growth (turbidity).

The Rideal-Walker test is performed in distilled water, which does not give any similarity of the disinfecting action under a practical condition, where much organic material is present.

If the phenol coefficient is 1 or less than 1, the chemical agent is said to be a good disinfectant or antiseptic.

Chick-Martin test. It is same as Rideal-Walker test, but done in the presence of organic matter such as feces or yeast.

Kelsey-Sykes Capacity Tests. Capacity tests measure the capacity of a disinfectant to retain its activity when repeatedly used microbiologically .These tests simulate practical disinfecting situations.

In Kelsey-sykes test, the test organism such as *Staphylococcus aureus*, *E.coli*, *Pseudomonas aeruginosa*, *Proteus vulgaris* is added to disinfectant in three successive lots at 0, 10 and 20 minutes. The organism is in contact with the disinfectant for 8 minutes, so that samples are transferred at 8, 18 and 28 minutes respectively to a nutrient medium. The disinfectant is assessed based on its ability to kill bacteria as judged by growth on nutrient medium. The test is carried out under both clean and dirty (in the presence of organic matter such as yeast or feces) conditions.

In-use Tests. These tests are used to monitor not only the performance of a disinfectant but also how it is being used.

In-use tests are realistic as they test a disinfectant's action in use in the hospital at the time of tests.

Samples of the disinfectant dilutions in use in the hospital are taken (usually 1 ml) and added to nutrient broth (usually 9 ml). This 1 in 10 dilution of disinfectant in nutrient broth is inoculated on to two agar plates using 10 drops of diluted disinfectant per plate, using a sterile Pasteur pipette. One plate is incubated at 37°C for 2-3 days and the other plate is incubated at room temperature.

If a few colonies appear, it does not imply the failure of in-use test, since disinfection is partial removal of organisms. However, if more than 5 colonies appear on the plate, it suggests that the disinfectant action is not effective.

Regular in-use tests are valuable for helping supervise the correct use of disinfectants in the hospital.

QUESTIONS

Essay Type Questions

1. Define disinfection. Name various disinfectants and describe in detail.
2. Give an account of testing antimicrobial potency of disinfectants and antiseptics.

Short Notes

1. Define disinfection.
2. Describe mode of action of disinfectants.
3. Pasteurization.
4. Name two uses of UV radiation.
5. Uses of aldehydes.
6. Uses of alcohols.
7. Phenols.
8. Chlorhexidine or Diguanides.
9. Halogens.
10. Quaternary ammonium compounds.
11. Oxidizing agents.
12. Testing of disinfectants.
13. Phenol coefficient (or) Rideal-walker test.
14. Chick-Martin test.
15. Kelsey-Sykes test.
16. In-use dilution test.

10

Culture Media

- *Definition*
- *Ingredients/constituents of culture media*
- *Classification of culture media*
- *Defined/synthetic media*
- *Semidefined media*
- *Simple media/Basal media*
- *Enriched media*
- *Enrichment media*
- *Selective media*
- *Differential media*
- *Indicator media*
- *Transport media*
- *Anaerobic media*
- *Sugar media/sugar fermentation test*
- *Culture media for fungi*

DEFINITION

Culture medium can be defined as an artificial food provided in the petriplates, test tubes, bottles to grow/cultivate, to isolate, to identify and to study growth, biochemical, antigenic and other characteristics of bacteria in the laboratory.

An ideal culture medium must give a rapid and good growth from a small inoculum and idealy from a single cell. It should make possible for all the characteristics of the isolate to be demonstrated.

INGREDIENTS/CONSTITUENTS OF CULTURE MEDIA

Many ingredients are incorporated to prepare culture media.

Water. Water is very essential for life as an hydrogen or electron donor in metabolism, and as a medium in which enzymatic activities takes place. Usually demineralized water or glass-distilled water is used in the preparation of culture media.

Electrolytes. NaCl or other electrolytes may be incorporated in the culture medium in optimum concentrations, as per the requirements of microorganisms.

Meat extract/lab lemco/beef extract. Meat extract is an essential ingredient in many culture media. It is prepared by boiling finely grinded meat or beef from which a soluble extract is obtained, which is concentrated by evaporation to a dark paste or powder. Commercially prepared meat extract is known as lab-lemco. It contains many water-soluble compounds and protein degradation products such as albumoses, gelatin, peptones, proteoses and amino acids; and other nitrogen compounds, creatine, purines etc. It also contains inorganic salts, growth factors and some carbohydrates.

Peptone. Peptone is a common ingredient of culture media. It provides nitrogen requirement of pathogenic bacteria. It is obtained by digestion of protein material with proteolytic enzymes such as pepsin, trypsin or papain. Peptone is a complex mixture of proteoses, polypeptides, amino acids, inorganic salts such as phosphates, potassium and magnesium and certain growth factors such as riboflavin and nicotinic acid.

Peptone is supplied as golden granular powder with a low moisture content. It is water soluble, does not coagulate on heating and can be incorporated in culture media, which are sterilized by heat (autoclaving). Commercially available digest broths can be used instead of peptone.

Different brands of peptone will have differences in composition and growth promoting properties. Also, there may be variations between different batches of the same brand. Special brands of peptone such as neopeptone, proteose peptone and mycological peptone are available for special uses.

Yeast extract. It is prepared from washed cells of baker's yeast or brewer's yeast. Yeast cells are allowed to undergo autolysis by mild heating at 55°C or hydrolysed with HCl on proteolytic enzymes. The extract is concentrated to thick paste or powder form by evaporation. Yeast extract contains a wide range of nutrients such as amino acids, inorganic salts, carbohydrates, vitamins and growth factors.

Blood. Blood is used to enrich culture media, to cultivate microorganisms with fastidious growth requirements. Usually 5–10% defibrinated sheep blood is used. Horse blood or Rabbit blood can be used. But human blood should not be used as it may contain antibodies, bactericidal and other inhibitory agents to human pathogens.

Gelatin. Gelatin is a protein of animal source. Initially gelatin was tried as a solidifying agent in culture media, but at incubation temperature at 37°C, it melts into liquid, hence its use was abandoned. Certain bacteria utilize and liquefy gelatin by producing gelatinase.

Agar-Agar. Agar powder is used as a solidifying agent to prepare solid culture media. It melts at 98°C and solidifies at 42°C and provides a smooth surface on solid medium. It is not used up as a nutrient by the bacteria (except a few marine bacterial flora). Hence, agar is most satisfactory and preferred solidifying agent.

It is prepared from sea weeds (Red Algae belonging to Rhodophyceae) such as *Gelidium*, *Pterocladia* and *Eucheuma* species. The main constituent of agar is a long-chain polysaccharide; in addition, it may contain inorganic salts and protein like materials. Agar is manufactured either in long shreds or in powder form. It varies in its composition from batch to batch. Special brands of agar such as NewZealand agar and Japanese agar are available for special purpose.

Routinely in culture media, agar is used at a concentration of 2% to prepare a good solid medium. When agar concentration is decreased to 0.2 to 0.5%, semisolid agar or sloppy agar is obtained, which enables motile organisms to spread. The agar concentration may be further decreased to 0.05 to 0.1% to prevent convection currents of air in thioglycollate media. The agar concentration can be increased to 6% to prevent swarming growth of *Proteus* and *Clostridium tetani*.

In gel diffusion 0.1 to 0.2% agar gel or agarose gel is used.

Table 10.1 Agar concentrations in different media.

Culture media	*Conc. of agar*	*Use*
Solid media	2%	solidifying agent
	6%	to prevent swarming of bacteria
Semi-solid media/ sloppy agar	0.2 to 0.5%	to enable motile organisms spread; to separate motile organisms from a mixture of motile and nonmotile organisms
Thiglycollate media (anaerobic medium)	0.02 to 0.01%	to prevent convection current in the medium

CLASSIFICATION OF CULTURE MEDIA

Culture media are classified in several ways.

I. Based on physical nature, culture media can be
- liquid media (broth)
- solid media
- semisolid media (sloppy agar)
- biphasic media (castaneda's medium)

II. Based on the oxygen tension maintained, culture media can be Aerobic or Anaerobic.

III. Based on the uses, culture media are classified into
- media for isolation and growth (Plating media)
- media for biochemical tests
- media for transport (Transport media)

IV. Based on the functions, culture media are classified into several types.
- simple media or ordinary media or basal media
- complex media
- synthetic or defined media
- semidefined media
- special media – they are further classified into
  - enriched media
  - enrichment media
  - selective media
  - differential media
  - indicator media
  - transport media
  - sugar media (carbohydrate media)
  - anaerobic media.

DEFINED MEDIA/SYNTHETIC MEDIA

These media are used to study metabolic requirements of the bacteria. These media are prepared from pure chemical compounds; hence, known as synthetic media. The exact chemical composition of the medium is known, hence called defined media.

SEMIDEFINED MEDIA

When the chemical composition of the medium is approximately known it is called semidefined or semisynthetic media *e.g.,* peptone water medium.

Peptone water. It is a simple, basal medium since it's chemical composition is approximately known, it is also called semisynthetic media. It contains peptone 1%; NaCl 0.5% and distilled water, with a pH adjusted to 7.4.

Uses. 1. It acts as a simple medium for the growth of many organisms, particularly Gram negative bacilli.

2. It is used to test indole production.

3. It is used to prepare sugar media.

4. Peptone water at an alkaline pH of 8.6; known as alkaline peptone water, used for enrichment of *Vibrio cholerae* from feces samples.

SIMPLE MEDIA/BASAL MEDIA

Simple media are those which contain only basic nutrients required for the growth of ordinary organisms, and used as a general purpose media. *e.g.,* peptone water, nutrient broth and nutrient agar. These simple media can be used as a base to prepare enriched media; hence known as basal media.

Nutrient broth. It is a simple basal liquid medium, supports growth of many organisms. It contains 1% peptone, 1% meat extract (lab lemco), 0.5% NaCl and distilled water, with a pH adjusted to 7.4.

Nutrient broth is used as a base to prepare many other culture media. It is also used to study growth curve.

There are three types of nutrient broth –

1. Meat infusion broth – It is an aqueous extract of lean meat to which peptone is added.

2. Meat extract broth – It is a mixture of meat extract and peptone.

3. Digest broth – It is an aqueous extract of lean meat, that has been digested with a proteolytic enzyme so that additional peptone need not be added.

Nutrient agar. Nutrient agar is the simplest and commonest medium used routinely in microbiology laboratories, to grow non-fastidious bacteria. It is prepared by adding agar at a concentration of 2% to the nutrient broth. Nutrient agar is commonly referred to as "agar medium".

Composition:

Peptone – 1%

Meat extract (lablemco) – 1%

NaCl – 0.5%,

Agar – 2%

Distilled water – 100 ml

pH 7.4.

Nutrient agar is used in the form of slopes, butts in test tubes or plates in petridishes.

Uses. Nutrient agar is used

1. to study colony characteristics
2. to detect pigment formation
3. to maintain stock cultures
4. for antibiotic sensitivity testing
5. pure growth of the bacterium on nutrient agar medium is used for slide agglutination and other tests.

Semi-solid agar. When agar concentration in agar medium is decreased to 0.2 to 0.5% a semisolid agar or sloppy agar is formed, which enables motile organisms to spread (by using craigie's tube). When agar concentration is further decreased to 0.05% to 0.1%, agar prevents convection currents and prevents the diffusion of air in thioglycollate media, used for the growth of anaerobic and microaerophilic organisms.

Firm agar. When agar concentration is increased to 6%; it prevents the swarming growth of *Proteus* species and *Clostridium tetani* and enable them to form discrete colonies.

ENRICHED MEDIA

They are prepared by adding blood, serum, egg, milk, glucose etc. to a basal medium. In other words, a simple basal medium is enriched by adding highly nutritious substances such as blood, serum, egg, milk glucose etc.

Enriched media are used for the cultivation of bacteria that possess fastidious growth requirements (complex growth requirements) or that are exacting in their growth requirements. *e.g.,*

1. Blood agar – It is used for the cultivation of Streptococci, pneumococci, *Hemophilus*.

2.Chocolate agar – It is used for the cultivation of *Hemophilus*, meningococci and gonococci.

3. Loeffer's serum slope – It is used for the cultivation of *Corynebacterium diphtheriae*.

4. Dorset's egg medium – It is used for the cultivation of *Mycobacterium tuberculosis* and *Corynebacterium diphtheriae*.

5. Milk agar – It is used to cultivate Staphylococci, to promote their pigment production.

6. Bordet – Gengou glycerine potato blood agar – It is used for the cultivation of *Bordetella pertussis*, which causes whooping cough (pertussis) disease.

7. Glucose broth – It is used for the cultivation of bacteria from blood specimens, known as blood culture.

8. Serum dextrose agar and serum potato infusion agar are used for the cultivation of *Brucella* species.

9. Yeast extract serum agar – It is used for the cultivation of *Mycoplasma*.

10. Wagatsuma agar (high salt blood agar) used for the cultivation of *Vibrio parahemolyticus*.

11. Egg yolk agar and serum agar are used for the cultivation of *Clostridium welchii* (also called as *Clostridium perfringens*) to demostrate Nagler's reaction.

12. Mannitol-egg-yolk-phenol red-polymyxin agar (MYPA) used for the isolation of *Bacillus cereus*.

13. Lowenstein-Jensen (LJ) medium used for the cultivation of *Mycobacterium tuberculosis*. Since LJ medium contains egg, it can be grouped under enriched media. But it also contains malachite green, a selective agent; hence widely referred to as selective media.

14. Charcoal blood agar for *Bordetella pertussis*.

Blood agar. It is a solid enriched medium, widely used in medical bacteriology, to isolate fastidious bacteria. It is prepared by adding 8–10% sheep blood or horse blood or rabbit blood or human blood to sterile melted nutrient agar at 50–55°C, defibrinated blood is preferred to citrated blood to prepare blood agar medium. It is used for the cultivation of bacteria such as Streptococci, pneumococci, gonococci and *Hemophilus* species. Blood agar can be used as an indicator medium to indicate hemolysis property of Streptococci and Staphylococci. It is also used as differential medium to differentiate alpha (α) hemolytic Streptococci, beta (β) hemolytic Streptococci and gamma (γ) hemolytic Streptococci.

Chocolate agar/heated blood agar. It is an enriched solid medium, suitable for the cultivation of H*emophilus influenzae*, pneumococci, meningococci and goncocci.

Chocolate agar is essentially the same as blood agar, except during preparation RBC are lysed releasing intracellular nutrients such as hemoglobin, hemin ("X" factor), and the co-enzyme NAD ("V" factor). Lysis of RBC gives the medium a chocolate-brown colour from which this medium gets its name. Chocolate agar is the most suitable medium for the cultivation of *Hemophilus influenzae*, because it requires "X" and "V" growth factors for its growth.

It is prepared by adding 8–10% defibrinated blood to sterile, melted nutrient agar at 50–55°C; in a boiling water bath at 75°C; by gentle agitation of blood and agar until the medium becomes chocolate-brown in colour. It can also be prepared by heating blood agar plates at 70–80° C for 10 minutes.

Loeffler's serum slope. It is an enriched solid medium preferred for the primary culture of *Corynebacterium diphtheriae*. In this medium, diphtheria bacilli grow very rapidly within 6 to 8 hours of incubation and luxuriant growth occurs within 12 to 18 hours. Further, smears from growth stained by Albert's or Ponder's or Neisser's method shows typical morphology with well formed metachromatic granules.

On Loeffler's serum slope, diphtheria bacilli form colonies which are small, circular white opaque discs at first, but enlarge on continued incubation and acquire a distinct yellow tint.

Loeffler's serum slope is also used for subculture diphtheria bacilli from potassium tellurite blood agar medium. It is used for growing pure cultures for toxigenicity testing.

Loeffler's serum slope is made up of sheep or horse serum, nutrient broth and glucose. It is sterilised and solidified simultaneously by inspissation.

Dorset's egg media. It is a solid enriched medium prepared by mixing egg and nutrient broth sterilised and solidified by inspissation.

Uses. 1. It is used for the cultivation of *Corynebacterium diphtheriae*.

2. Dorset's egg medium with glycerine is used as a selective medium for the cultivation of *Mycobacterium tuberculosis*.

3. It is used for the preservation of cultures, particularly to prevent S $\rightarrow$ R (smooth to rough) variation (*e.g., Salmonella typhi*).

Milk agar. It is an enriched solid medium prepared by adding 8–10% milk to nutrient agar. It enhances the pigment production by Staphylococci. The pigments of Staphylococci does not diffuse into the medium. Hence pigmented (colored) colonies are particularly marked against the opaque milky white background. *e.g.*,

1. *Staphylococcus aureus* produces golden-yellow colonies.
2. *Staphylococcus albus* (*epidermidis*) produces white colonies.

3. *Staphylococcus citreus* produces lemon-yellow colonies.

Pigment production can also be enhanced by the addition of 1% glycerol monoacetate into nutrient agar.

ENRICHMENT MEDIA

Enrichment media are essentially liquid media, containing specific nutrients required to enhance the growth of a particular bacterial pathogen, that may inhibitory to nonpathogenic commensals. In other words, some chemical substances are incorporated into liquid media, which cause enrichment of the required pathogenic bacterium and inhibits the growth of unwanted bacteria from a mixture of organisms such as feces, throat swab etc. *e.g.,*

1. Selenite F broth (F for feces) for enrichment of typhoid and paratyphoid bacilli from fecal samples.
2. Tetrathionate broth for enrichment of *Salmonella* species from feces.
3. Alkaline peptone water (pH 8.6) for enrichment of *Vibrio cholerae* from feces.
4. Monsur's taurocholate tellurite peptone water (pH 9.2) can also be used for enrichment of *Vibrio cholerae* from feces.
5. Bile broth used for isolation of *Salmonella* from blood.
6. Salt broth containing 8–10% NaCl is used for enrichment of *Staphylococcus aureus.*

Selenite F broth. It is an excellent and widely used liquid enrichment medium, used for the isolation of *Salmonella* from *feces*, sewage, food stuffs and other materials containing mixed bacterial flora. It is prepared from peptone, lactose, sodium acid selenite and phosphate buffer with pH adjusted to 7.1.

Feces sample is added to selenite-F broth (F for fecal) broth and incubated at 37°C for 6–8 hrs and subcultured on to solid media. Sodium selenite can be utilised by *Salmonella*, but toxic to *E.coli* and other enterobacteriaceae members. Selenite is reduced by *Salmonella* and produce alkali, that increases the pH decreasing toxicity. Hence, phosphate buffer is added to prevent this.

Selenite F broth is a brick red or orange colored liquid. A slight amount of red precipitate may form but this does not interfere with the enrichment.

Tetrathionate broth. It is a liquid enrichment medium used for the enrichment of Salmonellae from fecel samples. The medium contains nutrient broth, calcium carbonate, sodium thiosulphate and iodine. Phenol red is the indicator. These substances inhibit the growth of coliform bacilli, while permitting typhoid and paratyphoid bacilli to grow freely. Tetrathionate broth is not as efficient as selenite F broth for enrichment of *Salmonella*, because it may permit the growth of *Proteus* species. Feces is inoculated into tetrathionate broth and incubated for 6–18 hours and a subculture is made on Mac Conkey agar or DCA medium.

SELECTIVE MEDIA

Selective media are solid media, in which chemical substances are incorporated, which promotes the selective growth of required bacterial pathogens and suppress the growth of unwanted, commensal, non-pathogenic bacteria.

Selective media and enrichment media are essentially similar; the only difference is that selective media are solid, while enrichment media are liquid. *e.g.,*

1. Salt milk agar.
2. Mannitol salt agar
3. Ludlam's medium

} for the isolation of *Staphylococcus aureus.*

4. Thayer-Martin medium for the isolation of gonococci and meningococci.
5. LJ medium for the isolation of tubercle bacilli.
6. Potassium tellurite chocolate agar for the isolation of diphtheria bacilli.
7. Knisely's PLET (Polymyxion, tysozyme, EDTA, thallous acetate) – for the isolation of anthrax bacilli.
8. Wilson Blair's brilliant green bismuth sulphite agar medium – for the isolation of typhoid and paratyphoid bacilli.
9. Deoxycholate citrate (DCA) agar.
10. XLD (Xylose-Lysine-Deoxycholate) agar.
11. SS (Salmonellae-Shigellae) agar.

} for the isolation of *Salmonella* and *Shigella.*

12. TCBS (Thiosulphate, citrate, bilesalts, sucrose) agar.
13. Aronson's media.
14. Monsur's gelatin taurocholate trypticase tellurile (GTTA) agar.
15. Alkaline bile salt agar (BSA)

} for the isolation of *Vibrio cholerae.*

16. Skirrow's medium
17. Campy BAP medium

} for the isolation of *Campylobacter.*

18. Sabouraud's Dextrose agar (SDA) for the isolation of fungi.

Potassium tellurite blood agar/McLeod's medium. It is a selective medium used for the cultivation of *Corynebacterium diphtheriae*. This special medium is devised by Mc-Leod with heated Rabbit's blood and potassium tellurite (0.04%) and called it chocolate tellurite agar.

Potassium tellurite acts as a selective agent inhibiting the growth of other organisms, particularly commensals of throat. Diphtheria bacilli reduce tellurite to metallic tellurium, which gets incorporated in the colonies giving them a black or grey color. The growth may be slow and colonies appear on two days of incubation.

Based on colony morphology on potassium tellurite chocolate agar medium, Mc-Leod classified diphtheria bacilli into three biotypes:

1. Gravis – Daisy head colonies
2. Intermedius – Frog's egg colony
3. Mitis – Poached egg colony.

Wilson and Blair's bismuth sulphite agar. It is a selective medium for the isolation of typhoid and paratyphoid bacilli from feces samples. It is prepared by adding bismuth sulphite-phosphate-glucose mixture and iron-citrate-brilliant green mixture to nutrient agar. Brilliant green and bismuth sulphite act as selective agents and inhibit the growth of coliforms including *Shigella* and *Proteus* species.

Salmonella typhi and *Salmonella paratyphi* '*B*' reduce sulphite to sulphide in the presence of glucose and hence produce black colonies with a metallic sheen due to the formation of iron-sulphide

(H_2S positive). *Salmonella paratyphi* 'A' and *Salmonella cholera*-suis which does not forms H_2S, produce green colored colonies.

Fecal culture on Wilson and Blair's is particularly valuable in patients of enteric fever on antibiotics, as the drug does not eliminate the bacilli from the gut as rapidly as it does from the blood. Also, to trace carriers, swabs left in the sewage drainers (sewer-swab technique) or membrane filters through which sewage is filtered; can be cultured on this medium.

TCBS agar. Thiosulphate citrate bile sucrose (TCBS) agar is the most widely used selective plating medium for the isolation of *Vibrio cholerae* from feces. It gives good growth of *Vibrio cholerae* and *Vibrio parahemolyticus* and other vibrios, inhibits the growth of enterobacteria, and Gram positive bacteria.

The pH of the medium is alkaline 8.6. Bromothymol blue is the indicator. It appears dark green colored, transparent on which *Vibrio cholerae* produces large yellow convex colonies due to sucrose fermentation. *Vibrio parahemolyticus* does not ferment sucrose hence produce green colored colonies.

Lowenstein-Jensen (LJ) medium. It is a selective medium for the cultivation and differentiation of human and bovine types of tubercli bacilli and atypical mycobacteria.

It contains mineral salts, starch, glycerol, asparagine, malachite green and egg. Mycobacteria obtain their nitrogen from asparagine and the carbon from glycerol. Malachite green acts as a selective agent and inhibits contaminants. The medium is sterilised and solidified simultaneously by inspissation in inspissator. No agar is present in the medium. Coagulation of egg gives the solid surface. Clinical specimens are decontaminated and also concentrated for bacilli by Petroff's technique and then inoculated into the medium. Growth occurs in 4–6 weeks.

Mycobacterium tuberculosis grows luxuriantly and produces large, dry, rough, heaped up colonies with a wrinkled surface. It is called "Eugonic" growth. Colonies are creamy white initially, becoming yellowish or buff coloured later. In comparison, *Mycobacterium bovis* grows sparsely and produces small, flat, smooth, moist and small discrete colorless colonies known as "dysgonic" growth.

The most widely employed medium for routine culture is LJ medium, without starch, as recommended by International union against tuberculosis (IUAT).

Deoxycholate citrate agar. DCA is a selective medium suitable for the isolation of *Shigella* and *Salmonella*. It is prepared by adding sodium citrate, sodium thiosulphate, ferric citrate, lactose and a bile salt sodium deoxycholate to nutrient agar. Neutral red is the indicator. Bile salts inhibit the growth of Gram positive organisms and to a certain extent the coliforms. Some coliforms may grow and produce pink colonies due to lactose fermentation, whereas non-lactose fermenters (NLF) produce pale, colorless colonies. Medium contains ferric citrate and H_2S producing bacteria form iron sulphide and the colony shows a central black dot.

DIFFERENTIAL MEDIA

Differential media are those in which chemical substances are incorporated which enable it bring out different characteristics of different bacteria; so that colonies of one particular species can be differentiated visually from those of another. *e.g.*, MacConkey agar, Eosin-Methylene blue (EMB) agar.

MacConkey's agar/Bile salt lactose neutral red agar. It is a differential medium widely used in the primary isolation, identification and differentiation of Gram negative bacilli, belonging to family enterobacteriacease.

It contains peptone, meat extract, NaCl, bile salt, lactose and neutral red indicator. Bile salt inhibits the growth of Gram positive bacteria. Some bacteria ferment lactose and produce acid which decreases medium pH and causes the neutral red indicator to give a pink or red color to colonies. They are known as Lactose fermenters (LF). Non-lactose fermenters (NLF) form colorless, pale colonies. Some organisms ferment lactose late, and called as Late-Lactose fermenters (LLF).

LF-*e.g., Esch.coli, Klebsiellae* sp.

Colonies of *Esch.coli* are pink, moist, large, partially translucent or opaque discs.

Colonies of *Klebsiellae* are pink, large, dome shaped, mucoid with varying degrees of stickyness.

NLF – *e.g., Salmonella, Shigella.*

LLF – *e.g., Shigella sonnei.*

INDICATOR MEDIA

Indicator media are those which indicate a property of the bacterium. These media contain an indicator which changes color when a bacterium grows in it. *e.g.,*

1. MacConkey agar indicates lactose fermenting property. LF produce pink colonies and NLF produce colorless colonies due to neutral red indicator.
2. Wilson and Blair's bismuth sulphite agar medium indicates H_2S production due to the reduction of sulphite to sulphide in the presence of glucose. *S.typhi*, *S.paratyphi B* and *S.paratyphi C* produce black colonies with metallic sheen due to H_2S production whereas *S.paratyphi A* and *S.cholera-suis* form green colonies, as they do not produce H_2S.
3. Potassium tellurite chocolate agar indicates reduction of tellurite by forming tellurium metal, which accumulates in the colonies of diphtheria bacilli forming black colonies.

TRANSPORT MEDIA

When the patient is not close to the laboratory, there is a risk that the pathogen in a specimen may not survive or may be overgrown by non-pathogens during the time it takes to transport the specimen to the laboratory. For this purpose, special media have been devised termed as "transport media". Enrichment media can be used to transportation of specimens. Transport media can also be used for preservation of bacteria in clinical specimens. *e.g.,*

1. Stuart's transport medium for gonococci.
2. Sach's buffered glycerol saline for enteric bacilli in feces.
3. Pike's medium for *Streptococcus pyogenes*, pneumococci and *Hemophilus influenzae* in nose and throat swabs.
4. Cary-Blair medium for *Vibrio cholerae* and *Campylobacter.*
5. V-R fluid (pH 9.2) for *Vibrio cholerae.*
6. Alkaline peptone water (pH 8.6) for *Vibrio cholerae.*

ANAEROBIC MEDIA

They are used for the cultivation of anaerobic bacteria. These media contain a reducing substance which absorbs all the oxygen and creates an anaerobic condition, which favours the growth of anaerobes. *e.g.,*

1. Robertson's cooked (chopped) meat (RCM) broth.

2. Thioglycollate medium.

3. Smith-Noguchi medium – Nutrient broth containing fresh animal tissues such as Rabbit kidney, spleen, testes or heart.

4. Nutrient broth with red hot iron fillings and with a liquid paraffin layer.

RCM broth. (Robertson's cooked meat broth) – It is used for the cultivation of anaerobic bacteria; also used for the preservation of aerobic bacteria.

The medium contains meat infusion or nutrient broth, minced, cooked ox heart tissue. Broth is layered over by liquid paraffin to prevent the entry of air. Chopped meat contains unsaturated fatty acids which act as reducing agent and absorb oxygen; hematin catalyses this reducing action; and sulphydryl groups create a low redox potential; all these factors favour the growth of anaerobic bacteria. Particularly *Clostridium* species. The specimen is inoculated deep in the medium in contact with the meat.

RCM broth detects proteolytic and saccharolytic activities of anaerobic bacteria. Proteolytic Clostridia blacken the meat with the formation of foul smelling sulphur compounds *e.g., Clostridium histolyticum*. Saccharolytic *Clostridia* turn meat red slightly with sour smell. *e.g., Clostridium welchii (perfringens)*.

Clostridium tetani does not have saccharolytic property and shows only mild proteolytic activity and hence no change in the meat appearance. Only prolonged incubation give slight blackening.

Thioglycollate medium/broth. It is an anaerobic medium. The medium contains reducing agents such as sodium thioglycollate, glucose, vitamin-C (ascorbic acid), cysteine and agar at a concentration of 0.05%, with methylene blue.

Thioglycollate acts as a reducing agent and creates an anaerobic environment deeper in the tube, allows anaerobic bacteria to grow. Glucose and thioglycollate maintain the anaerobic condition. Agar (0.05%) prevents convection currents of air. Methylene blue act as an oxidation-reduction potential indicator. Methylene blue remains colorless throughout the medium except at the surface where oxygen may be present.

SUGAR MEDIA/SUGAR FERMENTATION TEST

Bacteria differ widely in their ability to metabolise/ferment carbohydrates, and produce either only acid or both acid and gas. Hence, carbohydrate fermentation is used for characterisation and identification of bacteria, particularly important in the study of Gram negative bacilli. Sugar media are used to test fermentation.

Carbohydrate media consists of peptone water, 1% sugar and Andrade's indicator. The sugars may be glucose, lactose, sucrose, maltose, xylose, mannitol etc. Andrade's indicator consists of acid fuchsin and NaOH. The medium is distributed in the test tubes and a small inverted tube called "Durham's tube" completely filled with liquid and containing no air bubbles is placed inside, and sterilised. The color of the medium is light yellow.

The test bacterium is inoculated and incubated. Acid production is indicated by the development of pink color. Gas accumulates in the inner Durham's tube.

Phenol red indicator can also be used then the original color of the medium is red and turns yellow on acid production.

Bromocresol purple indicator can also be used. Then the original color of the medium is purple and turns yellow on acid production.

To test sugar fermentation of bacteria with fastidious growth requirements, such as Streptococci, pneumococci, gonococci, meningococci and diphtheria bacilli, Hiss's serum water is used. It is a sugar medium enriched with serum. *e.g.,*

1. *Esch.coli, Klebsiellae* are lactose fermenters (LF).
2. *Salmonella, Shigella* are non-lactose fermenters (NLF).
3. Mannitol fermentation for *Salmonella* and *Shigella*.
4. Xylose and arabinose fermentation for differentiating *Salmonella paratyphi 'A'* and *S.paratyphi 'B'*.

Depending upon the species concerned, various end products are formed in sugar fermentation.

1. Organic acids – formic, acetic, propionic, butyric and lactic acids.
2. Neutral products – Acetone, ethyl alcohol, butyl alcohol and acetyl methyl carbinol.
3. Gases – chiefly carbondioxide and hydrogen.

CULTURE MEDIA FOR CULTIVATION OF FUNGI

Potato dextrose agar (PDA). It is used to cultivate saprophytic fungi.

Potato	–	200 g
Dextrose	–	20 g
Agar	–	20 g
Distilled water	–	1 lit.
pH	–	3.5–4.0

Scrub the potatoes, and cut into small cubes and boil in water for few minutes and squeeze as much of the pulp as possible through a fine sieve. To the filtrate add dextrose and agar and make up the volume to 1 lit. by adding distilled water. The pH is adjusted to 3.5 to 4.0 (acidic). The medium is dispensed (or) distributed in required amounts taking care to keep solids in suspension. The medium is sterilized by autoclaving and cooked to 50°C and poured into petridishes.

Sabouraud's dextrose agar (SDA). It is used for the cultivation of pathogenic fungi from clinical specimens. The medium was devised by a medical mycologist, Dr. Raymond Sabouraud, hence known as Sabouraud's dextrose agar medium. It is a selective medium for fungi, because of its high sugar content and acidic pH.

Dextrose	–	40 gm
Peptone	–	10 gm
Agar	–	20 gm
Distilled water	–	1 lit.
pH	–	5.4

The medium can be made further selective by adding antibiotics like chloramphenicol to prevent bacterial contamination and cycloheximide to prevent fungal contamination.

Fungal growth is noted by big flowery colonies or pigmented colonies.

Corn-meal agar. Corn-meal agar is low in nutrients. It suppresses vegetative growth while stimulating sporulation of many fungi. It can be used to produce the distinctive chlamydospores of *Candida albicans*. It is useful in the preparation of slide cultures and is generally useful in the study of sporulation in fungi.

Corn meal	–	40 g
Agar	–	15 g
Distilled water	–	1 lit.

The addition of 1% tween enhances the production of chlamydospores.

Boil the corn meal in 1 litre of water for an hour, filter through muslin and add the agar. Steam to dissolve, dispense in required amounts and sterilize by autoclaving. Allow to cool to 50°C and pour into petridishes.

Martin's rose bengal agar medium (MRBA). This medium is used to isolate fungi from soil and other specimens, since it becomes bacteria-free.

Peptone	–	5 g
Dextrose	–	10 g
KNO_3	–	1 g
KCl	–	0.05 g
$MgSO_4$	–	0.5 g
Agar	–	20 g
Rose bengal	–	0.003 g (1 in 30,000 dil.)
Distilled water	–	1 lit.
pH	–	4.0

Sterilize by autoclaving.

In another modification KCl and KNO_3 are replaced by KH_2PO_4 (1 gm) and streptomycin (3 mg per ml).

Czapek-Dox (CD) agar. It is used for the cultivation of fungi.

Sucrose	–	30 g
$NaNO_3$	–	3 g
KH_2PO_4	–	1 g
$MgSO_4.7H_2O$	–	0.5 g
KCl	–	0.5 g
$FeSO_4.7H_2O$	–	0.01 g
Agar	–	20 g
Distilled water	–	1 lit.
pH	–	4.0

Sterilized by autoclaving.

QUESTIONS

Short Notes

1. Meal extract/lab lemco.
2. Peptone.
3. Agar/Agar-agar.

4. Defined media/synthetic media.
5. Semidefined media.
6. Peptone water medium.
7. Simple media/ordinary media/Basal media.
8. Nutrient broth.
9. Nutrient agar.
10. Enriched media.
11. Blood agar-constituents, preparation and uses.
12. Chocolate agar.
13. Loeffler's serum slope.
14. Dorset's egg media.
15. Milk agar.
16. Name four commonly used enriched media and their uses.
17. Enrichment media.
18. Selenite F broth.
19. Tetrathionate broth.
20. Name any two enrichment media and their uses.
21. Selective media.
22. Name four commonly used selective media and their uses.
23. Wilson and Blair's medium.
24. Potassium tellurite blood agar.
25. TCBS agar.
26. Lowenstein - Jensen (LJ) medium.
27. Deoxycholate citrate agar (DCA).
28. What are the selective media used for *Staphylococcus aureus*, *Bacillus anthracis*, *Neisseria gonorrhoeae* and *Corynebacterium diphtheriae*.
29. Differential media.
30. MacConkey agar.
31. Indicator media.
32. Transport media.
33. Name four transport media and their uses.
34. Anaerobic media.
35. Name two anaerobic media and their uses.
36. RCM broth.
37. Thioglycollate medium/thioglycollate broth.
38. Sugar media/carbohydrate media/carbohydrate (sugar) fermentation.

11

Isolation of Bacteria, Cultivation Methods for Bacteria, Inoculation of Culture Media, Culturing Microorganisms

- *Inoculation*
- *Primary culture*
- *Isolate*
- *Subculture*
- *Axenic culture*
- *Inoculation wire loop*
- *Straight wire*
- *Spud/L-shaped wire*
- *Spreader*
- *Pasteur pipette*
- *Methods of cultivation*
  - *Streak culture/ surface plating*
  - *Stroke culture*
  - *Stab culture*
  - *Shake culture*
  - *Lawn/Carpet culture*
  - *Pour plate culture*
  - *Liquid culture*
  - *Sweep plate method*
  - *Cough plate method*
- *Anaerobic methods of cultivation*
  - *Glove boxes (anaerobic chambers)*
  - *Anaerobic bags/pouches*
  - *Reduction of oxygen in the media*
  - *Mc Intosh Field's anaerobic jar*
  - *Absorption of oxygen–chemcial method and Biological method*
  - *Candle jar method*

INOCULATION

The process of seeding bacteria (or) a specimen containing bacteria in to culture media is called "inoculation".

PRIMARY CULTURE

When an organism is isolated for the first time directly from a sample is called "Primary culture" or "Primary isolation". Primary cultures are usually done for the isolation of organisms. Thus isolation of microorganisms from pathological materials or natural sources such as sputurn, pus, throat swab, CSF, blood, faeces and aspirated fluid from pateints on agar media in pure cultures is known as "Primary isolation". Isolation of microorganisms from water, milk and soil samples is also called primary isolation.

ISOLATE

Each primary culture isolated/cultivated in pure culture from a natural source is called an isolate.

SUBCULTURE

The periodic transfer of cultures to fresh media under sterile, aseptic conditions and its subsequent growth is termed "Subcultures" or Secondary cultures", Where bacteria are transferred or cultured from one medium to another medium.

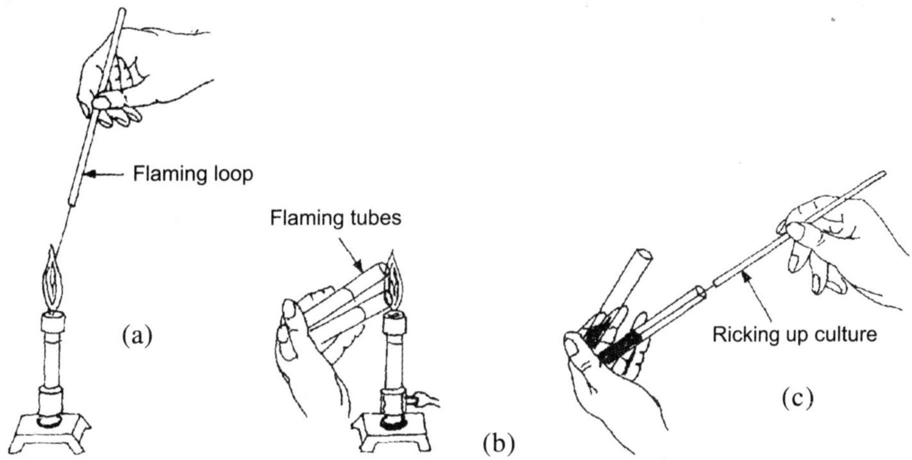

Fig. 11.1 The process of picking up inoculum from a culture tube for transfer to another slant (subculturing).

Subcultures are usually done

1. to obtain a pure growth of the bacterium
2. to study the characteristics/properties of the isolated organism
3. to maintain/preserve stock cultures

AXENIC CULTURE

It is a pure culture of an organism of a single species (*e.g.*, bacterium, fungus, protozoan etc.) growing in a medium free of other living organisms.

For inoculation of a specimen in to culture medium, the following instruments are used.

INOCULATION WIRE LOOP

It consists of a nichrome wire of thickness 23 SWG and of 3 inches length, mounted in a glass or metal holder. The other end of wire is drawn into a flat, circular, completely closed loop of 2–4 mm internal diameter. Instead of nichrome wire, platinum or Eureka may be used.

The wire loop is sterilized by holding it vertically in a Bunsen flame so that the whole length becomes red hot at the same time. The advantages of nichrome, platinum and eureka wires are that they get heated quickly and cooled quickly. It is allowed to cool down before touching any specimen or culture.

It is used for inoculation of clinical specimens on to the culture media or transfer of the material on to the slide to prepare smears etc. A standard wire loop for urine culture should deliver 0.01 ml of urine for quantitative estimation of bacteria in urine.

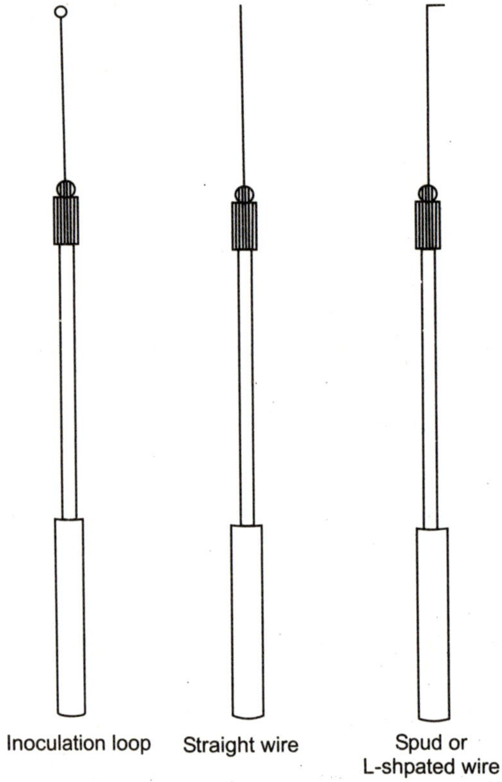

Fig. 11.2 Inoculation wire loop.

STRAIGHT WIRE

This inoculation wire is straight, without a loop and made of Nichrome or platinum or Eureka with a length of 4.5 inches. Straight wires are used for picking up single, exact colonies and for deep stab inoculation.

SPUD/L-SHAPED WIRE

It is a straight wire bent at right angles into L-shaped and tip is flattened. It is used to handle tenacious growths such as fungal colonies, to pick up sticky colonies of Actinomycetes and for scraping the medium.

SPREADER

It is a capillary tube bent at right angle. This is used for spreading or carpetting the liquid culture on the solid medium employed for antibiotic sensitivity testing and phage typing.

PASTEUR PIPETTE

It is single glass tube drawn into a long tapering end, as a capillary pipette. It is sterilised in hot air oven at 160°C for 1 hour. It is used with a rubber teat.

It is used for transferring liquid cultures, liquid media, antigen and antisera etc. It is used for inoculation of media for biochemical tests and for serological tests.

Bacterial cultivation serves three main purposes

1. to grow and isolate all bacteria present in an infection.
2. to determine which of the bacteria that grow are most likely causing infection and which are likely contaminants or colonizers
3. to obtain sufficient growth of clinically relevant bacteria to allow identification and characterization .

METHODS OF CULTIVATION

For culturing microorganisms or for inoculation of specimen into culture media, various methods are employed.

1. Steak culture/surface plating
2. Stroke culture
3. Stab culture
4. Shake culture
5. Lawn culture/carpet culture
6. Pour plate culture
7. Liquid culture
8. Sweep plate method
9. Cough plate method

Streak Culture/Surface Plating

It is the most efficient and easy way of isolating and enumerating microorganisms.

It is routinely employed conventional technique for the isolation of bacteria in pure culture from various clinical specimens. With a sterile wire loop, specimens such as sputum, pus, feces, CSF and aspirated fluid is transferred on to the surface of a well-dried plate, and spread over a small area at the periphery. It is known as inoculum (Primary inoculum). Then the wire loop is sterilized again and the inoculum is distributed thinly over the plate by streaking it with the loop in a series of parallel lines, in different segments of the plate. The wire loop should be heated and cooled (sterilized) between the different sets of streaks. Hence, this method is also called "Heating and subsequent streaking".

On incubation, growth may be confluent at the site of primary inoculum, but becomes progressively thinner, and well separated, discrete colonies appear over the final series of streaks.

Surface plating can also be done by successive or consecutive rubbing, and grid plate method.

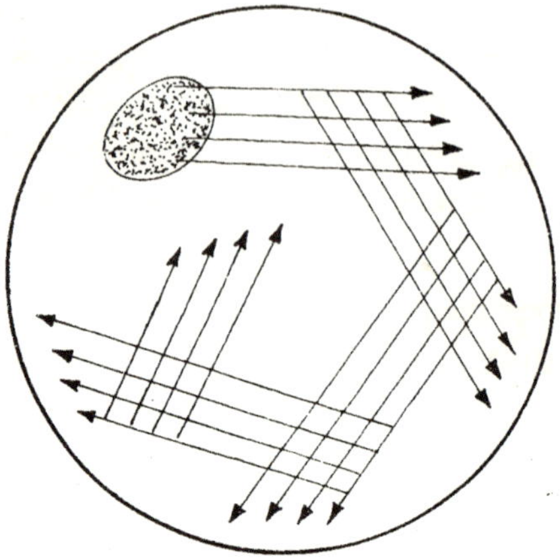

Fig. 11. 3 Streak culture.

Stroke Culture. Stroke cultures are made in test tubes or bottles containing agar slope or slant. The agar medium is allowed to set in tubes in a slanting position at 45° angle. The specimen or a colony is taken with a sterile wire loop and inoculated on to a slope by strokes, by holding the tube horizontally. If there is a butt, inoculation into butt is done by stabbing with a straight wire.

Stroke cultures are employed 1. for obtaining pure growth of the bacterium, 2. for slide agglutination tests, 3. for biochemical tests and other diagnostic tests.

e.g., Inoculation of Nutrient agar slant, Loeffler's serum slope, TSI agar and Sabouraud's agar medium etc.

Stab Culture. The agar medium for stab culture is allowed to set in upright position in test tubes providing a flat surface at the top of the medium.

A straight wire of 4.5 inches length is sterilized and the colony is picked up and inoculated by puncturing or stabbing deep in to the medium (such as nutrient gelatin or glucose agar).

Stab cultures are used

1. to test gelatin liquefaction or production of gelatinase, which liquefies gelatin.

2. to study the oxygen requirement of the bacterium to differentiate aerobic and anaerobic bacteria. Aerobic bacteria grow on the surface, where oxygen is available. Anaerobic bacteria grow deep in the medium, where oxygen is not available, whereas facultative anaerobes grow along the stab on the surface as well as deep in the medium.

3. for maintenance or preservation of stock cultures

4. to study the motility of bacteria in "semi-solid agar".

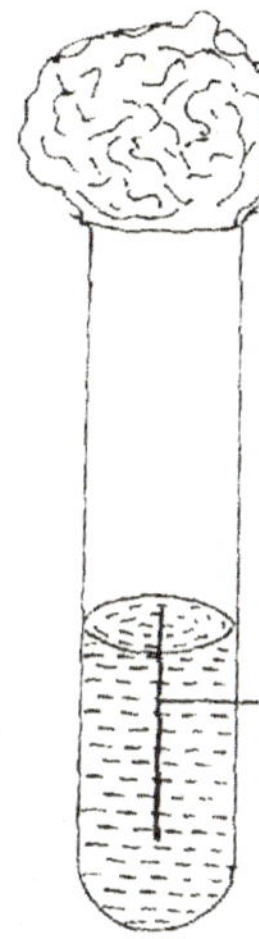

Fig. 11.4 Stab culture.

Shake Sulture

Shake cultures are made by melting nutrient agar in a test tube, heating it to 45°C in a water bath. The specimen is inoculated with a straight wire; liquid culture can be inoculated with a Pasteur pipette and the tube is rolled between the palms so that inoculum gets mixed with the molten agar and then allowed to set in upright position.

This method enables the growth of anaerobic and microaerophilic bacteria in the depths of media.

Shake cultures can be used as an alternate method to stab cultures.

To estimate BOD (biochemical oxygen demand) of water samples the specimen is inoculated into liquid media and incubated in BOD incubator with continuous shaking by mechanical shakers inside the BOD incubator.

Lawn Culture/Carpet Culture

Lawn cultures are prepared by flooding/spreading the surface of the agar plate with a liquid culture or bacterial suspension. The excess fluid can be pipetted out. Alternatively, a sterile swab soaked in bacterial culture can be rubbed over the entire surface of the medium.

The lawn culture provides a confluent, uniform surface growth of the bacterium and is useful for– 1. Antibiotic sensitivity testing by disc diffusion method, 2. Phage typing, 3. Obtaining a large amount of growth as in the preparation of large amount of bacterial suspensions to produce antigens or vaccines.

Pour Plate Culture

Pour plate cultures are used to estimate colony count or viable count or Standard Plate Count (SPC) of bacteria and fungi in water, milk and soil samples. Pour plate method is also useful for quantitative urine cultures.

The sample is diluted several times (serial dilutions) and a small volume (usually 1 ml) of the diluted sample is mixed with 10-15 ml agar medium in a test tube, that is molten and cooled to 45°C; and the mixtures are shaken or rolled between the palms (as in shake cultures) and poured immediately in to sterile petriplates. Most bacteria and fungi are not killed by a brief exposure to the warm agar. After the agar is hardened, each cell is fixed in its place and forms an individual colony upon incubation. The total number of colonies equals the viable microorganisms in the diluted sample the colonies can be seen trapped deep inside the medium.

The visible colonies can be counted with naked eye or in a colony counter and the number of colonies per ml of the sample is reported as the standard plate count (SPC) per ml.

$$\text{Number of cells per ml} = \frac{\text{Number of colonies}}{\text{Amount inoculated x dilution}}$$

Liquid Cultures

Liquid media in tubes, bottles or flasks may be inoculated with a sterile wire loop or by adding the inoculum with pipettes and syringes. Liquid cultures are preferred

1. When concentration of bacteria in inocula are expected to be small *e.g.*, sterility tests.
2. When large inocula are to be inoculated *e.g.*, blood culture.
3. For inocula containing antibiotics and other inhibitory substances, as these are rendered diluted and ineffective by dilution in the liquid media *e.g.*, blood culture.
4. When large yields are desired, the yield being enhanced by agitation, aeration *e.g.*, production of alcohols and antibiotics.
5. For biochemical tests *e.g.*, sugar fermentation and IMViC reactions.
6. For enrichment media *e.g.*, selenite F broth.
7. For presumptive coliform test in bacteriological analysis of water.

The major disadvantage of liquid culture is that it does not provide a pure culture from mixed inocula.

Sweep Plate Method

The edges of the petriplate with culture medium is rubbed over the cloth with the medium facing it. The dust particles along with microorganisms stirred up from the fabric and get settled on the culture medium. Colonies develop on incubation, which can be counted and viable counts made.

Cough Plate Method

Cough plate method is used to collect specimens directly from patients at bed side suffering from whooping cough (pertussis) caused by *Bordetella pertussis*.

Bordet-Gengou glycerine-potato-blood agar plate is held about 10-15 cm infront of the patient's mouth, during a spontaneous or induced paroxysm of coughing, so that respiratory exudates impinge directly on the medium. The plate is incubated for 48-72 hours. *Bordetella pertussis* produces colonies resembling mercury drops or bisected pearls when growth is confluent, silvery or aluminium paint like appearance is seen.

The colonies should be first examined by Gram's staining and then confirmed by slide agglutination test with specific antiserum.

ANAEROBIC METHODS OF CULTIVATION

Anaerobic bacteria do not require oxygen for their growth. In the presence of oxygen, hydrogen peroxide which is toxic to growth accumulates. The enzyme catalase which splits hydrogen peroxide is absent in anaerobes. Hence, special methods have been devised to process specimens and cultivate anaerobic bacteria in oxygen-free atmosphere.

Various anaerobic methods of cultivation are listed here below:

I. Gloves boxes (Anaerobic chambers).

II. Anaerobic bags/Anaerobic Pouches.

III. Anaerobic media/Reduction of oxygen in the media

(*i*) RCM broth.

(*ii*) Thioglycollate medium.

(*iii*) Smith-Noguchi's medium.

(*iv*) Nutrient broth with red hot iron pieces.

IV. Mc Intosh-Filds's anaerobic Jar

(*i*) Evacuation and replacement method or displacement of oxygen.

(*ii*) Displacement and combustion of oxygen.

(*iii*) Gas Pak

V. Absorption of oxygen

1. Chemical method

(*i*) Alkaline pyrogallol method

(*a*) Buchners's tube

(*b*) Spray anaerobic dish

(*c*) Ordinary Petri dish

(*ii*) Rosenthal (chromium + H_2SO_4) method

(*iii*) Phosphorous stick method

2. Biological method.

VI. Candle jar method

VII. Cultivation in vacuum

VIII. Shake cultures

IX. Stab cultures.

Glove Boxes/Anaerobic Chambers/Anaerobic Cabinets

Glove boxes are used for processing of specimens, incubation of cultures, periodic examination of culture plates, subcultures, and to make prereduction of media for anaerobic organisms in an oxygen-free atmosphere

They are made of plastic or metal with a front glass window. Specimens, cultures and other materials are placed in the chamber through an air lock. It has gloves or sleeves that form air-tight seals around the arms to handle items inside the chamber. A gas mixture of 5% CO_2 , 10% hydrogen and 85% nitrogen and a palladium catalyst maintain the anaerobic environment inside the chamber. Some cabinets use methylene blue as an indicator to monitor anaerobiosis.

Anaerobic Bags/Anaerobic Pouches

They are useful for laboratories processing small number of specimens. They can be used to transport specimens, and also to incubate one or two agar plates.

Reduction of Oxygen in the Media/Anaerobic Media

These media contain a reducing agent which absorbs all the oxygen and creates an anaerobic condition, which favours the growth of anaerobes.

(i) RCM broth. It contains meat infusion or Nutrient broth and minced, cooked beef heart tissue. Liquid paraffin is layered over the broth to prevent the entry of air. Chopped meat contains unsaturated fatty acids which act as reducing agent and absorb oxygen, hematin catalyses this reducing action, and sulphydryl groups create a low redox potential; All these factors favour the growth of anaerobic bacteria, particularly *Clostridium* species.

(ii) Thioglycollate medium. It contains reducing agents sodium thioglycollate, glucose, Vitamin-C, cysteine and agar at a concentration of 0.05%, with methylene blue as indicator.

Thioglycollate acts as a reducing agent and creates an anaerobic environment. Glucose and thioglycollate maintain the anaerobic condition. Agar (0.05%) prevents convection currents, which prevents diffusion of air in to the medium.

(iii) Smith-Noguchi medium. Nutrient broth containing fresh animal tissues such as Rabbit kidney, spleen, testes or heart, is used as anaerobic media.

(iv) Nutrient broth with red hot iron pieces and layered with a liquid paraffin, can be used as a simple anaerobic medium.

McIntosh-Filde's Anaerobic Jar.

To grow anaerobes on the surface of solid media it is necessary to provide an atmosphere free of oxygen. This is achieved by the use of anaerobic jars, such as McIntosh-filde's and Baird and Tatlock anaerobic jar.

It consists of a metal or heavy plastic jar with a metal lid that can be clamped down on a gasket to make it air-tight with a screw-clamp. The lid has two tubes with taps, one acting as the inlet and the other as the outlet. The lid has two terminals, connected to an electric supply. One or more capsules containing palladiumized alumina pellets are suspended under the lid with wires and connected to electric terminals on the lid for heating. Alternatively room temperature catalyst, called Deoxo pellets, in which palladium is coated on alumina can be used.

Inoculated culture plates are placed inside the jar with medium upside and lid downwords, as soon as they are seeded, and the lid is clamped air-tight. Following procedures are adopted to provide anaerobiosis in anaerobic jars, with an increased CO_2 concentration, as CO_2 enhances the growth of many anaerobes.

(i) Displacement of oxygen or evacuation-replacement method. The outlet valve is connected to a vacuum pump and the air is removed from the sealed jar by drawing a vacuum of 25 inches of mercury (62.5 cm or 625 mm of Hg). This process is repeated two times, filling the jar with an oxygen-free gas such as nitrogen, between evacuations. Finally, the jar is filled with a gas mixture containing 80% nitrogen, 10% hydrogen and 10% CO_2 (or 90% hydrogen and 10% CO_2). The inlet valve is then closed and the jar is incubated at 37°C when room temperature catalyst is used, there is no need of heating.

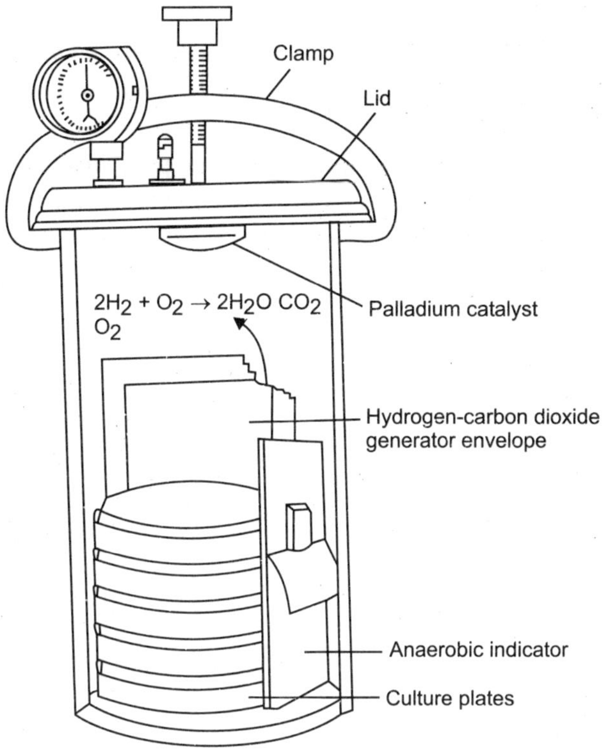

Fig. 11.5. Mc-Intosh-Filde's Anaerobic Jar.

(ii) Displacement and combustion of oxygen. The electric terminals are connected to a current supply so that palladiumized asbestos is heated. This acts as a catalyst for the combination of hydrogen with residual oxygen present in the jar. This method of displacement of oxygen combined with combustion ensures complete anaerobiosis, but rarely carries the risk of explosion.

(iii) Gas pak system. It is devised by Brewer and Allgeier (1966). The Gas pak is at present the method of choice for producing anaerobiosis in anaerobic jars.

It is a disposable aluminium foil packet, commercially available, containing pellets of sodium borohydride and cobalt chloride and of citric acid and sodium bicarbonate. They generate hydrogen and CO_2 on addition of water, hence known as 'hydrogen and CO_2 generator envelope".

The Gas pak envelope is kept in the jar, with water added along with inoculated plates and the lid is tightened. The Gas pak chemicals generate H_2 and CO_2 and the presence of a catalyst enables the combination of H_2 and oxygen to produce anaerobic environment. Production of heat within a few minutes and subsequent development of moisture on the walls of the jar are indications that the catalyst and Gas pak envelope are functioning properly.

However Methylene blue or resazurin indicators can be used to verify anaerobiosis. Methylene blue becomes colorless in the absence of oxygen; whereas it becomes blue colored when exposed to oxygen.

Gas kit, another disposable envelope, similar to Gas pak, is also used to produce anaerobiosis.

Absorption of oxygen. Anaerobiosis can be produced by absorption of oxygen from closed systems either by chemical method or biological method.

Chemical Methods

(*i*) ***Alkaline pyrogallol.*** It absorbs oxygen. It is used in various modifications.

(*a*) ***Buchner's tube.*** Pyrogallic acid added to a solution of NaOH in a large test tube placed inside an air-tight jar provides anaerobiosis.

(*b*) ***Spray anaerobic dish.*** It is a glass dish with its bottom partitioned into two halves, and the top accommodating one half of a Petri dish carrying the medium. Pyrogallic acid and NaOH are placed in the separate halves at the bottom of the dish. The inoculated culture plate is inverted on the top of the dish and sealed air-tight. The dish may be tilted slightly to mix the chemicals.

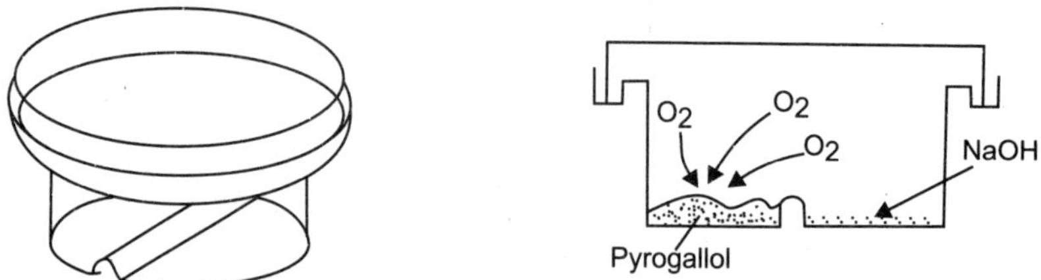

(a) (b)

Fig. 11.6. The spray plate.

(*c*) ***Alkaline pyrogallol in an ordinary petri plate.*** This method employs a disc of filter paper having the same diameter as a Petri dish. It is placed on top of one half of the dish, and pyrogallol and sodium carbonate in dry powder form is spread on it. The inoculated plate is inverted over the filter paper and sealed tight with molten wax. The dry pyrogallol and sodium carbonate is activated by the moisture within the closed system, and complete anaerobiosis develops within about two hours.

(*ii*) ***Rosenthal method.*** Anaerobiosis within jars can be produced with a mixture of chromium and sulphuric acid. Oxygen is reduced to water.

(*iii*) ***Phosphorous stick method.*** Inoculated plates are kept in a closed air-tight jar. Yellow phosphorous sticks are burnt in the jar to absorb oxygen. The phosphorous continues to burn till all the oxygen gets exhausted and ultimately only the inert gases and partial vacuum remain. A small container of water should be kept to absorb phosphorous pentoxide formed due to phosphorous burning.

Biological Method

Absorption of oxygen from jars is attempted by incubating cultures with germinating seeds, chopped vegetables (Potatoes), and aerobic organisms such as *Pseudomonas aeruginosa* and *Serratia marcescens*. Anaerobiosis produced by biological methods is slow and ineffective.

Candle Jar Method

It is most widely used method. This method also provides a concentration of CO_2 which stimulates the growth of most bacteria. Inoculated culture plates are placed inside a large air-tight container and a lighted candle kept in it, and the lid is sealed with molten wax.

The burning candle uses up all oxygen inside the jar before it is extinguished, and creates anaerobic condition. But candle jar method is ineffective, some oxygen is always left behind.

Cultivation in Vacuum

Cultivation in vacuum was attempted by incubating cultures in a vacuum desiccator but the method has some disadvantages (*i*) Some oxygen may be left behind,

(*ii*) Fluid cultures may boil over in vacuum,

(*iii*) Media may get detached from culture plates in vacuum.

Shake Cultures

Shake cultures are made by melting nutrient agar in a test tube, cooling it to 45°C in a water bath. The specimen or culture is inoculated and the tube is rolled (shaken) between the palms so that inoculum gets mixed with the molten agar and then allowed to set in upright position. This method enables the growth of anaerobic and microaerophilic bacteria in the depths of media.

Stab Cultures

The agar medium for stab culture is allowed to set in upright position, providing a flat surface at the top of the medium. The colony picked up with a straight wire and inoculated by puncturing or stabbing deep into the medium. Anaerobic bacteria grow deep in the medium, whereas aerobic bacteria grow on the surface.

QUESTIONS

Essay Type Questions

1. Give an account of various methods of anaerobic culture of bacteria.
2. Enumerate the growth requirements of bacteria. Describe in detail the anaerobic methods of cultivation.

Short Notes

1. Inoculation wire loop.
2. Spud.
3. Pasteur pipette.
4. Surface plating/streak cultures.
5. Stroke culture.
6. Stab culture.
7. Shake cultures.
8. Lawn culture/carpet culture.
9. Pour plate method.
10. Liquid cultures.
11. Cough plate method.
12. Primary cultures.
13. Subculture.
14. Axenic culture.
15. Anaerobic culture methods/culture of anaerobic bacteria.
16. Mc Intosh-Field's anaerobic jar.
17. Draw a neat labeled diagram of Mc Intosh-Field's anaerobic jar.
18. Anaerobic cabinets/Glove boxes/Anaerobic chamber.
19. Gas pak.
20. Alkaline pyrogallol method.
21. Candle jar.
22. RCM broth.
23. Thioglycollate medium.

12

Biochemical Tests for the Identification of Bacteria

- *IMViC Reactions*
  - *– Indole test*
  - *– Methyl red test*
  - *– Voges-Proskauer test*
  - *– Citrate utilization test*
- *Urease test*
- *Catalase test*
- *Oxidase test*
- *Phynyl alanine deaminase test*
- *TSI agar*
- *Oxidation-Fermentation test/Hugh & Leifson's test*

IMViC REACTIONS

IMViC is a sigla, refers to Indole test, Methyl Red test, Voges-Proskauer test and Citrate utilization tests. '*i*' is added for the easiness of pronounciation. IMViC reactions are widely used for the identification and differentiation of intestinal Gram negative bacilli.

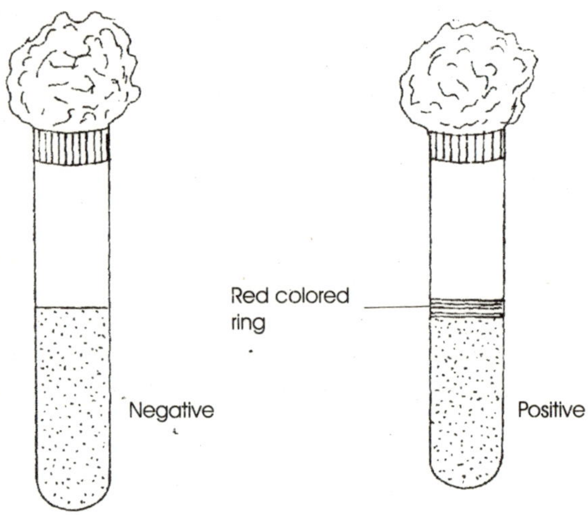

Fig. 12.1 Indole test.

Indole Test

Some bacteria decompose the amino acid tryptophan to form indole, which is tested for by a colorimetric reaction with Kovac's (or Ehrlich's) reagent.

The test bacterium is inoculated into peptone water medium and incubated at 37°C for 1-2 days. To this culture add few drops of Kovac's reagent or Ehrlich reagent and shake gently. A red color ring in the top alcohol layer indicates a positive reaction.

Kovac's reagent is composed of p-dimethyl amino benzaldehyde, Amyl or isoamyl alcohol, conc. HCl.

E.coli and *Vibrio cholerae* are indole positive, whereas *Klebsiella* and *Salmonella* are indole negative.

Methyl Red Test

The test is employed to detect the production of acid during the fermentation of glucose and maintenance of a pH below 4.5 in an old culture, tested by Methyl Red reagent.

The test bacterium is inoculated into glucose phosphate peptone water medium and incubated at 37°C for 1-2 days. Add a few drops of methyl red reagent, mix and read. Positive tests are bright red and negative are yellow. If the results are equivocal, the test can be repeated with cultures incubated for 5 days. For some organisms, incubation at 30°C for 5 days may be preferable.

Voges-Proskauer Test/Acetoin Production

Some bacteria ferment carbohydrates with the production of acetyl methyl carbinol (acetoin) or its reduction product 2, 3 butylene glycol, which is oxidized to diacetyl. It is tested by a colorimetric reaction with a guanidine group under alkaline conditions.

The test bacterium is inoculated in to Glucose phosphate peptone water medium and incubated at 37° C or 30°C for 1-2 days only.

Add 1 ml of 40% Potassium hydroxide and 3 ml of a 5% solution of α-naphthol in absolute alcohol (Barrit's reagent). A positive reaction is indicated by the development of a pink color in 2-5 minutes, becoming crimson in 30 minutes.

This test is usually done in conjunction with methyl red test, since the production of acetyl methyl carbinol or 2:3 butylene glycol leads to less acid production. An enterobacterial organism is usually either methyl red positive and Voges-Proskaver negative or methyl red negative and Voges-Proskauer positive.

Citrate Utilization Test

The test is based on the ability of an organism to utilize citrate (sodium citrate) as the sole carbon and energy source for growth and an ammonium salt (Ammonium dihydrogen phosphate) as the sole source of nitrogen.

For citrate utilization test, Koser's liquid citrate medium or Simmon's citrate agar may be used to inoculate test bacterium and incubated at 37°C for 1-2 days.

Koser's liquid citrate medium –

Positive reaction = turbidity (growth)

Negative reaction = no turbidity

Simmon's citrate agar medium –

Positive reaction = blue color and streak of growth. Utilization of citrate changes the pH of the medium to alkaline (formation of NaOH) which is indicated by color change from green to blue (bromothymol blue indicator).

Negative reaction = Original green color and no growth.

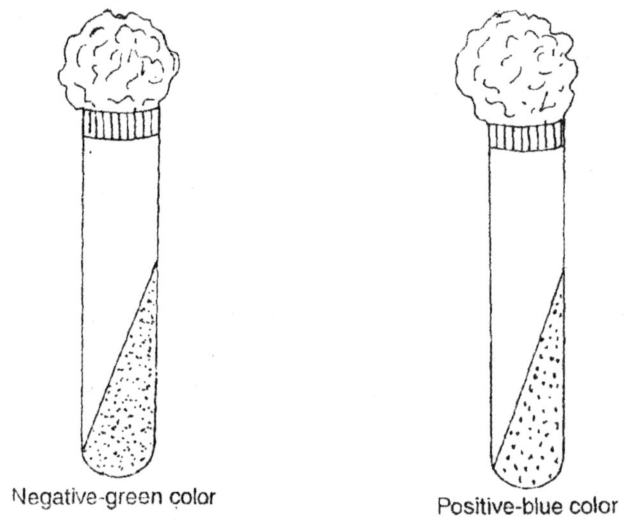

Fig. 12.2. Citrate utilization test (Simmon's citrate agar).

UREASE TEST/CHRISTENSEN'S AGAR MEDIUM

Some bacteria are able to decompose urea to form Ammonia and Carbon dioxide by means of the enzyme urease.

The test is done in Christensen's agar medium. It is composed of peptone, sodium chloride, dipotassium hydrogen phosphate, Phenol Red indicator, Urea, glucose and agar by dissolving in distilled water with a pH of 7.0. The medium can be used as liquid by omitting the agar.

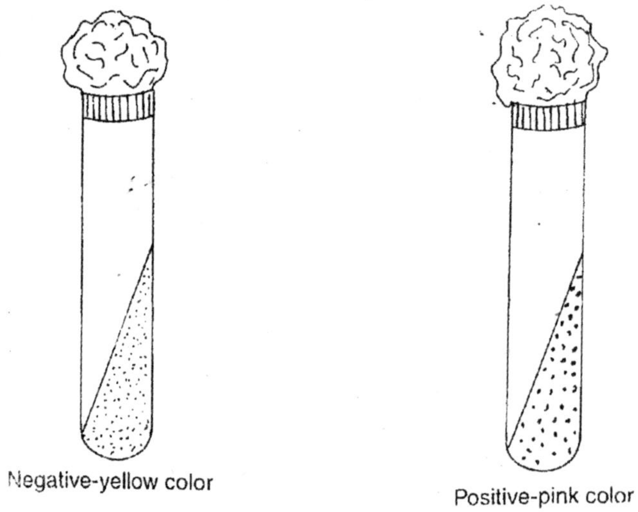

Fig. 12.3. Urease test (Christensen's agar medium).

The test bacterium is inoculated on to slope and incubated at 37°C. Examine after overnight incubation, No test is reported negative until after 4 days incubation.

Breakdown of urea with production of ammonia is indicated by the change in color of the medium from yellow to pink, due to phenol red indicator.

Proteus, *Klebsiella* and *Ureaplasma* are urease positive. *Helicobacter pylori* produces abundant urease, which is utilized as a rapid diagnostic test.

CATALASE TEST

Some bacteria produce catalase enzyme, which catalyzes the release of oxygen from hydrogen peroxide (H_2O_2).

$$H_2O_2 \xrightarrow{\text{Catalase}} H_2O_2 + \frac{1}{2} O_2$$

A small amount of culture to be tested is taken with a sterile wire loop or thin glass rod and is inserted into hydrogen peroxide solution, held in a small tube. Production of gas bubbles indicates catalase production. Alternatively a loop full of hydrogen peroxide may be added to colonies on nutrient agar. Prompt effervescence indicates catalase production. *Staphylococcus aureus* and Enterobacteriaceae members are catalase positive.

Since blood contains catalase, cultures from media containing blood are not suitable for catalase test.

Nichrome wire loop should never be used to pick up colonies because iron component of nichrome wire loop will give false positive reaction.

OXIDASE TEST

Oxidase test depends on the presence of oxidases in bacteria that will catalyze the transport of electrons between electron donors in the bacteria and a redox dye (tetramethyl-p-phenylene diamine). The dye is reduced to a deep purple color.

The test can be done in two ways.

1. Plate method– A freshly prepared 1% solution of tetra methyl-p-phenylene diamine dihydrochloride is poured over the colonies on agar plates. The oxidase positive colonies rapidly develop a purple color.
2. Filter paper method or Kovac's method-strips of whatman's No. 1 filter paper are soaked in a freshly prepared 1% solution of tetramethyl-p-phenylene diamine dihydrochloride, and laid in a Petri dish. The colony to be tested is smeared over it. A positive reaction is indicated by a deep purple color, within 5-10 seconds and a negative reaction by absence of coloration.

Neisseria, Alcaligenes, Aeromonas, *Vibrio*, *Campylobacter*, *Pseudomonas* and *Hemophilus* are oxidase positive, whereas enterobacteriaceae species give negative reactions.

PHENYL ALANINE DEAMINASE TEST

This test indicates the ability of bacteria like *Proteus* to deaminate phenyl alanine with production of phenyl pyruvic acid which will react with ferric salts to give a green color.

Test bacterium is inoculated into Nutrient agar or Yeast extract agar containing DL-phenyl alanine and incubated at 37°C for 4-24 hrs. Add a few drops of 10% ferric chloride solution to run down on to the slope. If the test is positive, a green color will develop in the fluid and in the slope.

TRIPLE SUGAR IRON AGAR (TSI AGAR)

It is used for differentiation and preliminary identification of Gram negative bacilli, originally designed as a multi-test medium, now mainly used as a standard test for H_2S. It is a composite medium consisting glucose, lactose, sucrose with phenol red indicator to detect gas production and ferric ammonium citrate to demonstrate hydrogen sulphide (H_2S) production. The medium is distributed in tubes with a butt and slant.

After inoculation of test bacterium and overnight incubation

1. If the slant remains red (alkaline) and butt becomes yellow; glucose is fermented, but sucrose and lactose are not fermented.
2. If both slant and butt become yellow (acid) all sugars are fermented.
3. If both slant and butt remain red (alkaline) all sugars are not fermented.
4. Air bubbles in the butt indicates gas production.
5. Blackening of the medium indicates H_2S production.

OXIDATION-FERMENTATION (O.F) TEST/HUGH AND LEIFSON'S TEST

This test is done to detect whether a bacterium utilizes glucose oxidatively or fermentatively in Hugh and Leifson's (O.F) semisolid medium containing carbohydrate (usually glucose) and pH indicator, bromothymol blue.

The test bacterium is stab-inoculated into duplicate tubes of medium; the medium in one tube is covered with sterile liquid paraffin; both the tubes are incubated. If acid is produced only at the surface of the medium, where conditions are aerobic, the metabolism of glucose is oxidative. If acid is found throughout the tube; including the lower layers where conditions are anaerobic, the metabolism is fermentative.

Fermentative organisms such as Enterobacteriaceae, *Aeromonas, Vibrio* produce acid reaction throughout the medium in the covered (anaerobic) as well as the open (aerobic) tube.

Oxidizing organisms such as *Pseudomonas* produce an acid reaction only in the open tube.

Organisms such as *Alcaligenes fecalis* that cannot break down the carbohydrates aerobically or anaerobically produce an alkaline reaction in the open tube and no change in the covered tube.

QUESTIONS

Short Notes

1. IMViC reactions.
2. Indole test.
3. Methyl red test.
4. Citrate utilisation test.
5. Urease test.
6. TSI agar.
7. O-F test.
8. Gelatin liquefaction test.

13

Preservation of Cultures/ Maintenance of cultures

- *Introduction*
- *Regular subcultures*
- *Liquid paraffin or mineral oil method*
- *Cold storage or refrigeration*
- *Deep freezing*
- *Preservation by drying*
- *Freeze-drying in vacuum or lyophilization*
- *Preservation in soil*

INTRODUCTION

All established microbiology laboratories usually maintain stock of various identified cultures for the use of students as well as for research purposes and epidemiological studies, and for experimentation.

Bacterial species differ in the ability of their cultures to remain alive after the completion of growth. Some species have poor viability (*e.g.*, gonococci) and their cultures usually die out within a few days, whether kept at 37°C, at room temperature or at 4 –5°C in refrigerator. Hence, they must be subcultured every 2 to 4 days for maintaining them. Spore-forming bacteria may remain viable for many years. Nonsporing Gram negative bacilli (*e.g.*, enterobacterioaceae), under suitable conditions, may remain viable for many months.

The preservation of bacterial cultures requires the following:

1. Drying of the culture should be prevented by hermetic sealing of the tube or bottle or ampoule.
2. Cultures should be stored in the dark, preferably at 4 – 5°C, but not at 37°C.
3. Culture should be grown in or on a suitable preservation medium or as a nutrient agar stab culture or slant culture. For example, enterobacteriaceae organisms may be kept alive on egg-saline medium for several years.

There are several methods available for maintenance of pure cultures; the choice of the method to be used depends upon the purpose, size of collection and the laboratory.

Some of the commonly used methods are as follows:

1. Regular subcultures

2. Liquid paraffin or mineral oil method
3. Cold storage (Refrigeration)
4. Deep freezing
5. Drying
6. Lyophilisation or freeze-drying in vacuum
7. Preservation in soil.

REGULAR SUBCULTURES

Certain bacteria that do not readily withstand freezing and/or drying must be subcultured regularly either in stab or slant cultures. *e.g.*, Gonococci. But over a period of time, regular subcultures may cause changes in original culture, due to (*i*) contamination, (*ii*) mutations, (*iii*) change in the name or number on the culture due to misinterpretation of writing, (*iv*) overgrowth by another organism which was there in small numbers in the original culture, (*v*) smooth to rough (S $\rightarrow$ R) variation.

LIQUID PARAFFIN *OR* MINERAL OIL METHOD

The frequency of regular subcultures can be reduced by lowering the metabolism of the organism by growing it on a media such as semisolid nutrient agar stabs and egg saline slopes and then sealing the surface of the medium with sterile liquid paraffin or mineral oil to exclude air, to reduce dehydration and ensures anaerobic conditions so that microorganisms remain in a dormant state. The culture is then stored at 4 – 5°C in a refrigerator.

This is a simple and most economical method of preserving bacteria and fungi where they remain viable for several years. The culture tubes may be dipped in molten wax alongwith cotton plug, so that the mouth of culture tube is sealed.

COLD STORAGE *OR* REFRIGERATION

Live cultures on a culture medium or slant or stab culture can be successfully stored in refrigerators or cold rooms maintained at 4°C. At this temperature, the metabolism of the organisms is lowered, but it is not low enough to stop metabolism completely. This, even at 4°C growth occurs slowly, nutrients will be utilized and waste products produced, which may lyse microorganisms. So, even, when preserved by refrigeration, regular subcultures are necessary, for bacteria, it ranges from 2 – 3 weeks and for fungi 3 – 4 months.

DEEP FREEZING

The culture slants, plates, broths and saline suspensions can be stored in a refrigerator in the freeze chamber at – 20° C or in a deep freeze at – 60°C or – 70°C. However, frequent freeze thawing kills the cultures. There are several ways of preserving cultures in a deep freeze.

1. Cultures can be preserved for several years in glycerol at –20°C to –40°C in a domestic deep freezer.

2. Cultures can be preserved at –70°C in solid carbondioxide. Suspensions of organisms in glucose broth, serum or skimmed milk are placed in ampoules and are frozen rapidly by immersion in a mixture of solid carbondioxide and alcohol to –70°C. If required, they may be dried by means of a vacuum pump and sealed. These ampoules with culture suspensions can be stored in a deep freezer at –70°C. For

subcultures, the ampoules may be warmed in a water bath at 45°C for few seconds and then inoculated into appropriate media.

3. Cultures may be preserved at –80°C in an ultra deep freezer, in which the cultures are protected by adding stabilizing agents such as sugars, glycerol or dimethyl sulphoxide into the suspending medium or by using a suspension of dried milk. These stabilizing agents prevent the formation of ice crystals which may kill frozen cells.

4. Culture are also preserved by freezing in liquid nitrogen at –190°C. This method may be used for a wide range of bacteria, viruses and many biological cells, which survive unchanged for long periods.

PRESERVATION BY DRYING

Preservation of bacterial cultures is highly useful in laboratories, that cannot afford expensive equipment or where preservations of cultures is infrequent.

Several methods for drying suspension of bacteria for preservation have been developed.

1. Paper discs. A thick suspension of bacteria is placed on sterile discs of thick absorbent paper which are then dried over phosphorous pentoxide (P_2O_5) in a desiccator under vacuum.

2. Gelatin discs. A thick suspension of bacterial culture is emulsified in nutrient gelatin and a few drops of it are placed on a sterile waxed paper or on a plastic petridish and then dried over phosphorous pentoxide under vacuum.

3. Pre-dried plugs. A thick suspension of bacteria are prepared and drops of it placed on sterile cellophane or on pre-dried plugs of peptone, starch or dextran, dried in a desiccator over phosphorous pentoxide in a vacuum.

4. L-drying. This method is described by Lapage et al, hence known as L-drying.

Bacteria in small ampoules are dried from the liquid state using a vacuum pump and desiccant.

5. Sordelli's method. The culture is emulsified in horse serum and is deposited on the inner wall of the small sterile tube, which is placed into another large sterile tube. A small quantity of phosphorous pentoxide is placed in the bottom of the outer tube over which the small tube is placed. The outer tube is then evacuated with a vacuum pump and then sealed, so that the culture in inner tube is dried over P_2O_5 in vacuum.

This method can be safely used when the samples to be preserved are small in quantity.

FREEZE-DRYING IN VACUUM *OR* LYOPHILISATION

The term "lyophilisation" means the rapid drying (dehydration) in high vacuum from the frozen state. The culture is frozen and then dried by sublimation of ice as vapors. Because of dehydration, microorganisms remain in dormant state (as metabolism requires water) and can retain viability for many years. Usually dehydration results in damage to cell, but in freeze-drying the culture is not in liquid state because dehydration is done in frozen state and does not result in damage to cell.

Lyophilisation is used to reserve stock cultures of bacteria, viruses, antisera, antibiotics, vaccines, human plasma, guinea pig complement serum. Freeze-drying involves several steps.

Suspending media for lyophilisation. The survival of bacteria during freeze-drying is influenced by the nature of the medium, in which they are suspended. Nutrient broth is usually satisfactory for most resistant organisms. Special protective suspending media containing sugar, peptone, skimmed milk, serum or a colloids such as peptone or dextran either glucose broth or nutrient broth with Rabbit or horse serum can be preferred.

Preparation of ampoules. Ampoules or vials or tubes made of neutral soft glass with an internal diameter of 6 mm with a little constriction at mouth are used for lyophilisation. Ampoules are disinfected with 2% HCl, rinsed with distilled water and dried. A small strip of Whatman No. 1 filter paper on which the number or name of the culture is typed/written is introduced as a label into ampoule. Then the ampoules are plugged and sterilized by autoclaving.

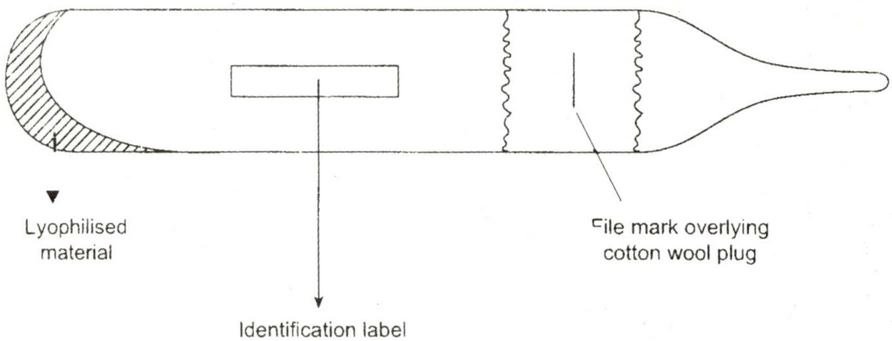

Fig. 13.1. An ampoule of lypophilised culture.

Harvesting the culture. Cultures grown on agar slants should be harvested 3–5 days after incubation. A few ml (2 ml) of suspending fluid such as nutrient broth, glucose broth or serum is added over agar slope and emulsified by gentle rubbing with pasteur pipette and transferred into ampoules. Each ampoule usually contains 0.1 to 0.2 ml of culture. The time interval between filling ampoules and freeze drying can be within minutes and should not exceed one hour; otherwise it may lead to renewed growth or germination of spores.

Primary drying. The ampoules are placed in the vertical holes of the constant speed centrifuge and covered with the bell-jar firmly. Switch on the centrifuge and then the vacuum pump and allow to run till pressure reaches 0.1 mm Hg, usually in about 5–10 minutes. The culture will be frozen as a thin layer on the inner wall of the ampoule. Immediately the centrifuge is switched off to avoid overheating.

The jar is lifted and the ampoules are removed and plugged with pre-sterilized non-absorbent cotton wool. The top of the cotton plug is cut and the plug is pushed inside some distance from the mouth of the ampoule. The upper part of the ampoule is then pulled out in a small flame to give a narrow constriction about half an inch above the plug.

Secondary drying. The ampoules are thoroughly checked for any cracks, leaks or damage and immediately placed in a secondary dryer which consists phosphorous pentoxide and the vacuum pump is switched on for 10 min., until the pressure is 0.05–0.01 mm Hg to ensure complete drying. The ampoules are checked for vacuum and then sealed with flame, and stored at 4°C.

Reconstitution of cultures from ampoules. For opening of the ampoules, mark the ampoule with a file transversely over the cotton-wool plug. Heat the tip of a glass rod red hot in Bunsen flame and apply it firmly to the filed mark on the ampoule, which should crack at that point. Allow time for air to enter via plug, then carefully remove cotton wool plug.

A small amount of sterile broth is added to ampoule aseptically and cultured on to a solid medium and incubated to obtain the pure culture.

PRESERVATION IN SOIL

Soil bacteria and fungi can be stored in their natural habitat, the soil. A small amount of soil is autoclaved, cooled and saturated with 1% sterile dextrose solution and inoculated with aqueous suspension of cells or spores. The microorganism is allowed to grow for 10 days and this soil culture is stored in a refrigerator. Microorganisms tend to undergo less variation in soil than in agar cultures.

QUESTIONS

Essay Type Questions

1. Describe the various methods of preservation of bacterial cultures in the laboratory.

Short Notes

1. Lyophilisation.
2. Freeze-drying in vacuum.

14

Classification of Microorganisms/ Microbial Taxonomy

- *Taxonomy*
- *Nomenclature*
- *Species concept and intraspecies classification*
- *Taxonomy ranks*
- *Role of taxonomy in diagnostic microbiology*
- *Kingdoms of organisms*
- *Differences between prokaryotes and eukaryotes*
- *Methods of classification*
  - *Phylogenetic*
  - *Based on staining reaction*
  - *Based on chemical composition*
  - *Biochemical classification*
  - *Nutritional*
  - *Morphological*
  - *Serological*
  - *Adansonian*
  - *Genetic analysis*
  - *Molecular*
- *Bergey's manual classification*

TAXONOMY

Taxonomy is concerned with the systematic arrangement of organisms into groups or categories called "Taxa" or "Divisions". The term "systematics" often used for taxonomy. The science of taxonomy can be divided into three parts.

1. Classification — The orderly arrangement of units into groups of larger units.

2. Nomenclature — The naming of units, characterised by classification.

3. Identification — Microorganisms are identified by comparing the characteristics of an "unknown" to the "known" units.

The major characteristics of microorganisms that have to be observed or determined to classify microorganisms include morphological, cultural, physiological, metabolic, antigenic, genetic and chemical composition.

NOMENCLATURE

Two kinds of names are given to bacteria.

1. Common name or casual name may vary from place to place and useful for communication at the local level.

2. Scientific name or international name is given by using the bionomial system of Linneaus according to International code of nomenclature of bacteria, prepared by the International committee on systematic bacteriology. The first part of the name begins with capital letter, indicates 'Genus' name, which is usually Latin or Greek noun. Genera may be masculine (ending in – us), feminine (ending in – lla, ada) or neuter (ending in – um). Second part is "species" name, which is a specific epithet and uncapitalized.

Table 14.1 Common and Scientific names of some bacteria

Common name	*Scientific name*
Gonococcus	*Neisseria gonorrhoeae*
Tubercle bacilli	*Mycobacterium tuberculosis*
Diphtheria bacilli	*Corynebacterium diphtheriae*
Typhoid bacilli	*Salmonella typhi*
Tetanus bacilli	*Clostridium tetani*

A satisfactory binomial system of nomenclature has not been evolved for viruses even today.

SPECIES CONCEPT IN MICROBIOLOGY/INTRA-SPECIES CLASSIFICATION

The basic taxonomic group in biology is the "Species". **Species** is defined as a group of individuals that are similar in characters, adopted to a particular ecological habitat and a way of life, and are capable of interbreeding freely and producing fertile offspring.

The above definition of species is most suitable for plants and animals which reproduce sexually. But it cannot satisfy the condition in prokaryotes and some lower eukaryotes, which are haploid and reproduce by asexual methods. Therefore, in microbiology the term "species" is defined as a collection of "strains" that share many stable properties in common and differ significantly from one another in many ways. However, a species may be divided into two or more "subspecies" based on minor but consistent phenotypic variations within the species or on genetically determined clusters of strains within the species.

A **"STRAIN"** is a population of organisms that descends from a single organisms or pure culture isolate or from a particular source, such as patient.

Strains within a species may differ slightly from one another in many ways. They are named according to the differences they exhibit *e.g.*,

Table 14.2 Classification of species

Biotypes	– strains with biochemical or physiological differences.
Serotypes	– possess distinctive antigenic characters.
Phagotypes	– differ in susceptibility to bacteriophages.

Morphotypes	– differ morphologically.
Pathotypes	– differ in pathogenicity to certain hosts.
Colicin types	-- differ in their ability to produce bacteriocins.

One strain of a species is designated as the **"Type strain"**. It is usually one of the first strains studied and is often more fully characterized than other strains. Only those strains very similar to the type strain are together form a species. Type strains are generally deposited in "Type culture collection centre" as a reference and maintained in International reference laboratories.

TAXONOMIC RANKS

Microorganisms are grouped into various "taxa", based on resemblances and relatedness. Kingdoms are divided successively into divisions, classes, orders, families, tribes, genera and species.

"GENUS" is a collection of similar species, one of them being the type species, which serves as a permanent example of the genus. A group of similar genera form a "Family", a group of similar families an "order", a group of similar orders a "class", a group of similar classes a "division" and a group of similar divisions a "kingdom", and thus goes the taxonomic hierarchy.

Table 14.3 Taxonomic ranks

Taxonomic rank	*Examples*		
Kingdom	Prokaryotae	Prokaryotae	Prokaryotae
Division	Gracilicutes	Gracilicutes	Tenericutes
Class	Scotobacteria	Scotobacteria	Mollicutes
Order	Eubacteriales	Spirochaetales	Mycoplasmatales
Family	Enterobacteriaceae	Leptospiraceae	Mycoplasmataceae
Genus	*Escherichia*	Leptospira	*Mycoplasm*a
Species	*Escherichia coli*	*Leptospira icterohaemorrhagiae*	*Mycoplasma pneumoniae*

ROLE OF TAXONOMY IN DIAGNOSTIC MICROBIOLOGY AND INFECTIOUS DISEASES

Taxonomy, in clinical microbiology facilitates communication among microbiologists and physicians to assign names and to maintain a record of characteristics of clinically relevant microorganism. This is necessary for

1. to establish an association of particular disease with specific microorganism.
2. to gather knowledge regarding the management and outcome of disease associated with specific microorganisms.
3. to establish patterns of resistance to antimicrobial agents.
4. to understand the mechanisms of drug resistance.
5. to recognize new and emerging pathogenic microorganisms.
6. to recognize changes in the types of infections or diseases caused by familiar microorganisms.
7. to develop new methods to detect and identify infectious agents.
8. to develop new antiinfective therapies.

KINGDOMS OF ORGANISMS

Linnaeus (1735) divided all organisms into two kingdoms – plant and animal. Linnaeus put protozoa in the animal kingdom, and the other microorganisms with the plants. But this classification was impractical for microorganisms, some of which are plant-like, others animal-like, and others with characteristics of both.

Ernst Haeckel (1865) established a third kingdom, called **protista**, to include microorganisms having characteristics of both plants and animals.

Microorganisms are divided into two categories, based on the nuclear structure.

1. **Prokaryotes** (pro=first, primitive; karyon=nucleus) *e.g.,* Bacteria, blue green algae (cyanobacteria)
2. **Eukaryotes** (Eu = advanced, well developed) *e.g.,* Algae, fungi, protozoa.

Table 14.4 Major schemes of classification

Kingdom	*Organisms included*	
Linnaeus (1735)	1. Plantae	Bacteria, fungi, algae, plants
	2. Animalia	Protozoa and higher animals
Haeckel (1865)	1. Plantae	Multicellular algae and plants
	2. Animalia	Animals
	3. Protista	Microorganisms
Whittaker (1969)	1. Plantae	Multicellular algae and plants
	2. Animalia	Animals
	3. Protista	Protozoa and single celled algae
	4. Fungi	Molds and yeasts
	5. Monera	All bacteria (prokaryotes)
Woese (1977)	1. Archaeobacteria	Bacteria that produce methane gas, require high levels of salt, or high temperature
	2. Eubacteria	All other bacteria, including disease causing bacteria, soil and water bacteria and photosynthetic bacteria
	3. Eukaryotes	Protozoa, algae, fungi, and animals

Table 14.5 differences between prokaryotes and eukaryotes

Feature	*Prokaryotes*	*Eukaryotes*
Group of organisms	Bacteria, Blue green algae	Algae, Fungi Protozoa
NUCLEUS		
– Nuclear membrane	Absent, genetic material free	Present
– Nucleolus	Absent	Present
– Chromosomes	Single, circular	More than one, linear
– Nuclear division	By simple fission, mitosis and meiosis absent	Mitosis and meiosis present

– Deoxyribonucleoprotein (histones)	Absent	Present
CYTOPLASM		
– Cytoplasmic streaming	Absent	Present
– Pinocytosis	Absent	Present
– Lysosomes	Absent	Present
– Golgi bodies	Absent	Present
– Endoplasmic reticulum	Absent	Present
– Mitochondria	Absent	Present
– Mesosomes	Present	Absent
– Ribosomes	70S (50S + 30S) Dispersed in cytoplasm	80S (60S + 40S) attached to ER
CHEMICAL COMPOSITION		
– Sterols	Absent	Present
– Muramic acid	Present	Absent
– Diaminopimelic acid	Present in some	Absent
FLAGELLAE		
	Each flagellum composed of one fibril of molecular dimensions	Each flagellum composed of 20 fibrils in a distinct pattern $(2 \times 9) + 2$

METHODS OF CLASSIFICATION/CLASSIFICATION SCHEMES/ CLASSIFICATION SYSTEMS

There are several approaches to bacterial classification and various schemes have been devised.

Phylogenetic (Evolutionary) Classification

During Post Darwinian period organisms are classified according to their evolutionary relationships. Haeckel placed all the microorganisms under protista kingdom, by separating them from plant and animal kingdoms. R.H. Whittaker developed a phylogenetic five kingdom classification of living forms – Monera, protista, fungi, plantae and animalia. Microorganisms are included in the first three kingdoms, while all prokaryotes are included under monera.

Classification Based on Staining Reaction

Based on Gram's staining, bacteria are divided into Gram positive and Gram negative bacteria. This is an important medical classification that depends on the cell wall composition.

Similarly, based on acid-fast staining, bacteria can be divided into acid fast bacilli and non-acid fast bacilli.

Classification Based on Chemical Classification

Based on chemical composition microorganisms can be classified. For example, the prokaryotic cell wall contains N-acetyl muramic acid, which is absent in eukaryotic cell wall. Similarly, sterols are present in eukaryotic cell membrane, while they are absent in prokaryotic cell membrane.

Biochemical Classification

Microorganisms can be classified based on various biochemical properties. *e.g.,*

1. Based on lactose fermentation, enterobacteriaceae members can be classified into lactose fermenters (LF), non-lactose fermenters (NLF) and late lactose fermenters (LLF).

2. Production of Indole, H_2S when grown on appropriate media may be useful for identification.

3. Production of specific enzymes like catalase, oxidase, urease, gelatinase, lecithinase are also used in the identification of bacteria.

Nutritional Classification

Based on energy requirements, bacteria are classified into two types – phototrophs and chemotrophs.

Similarly, based on the ability to synthesize essential metabolites, bacteria are classified as Autotrophs and heterotrophs.

Based on oxygen requirement, bacteria are classified as aerobes and anaerobes.

Similarly based on temperature required for growth; bacteria may be classified as psychrophiles, mesophiles and thermophiles.

Morphological Classification

Based on morphology bacteria are divided into various groups, as follows:

I. Filamentous bacteria or higher bacteria *e.g.,* Actinomycetes, Mycobacteria

II. True bacteria or lower bacteria – *e.g.,*

1. Gram positive bacilli : Aerobes – *Corynebacterium, Bacillus, Listeria.*
   Anaerobes – *Clostridium, Lactobacillus, Eubacterium.*
2. Gram positive cocci : Staphylococci, Streptococci, Enterococci, pneumococci
3. Gram negative cocci : Aerobes – *Neisseria* (gonococci and meningococci)
   Anaerobes – *Veillonella.*
4. Gram negative bacilli : Aerobes – Enterobacteria – *Escherichia, Klebsiella, Proteus, Salmonella, Shigella*
   Pseudomonads – *Pseudomonas, Alcaligenes*
   Parvobacteria – *Hemophilus, Bordetella, Brucella, Pasteurella, Yersinia*
   Anaerobes – *Bacteroides, Fusobacterium*
5. Gram negative vibrios : *Vibrio, spirillum, Campylobacter, Helicobacter*

III. Spirochetes – *Borrelia, Treponema, Leptospira.*

IV. Mycoplasmas – *Mycoplasma, Ureaplasma.*

V. Rickettsiae – *Rickettsia, Coxiella, Bartonella.*

VI. Chlamydiae – *Chalmydia.*

Serological/Antigenic Classification

Microorganisms possess many different kinds of antigens. Microorganism or some part of the organism is injected into an animal and subsequently the blood serum of the animal is tested for the presence of antibodies.

Species and types of microorganisms can be identified by specific antigen-antibody reactions. The specificity of these tests is greatly improved due to the availability of monoclonal antibodies.

Seological techniques include agglutination, precipitation (gel diffusion, counter immunoelectrophoresis), latex agglutination, neutralisation tests, complement fixation, immunofluorescence and ELISA.

Adansonian Classification/Numerical Taxonomy/Phenetic System of Classification/Taxometrics

It was first suggested by Michael Adanson, the 18th century botanist, hence called Adansonian taxonomy. It proved to be a powerful tool in microbial taxonomy as it is more useful for classification of strains within a larger group that shares major characteristics. The use of computers extended the scope of numerical taxonomy.

This system determines the degree of relationship between strains by a statistical coefficient by scoring a large number of phenotypic characters such as morphological, cultural, biochemical, physiological, serological and ecological etc., all of which are given equal weight. Hence, it is called "phenetic system".

"Similarity coefficient" is obtained when shared positive characters are considered. It does not take into account negative characters. Whereas a "Matching coefficient" is obtained when both positive and negative shared characters (matches) are taken into account. These matches can be expressed as a percentage as S_M (simple matching coefficient) which can be expressed as follows:

$$S_M = \frac{N_S}{N_S + N_D} \times 100 \qquad S_M = \text{Simple matching coefficient}$$

N_S = Number of shared (similar) characters

N_d = Number of different characters.

The similarities are analysed by computers to indicate degrees of similarity for a group of different microorganisms to yield "groups or clusters" and the strains are arranged into "phenons (phenetic groups)". These similarity values between measured characters yield a check board of entries, a square table of similarities known as "**Similarity matrix** (S-matrix) or **dendrogram** or phenogram". Thus dendrogram shows heirarchial relationships between organisms.

Genetic Analysis as a Basis of Classification

The study of chromosomal gene exchange through transformation, transduction and conjugation in prokaryotes is sometimes useful in their classification. Based on susceptibility to bacteriophages, bacterial species can be divided into several phage types.

Plasmids are also important in taxonomy because they are present in most bacteria and carry genes coding for phenotypic traits.

Macromolecular Classification/Molecular Classification

Comparison of macromolecules such as proteins, enzymes and nucleic acids indicate relatedness between organisms and is useful in taxonomy.

1. ***Comparison of proteins.*** The amino acid sequences of proteins reflect mRNA sequences and therefore closely related to the structures of the genes coding for their synthesis. Hence, comparisons of proteins from different microorganisms are very useful taxonomically.

The physical, kinetic and regulatory properties of enzymes have been employed in taxonomic studies.

2. *Nucleic acid (DNA) base composition.* In double-stranded DNA, three hydrogen bonds join guanine and cytosine (G≡C) base pairs, and two bonds connect adenine and thymine (A=T) base pairs. As a result, DNA with a greater G + C content will have more hydrogen bonds, and its strands will separate only at higher temperature, that is, it will have a higher melting point. DNA melting can be followed spectrophotometrically because the absorbance at 260 nm UV light by DNA increases during strand separation.

$$\text{Mol \% G + C} = \frac{G + C}{G + C + A + T} \times 100$$

G + C content is determined by acid hydrolysis method, thermal denaturation (melting temperature) method and Buoyant density method. By measuring the G+C content of bacteria, it can be shown that there is a wide range in the G + C component of DNA varying from about 25 to 80 moles % in different genera. However, for any; one species, the G + C content is relatively fixed, which provides a basis for classification.

3. *Nucleic acid hybridization/DNA homology.* DNA homology experiments are used for detecting similarities between closely related organisms, whereas RNA homology experiments are used to detect more distantly related organisms. They indicate taxonomic and phylogenetic relationships.

If a mixture of single-stranded DNA formed by heating dsDNA is cooled (annealing), strands with complementary base sequences will reassociate to form stable dsDNA. Single strands of DNA from two bacterial species can be compared by hybridization in vitro.

4. *Ribosomal RNA (rRNA) sequencing.* The structure of ribosomal RNA (rRNA) appears to have been highly conserved during the course of evolution and close similarities in nucleotide sequences reflect phylogenetic relationships. Investigation of similarities in oligonucleotides derived from rRNA are increasingly used in taxonomic studies.

BERGEY'S MANUAL OF SYSTEMATIC BACTERIOLOGY

It is well known as "Bible of Microbiology". Chester (1899-1901) published a manual of determinative bacteriology, which embodies classification of bacteria. This was modified by David Bergey into what is popularly now called "Bergey's manual of determinative bacteriology". The first edition was published in 1923. This has been updated and eighth edition was released in 1974.

Bergey's manual has been updated again in 1984 into "Bergey's Manual of Systematic Bacteriology" published in four volumes by R.G.E. Murray et al. In this edition, prokaryotes are classified into four divisions as, shown below:

Division I – Gracilicutes

Division II – Firmicutes

Division III – Tenericutes

Division IV – Mendosicutes

All the bacteria are divided in these divisions into 33 sections. Volume I has 11, Volume II has 6, Volume III has 8 and Volume IV has 8 sections.

QUESTIONS

Essay Type Questions

1. Explain different methods of classification of bacteria.

Short Notes

1. Species concept in microbiology.
2. Strain.
3. Role of taxonomy in infectious diseases.
4. Prokaryote.
5. Differences between prokaryotes and eukaryotes.
6. Morphological classification of bacteria.
7. Adansonian classification/numerical taxonomy/phenetic system of classification.
8. Dendrogram/similarity matrix.
9. G + C content/G + C ratio.
10. Nucleic acid hybridization.
11. Bergey's manual classification.

15

Antibiotics and Antibiotic Sensitivity Tests

- *Definitions*
  - *Antimicrobial agent*
  - *Chemotherapeutic agent*
  - *Chemotherapy*
- *Chemotherapeutic Index*
- *Antibiotics*
- *Spectrum of activity of antimicrobial agents*
  - *Narrow spectrum antibiotics*
  - *Broad spectrum antibiotics*
- *Mode/mechanism of action of antimicrobial agents*
- *Some antibiotics used for chemotherapy of bacterial and fungal infections*
- *Synergism/synergistic effect of antibiotics*
- *Antagonism/antagonistic action of antibiotics*
- *Bacteriostatic and bactericidal antibiotic*
- *Antibiotic sensitivity tests*
  - *Dilution methods*
  - *Tube (broth) dilution method*
  - *MIC*
  - *MBC*
  - *Agar dilution method*
  - *Diffusion tests*
  - *Disc-diffusion (Kirby-Bauer) test*
  - *E-test*
  - *Stokes method*
- *Antibiogram*
- *Assay of antibiotics*
  - *Chemical assay*
  - *Microbiological assay*
- *Non-medical uses of antibiotics*
- *Phage therapy*
- *Bacteriocins*

DEFINITIONS

Antimicrobial Agent

Any chemical substance which inhibits the growth or causes death of a microorganism is known as antimicrobial agent.

Chemotherapeutic Agent

Synthetic chemicals that are used to kill or inhibit the growth of microorganisms in the body tissues are called chemotherapeutic agents. In other words, chemotherapeutic agents are synthetic chemicals used in the treatment of microbial infections.

Chemotherapy

The term chemotherapy is introduced by Ehrlich, to denote the treatment of a microbial disease by the administration of the drug which kills or inhibits the growth of pathogen, without any toxic action on the tissues, in therapeutic concentrations.

CHEMOTHERAPEUTIC INDEX

Chemotherapeutic agent must possess selective toxicity against the pathogen and should act at a concentration that can be tolerated by the host tissues; this selective toxicity is expressed in terms of "chemotherapeutic index", which compares the maximum dose that can be tolerated by the host without causing death, known as "maximum tolerated dose", with the minimum dose that cures the particular infection, known as" minimum curative dose".

$$\text{Chemotherapeutic index} = \frac{\text{Maximum tolerated dose}}{\text{Minimum curative dose}}$$

The chemotherapeutic index provides a rough guide to the degree of selective toxicity, and therapeutic value of a chemical. A high value of chemotherapeutic index indicates that the chemotherapeutic agent is highly efficient against the pathogen and less toxic to the host.

ANTIBIOTICS

Antibiotics are defined as natural antimicrobial agents produced by microorganisms, that is capable in small concentractions to kill or inhibit the growth of other microorganisms.

The ability to produce antibiotics is particularly common among soil microorganisms and therefore, antibiotics are widely distributed in nature; where they play an important role in regulating the microbial population of soil, water, sewage and compost. Of many antibiotics that have been purified, only a few have been nontoxic to be of use in medical practice. Those that are currently of greatest use have been derived from a small group of microorganisms belonging to genera *Penicillium*, *Streptomyces*, *Cephalosporium*, *Micromonospora* and *Bacillus*.

SPECTRUM OF ACTIVITY OF ANTIMICROBIAL AGENTS

Based on the spectrum of activity, antibiotics are classified into two types.

1. Narrow Spectrum Antibiotics are those which can kill or inhibit the growth of only a few species of microorganisms. *e.g.*, Penicillin—mainly active against Gram positive bacteria. Aminoglycosides, such as gentamycin and streptomycin are mainly active against Gram negative bacteria. Metronidazole-mainly active against anaerobic bacteria and some protozoans.

2. Broad spectrum antibiotics are those which can kill or inhibit the growth of many different species of microorganisms, including both Gram positive and Gram negative bacteria. *e.g.*, Tetracyclines, ampicillin, cephalosporins, and quinolones. They are often used for the "blind" treatment of infections. Unfortunately there is much abuse of broad spectrum antibiotics in clinical practice.

MODE/MECHANISM OF ACTION OF ANTIMICROBIAL AGENTS

Antimicrobial agents kill or inhibit microorganisms by several mechanisms –

1. Inhibition of cell wall synthesis.

   e.g., Penicillins, bacitracin, cephalosporins, cycloserine, vancomycin and ristocetin

2. Inhibition or alteration of cell membrane permeability.

   e.g., Amphotericin B, colistin, imidazoles, nystatin, polymyxins.

3. Inhibition of protein synthesis.

   e.g., Chloramphenicol, erythromycins, lincomycins, tetracyclines, Aminoglycosides – Amikacin, Gentamycin, Kanamycin, neomycin, netilmycin, streptomycin, Tobramycin, etc.

4. Inhibition of transcription and nucleic acid synthesis.

   e.g., Nalidixic acid, novobiocin, pyrimethamine, rifampin, sulfonamides, trimethoprim.

5. Antimetabolite action (antagonistic to metabolites).

   e.g., Sulfonamides, sulfones, trimethoprim and PAS (paraamino salicylic acid)

Table 15.1 Some antibiotics used for chemotherapy of bacterial and fungal infections

Antibiotic	*Produced by*	*Active against*	*Mode of action*
β-lactams			
Penicillins	*Penicillium sp*	Gram positive bacteria	Inhibit cell wall synthesis
Cephalosporins	*Cephalosporium* sp	Gram negative bacteria	
Monobactams	*Chromobacterium violaceum*	Causing respiratory, intestinal, and urinary tract infections; penicillinase producing bacteria	
Carbapenems	*Streptomyces cattleya*		
Aminoglycosides			
Streptomycin	*Streptomyceus griseus*	Tuberculosis	Induce abnormal protein synthesis
Spectinomycin	*Streptomyces* sp.	Penicillin-resistant gonococci	
Neomycin	Strept. fradiae	inhibits intestinal bacteria	
Kanamycin	*Strepto, kanomycetius*	Most gram negative bacteria	

Antibiotic	Produced by	Active against	Mode of action
Gentamycin	*Micromonospora purpurea*	except Pseudomonas.	
Tetracyclines	*Streptomyces* sp.	Active against a variety of Gram positive and Gram negative bacteria including Pseudomonas	Interfere with protein synthesis
Macrolides		Broad spectrum–Many gram positive and gram negative bacteria; also organisms such as *Mycoplasma, Rickettsia*, and *Chlamydiae*	
Erythromycin	*Strepto.erythreus*		Interfere with protein synthesis
Lincomycin	*Strepto. lincolensis*	Gram positive bacteria	
Chloramphenicol	*Strept.venezuelae*	Gram positive bacteria	Interfers with protein synthesis
(Chloromycetin)		Broad spectrum-severe	
Polypeptides		Gram negative infections	
Colistin	*Bacillus colistinus*	Gram negative bacteria including *Pseudomonas*	Deterioration of cell membrane
(Polymyxine E) Polymyxin B	*Bacillus polymyxa*	Gram negative bacteria; less effective than colistin	Deterioration of cell membrane
Bacitracin	*Bacillus subtilis*	Gram positive, but not gram negative bacteria	Inhibits, cell wall formation
Vancomycin	*Streptomyces orientalis*	Gram positive bacteria, including penicillinase-producing *Staphylococci* and *Enterococci*	Interferes with protein synthesis
Rifamycin	*Strept. mediterranei*	Tuberculosis	Interferes with protein synthesis
Viomycin	*Strept. griseus* var. purfureus	Tuberculosis	Interferes with protein synthesis.
Antifungal antibiotics	*Strept. noursei*	Fungal infections particularly oral, skin, intestinal and vaginal lesions due to candida deep-seated mycotic infections	Damages cell membrane
Polyenes Nystatin Amphotericin-B	*Strept. nodosus*		
Griseofulvin	*Penicillium griseofulvin*	Fungal infections	Interferes with membrane function damages cell membrane

SYNERGISM/SYNERGISTIC EFFECT OF ANTIBIOTICS

Synergism is referred to as correlated action or cooperation on the part of two or more drugs, so that a greater effect is achieved.

Antibiotics are frequently given to patients in a combination of two or three drugs, to prevent the development of resistance (as in the treatment of tuberculosis), and also to achieve a synergistic effect.

Synergism of bactericidal action can be seen with certain combinations of drugs such as penicillin and streptomycin; a low concentration of one drug promotes the lethal action of the other. Sublethal pretreatment with penicillin increases sensitivity to streptomycin because damage to the cell wall caused by penicillin facilitates subsequent entry of streptomycin.

e.g., Treatment of infections with *Streptococcus fecalis* with a combination of penicillin and streptomycin; *Pseudomonas aeruginosa* infections with a combination of polymyxin and carbenicillin, synergistic effect of antibiotics can be seen.

ANTAGONISM/ANTAGONISTIC ACTION OF ANTIBIOTICS

Certain antibiotics may antagonize the action of others. Bacteriostatic drugs such as chloramphenicol and tetracyclines have been found to inhibit the bactericidal action of penicillin and streptomycin. The antagonism of bactericidal drugs by bacteriostatic drugs may occur as a result of combined therapy under clinical conditions. Hence, a combination of these two kinds of drugs is contraindicated.

BACTERIOSTATIC AND BACTERICIDAL ANTIBIOTICS

When an antibiotic causes cessation (inhibition) of growth of the bacterium, which is reversed when the antibiotic is removed, it is called "Bacteriostatic". If an antibiotic kills the bacterium, it is called "Bactericidal".

This distinction is often arbitrary and depends on the concentration of the drug. A bacteriostatic agent may become bactericidal, if the concentration is increased.

Table 15.2 Bacteriostatic and Bactericidal antibiotics

Bacteriostatic	***Bactericidal***
(Depends and varies according to the conc. of drug)	
Chloramphenicol	Aminoglycosides
Erythromycin and other macrolides	Beta-lactams (Penicillins), cephalosporins
Clindamycin, Lincomycin	Vancomycin
Sulphonamides	Quinolones
Trimethoprim	Rifampin
Tetracyclines	Metronidazole
Nitrofurans	Co-trimoxazole

MICROBIAL SUSCEPTIBILITY TO CHEMOTHERAPEUTIC AGENTS (OR) ANTIBIOTIC SENSITIVITY TESTS

Strains of microorganisms differ in their degree of susceptibility to antibiotics and chemotherapeutic agents. The susceptibility of an organism may change with time. It is therefore important for the physician to know the identity of the microbe causing the infection, as well as its susceptibility to antibiotics, so that the specific, correct antibiotic can be selected for treating the infection.

The susceptibility of the pathogen to various antibiotics and chemotherapeutic agents is determined by two methods.

1. Dilution tests
2. Diffusion tests.

1. Dilution Method

It is of two types: 1. Tube dilution or broth dilution method, and, 2. Agar dilution method. Dilution tests are generally used-when therapeutic dose is to be regulated as in the treatment of endocarditis, for tests on slow growing bacteria such as tubercle bacilli, and when small degrees of resistance are to be demonstrated.

1. *Tube Dilution Method or Broth Dilution Technique.* It is used to determine the minimum inhibitory concentration (MIC) and the minimum bactericidal concentration (MBC) of an antibiotic for a pathogen.

The tube dilution method uses a series of test tubes containing sterile culture medium, usually Mueller-Hinton broth and various concentrations of each of a variety of antibiotics. All tubes are inoculated with the microorganism to be tested and then incubated. Control consists of drug-free broth. Then the tubes are examined to see which antibiotics have inhibited the growth of the organism. For each antibiotic MIC is determined.

Minimum inhibitory concentration (MIC) is defined as the lowest concentration (or highest dilution) of the drug/antibiotic that inhibits the growth, as determined usually by the lack of turbidity. The antibiotics having the lowest MIC values would have the highest antimicrobial activity.

Minimum bactericidal concentration (MBC) is defined as minimum concentration of an antibiotic required to kill a defined per cent (usually 99.9%) of bacteria when a mixture of bacteria and antibiotic are incubated together.

The MBC is determined by inoculating a drug-free medium from each test tube that showed no growth in MIC determination. The MBC is determined by the growth pattern seen after incubation. The MBC may be equal to or greater than the MIC.

Determination of MBC is not routinely performed but is indicated in the treatment of endocarditis by Streptococci and other organisms, to adjust the dose and combination of antibiotics.

Broth dilutions can be performed in a microtitre plate. The technique has been highly automated.

2. Agar Dilution Technique

It is more convenient when several strains are to be tested at the same time. In this method serial dilutions of the drug are prepared in Mueller-hinton agar, melted to 45°C and then poured into plates. Several strains can be inoculated on each plate containing antibiotic. Following incubation, the MIC, lowest concentration of the drug that inhibits colony formation is determined.

Diffusion Tests

In diffusion tests, the drug is allowed to diffuse through a solid medium so that a concentration gradient is established, the concentration being higher near the site of the drug and gradually decreases with distance. The test strain is inoculated on the medium and on incubation, its sensitivity to the drug is determined from the inhibition of its growth.

Various methods can be used for application of the drug. The drug may be added to.

1. Ditches or holes cut in the medium.
2. Hollow cylinders (or) bottomless cylinders, called Heatley cups.
3. Porous cups.
4. The most commonly employed method is use of discs of antibiotic impregnated filter paper known as disc-diffusion test. The concentration of drug in discs may be as per Kirby-Bauer or I.C.S. recommendations.

Disc-Diffusion Test/Bauer-Kirby Disc Diffusion Method

It is a qualitative method to determine susceptibility of bacteria to drugs, employing discs made of filter paper (Whatman No. 2 filter paper) or special quality absorbent paper about 6 mm in diameter, impregnated with appropriate concentrations of the drug, as per Kirby-Bauer or I.C.S. methods. The discs are stored dry with a desiccant, in the cold (Refrigerator). The potency of the discs is periodically tested, using control standard strains of known sensitivity, such as *Staphylococcus aureus*, oxford strain NCTC 6571.

Preparation of Inoculum. The colonies of test strain may be inoculated into peptone water or nutrient broth or tryptone soy broth and incubated at 37°C for 4 – 8 hours, till light to moderate turbidity develops. The inoculum may be adjusted to give a uniform, dense but not confluent growth. The turbidity of inoculum can be adjusted against Mac farland standard tube (0.5 ml 1.175% $BaCl_2$. $2H_2O$ sol. + 99.5 ml 0.36 N (1%) H_2SO_4) with physiological saline or broth.

Antibiotic sensitivity medium. To determine susceptibility to antibiotics, usually Mueller-Hinton agar medium is used as a standard sensitivity medium. Nutrient agar is also routinely used, but it should not be preferred as it contains inhibitors of sulphonamides, trimethoprim and other sulphur containing drugs. These inhibitors may be neutralized by the addition of lysed horse blood. For fastidious pathogens such as Streptococci and pneumococci, blood agar plates may be used.

Inoculation. Inoculation on to Mueller-Hinton agar may be done by two methods-

1. The broth culture of inoculum may be poured on to the surface of solid medium and the plate is tilted for uniform spreading; and then excess fluid may be pipetted off.
2. A sterile cotton swab is soaked in inoculum, and pressed against the upper inside wall of the tube to remove excess fluid and rub it over the surface of solid medium three times, turning the plate 60° angle between each swabbing.

Application of discs. Antibiotic-impregnated filter paper discs are applied gently under sterile conditions with a sterile forceps. Discs are placed flat on the surface and firmly applied to ensure adhesion. The discs should preferably be deposited with centres at least 25 mm to 30 mm apart.

Mechanical devices of disc dispensers are available, which deliver all discs simultaneously on to the surface of solid medium.

Incubation. For most organisms incubation at 35°C to 37°C for 18 hrs or over night is sufficient. In case of fastidious pathogens the incubation may be done in the presence of increased CO_2 concentration. The incubation time may be increased beyond 18 hrs to enhance detection of certain resistance patterns *e.g.*, Methicillin resistance in Staphylococci and vancomycin resistance in Enterococci. Anaerobic bacterial sensitivity tests are incubated under anaerobic conditions.

Reading results. After incubation, the plates are examined for zones of inhibition of growth, around the discs. Growth will be inhibited around discs containing antibiotics to which the bacterium is susceptible, but not around those to which it is resistant. The diameter of the zone of inhibition may be measured with a ruler or Vernier calipers in millimeters (mm).

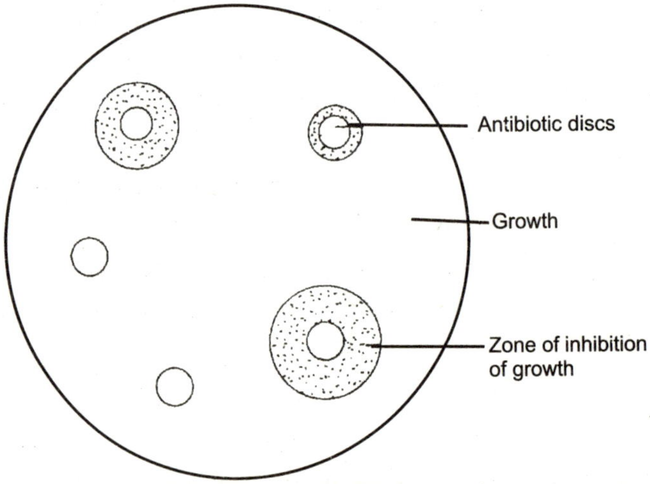

Fig. 15.1. Disc diffusion test.

Interpretation of results. The results are interpreted and reported as "sensitive," "moderately sensitive" and "resistant" by referring the diameter of zone inhibition with standard interpretation tables.

Factors affecting disc diffusion test. The accuracy of disc diffusion test depends on

- disc concentration,
- diffusibility of the drug,
- stability of the drug,
- nature, composition and depth of the medium,
- pH of the medium,
- size of inoculum,
- incubation temperature,
- incubation period or length of incubation,
- metabolic activity of the organisms.

E-Test. It is used for quantitative estimation of susceptibility of bacteria to drugs. It uses plastic strips, one side of the strip contains the antimicrobial agent concentration gradient and the other contains a numeric scale that indicates the drug concentration.

Mueller-Hinton agar plates are inoculated as for disc diffusion and the strips are placed on the inoculum lawn. Several strips may be placed radially on the same plate so that many drugs can be tested on a single isolate. Following overnight incubation, the plate is examined and the number present at the point where the border of growth inhibition intersects the E-strip is taken as the MIC.

E-test provides MIC of various drugs, which is useful in situations in which the level of resistance can be clinically important *e.g.*, Penicillin or cephalosporins against Pneumococci.

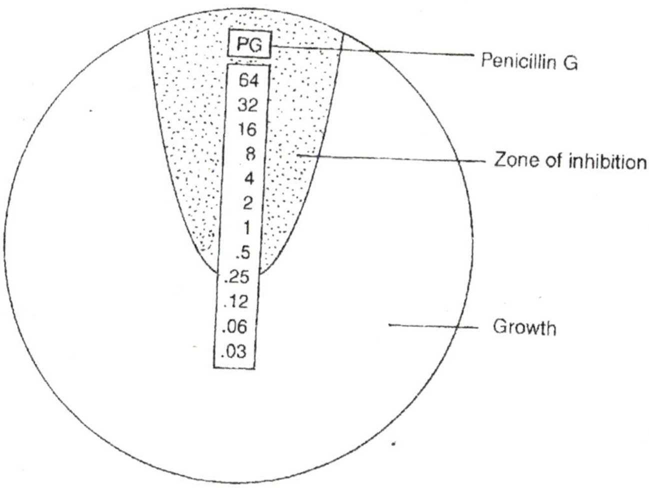

Fig. 15.2. E–Test.

Stokes method. In stokes method, the control culture is applied and spread evenly by a sterile swab in two bands on either side of the plate leaving an uninoculated central band. For organisms isolated from urine sample, the controls are *E.coli* NCTC 10418; for organisms isolated from other materials, *Staph.aureus* NCTC 6571; and for Pseudomonads *Pseudo.aeruginosa* NCTC 10662.

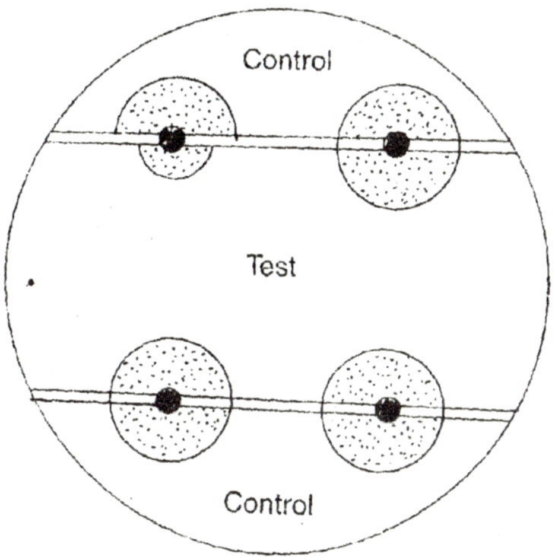

Control culture inoculated on either side of the test culture

Fig. 15.3. Stokes method.

The test organism is seeded evenly in the central band by rubbing with a swab dipped in inoculum.

Antibiotic discs are applied with forceps on the line between the test and control organisms and pressed gently to ensure contact with the medium. Four or six discs can be accommodated in a petriplate, depending on its size; The plates are incubated overnight at 35–37°C (or) if methicillin discs are used, incubate at 30°C.

Zone of inhibition formed around each disc are composed of control and test bacteria. Zone of inhibition are measured from the edge of the discs to the edge of the zone. As the control and test organisms are adjacent on the same plate, the difference between the respective zone sizes can be directly measured. Each zone of inhibition is interpreted as follows:

Sensitive – zone size equal to, wider than or not more than 3 mm smaller than the control.

Intermediate (Moderately sensitive) – zone size greater than 3 mm, but smaller than the control by more than 3 mm.

Resistant – zone size 3 mm or less.

In a rotary plating method, the control organism is inoculated in the centre and the test organism at the periphery of the plate leaving a gap of 2-3 mm between test and control inocula, where antibiotic discs are applied.

ANTIBIOGRAM

The sensitivity pattern of a microorganism to a series of antibiotics is called antibiogram. This antibiogram is useful –

– as a guide for antibiotic therapy

– as a marker in the identification of an organism, usually in epidemiological studies .It may be used as a preliminary to phage typing in the investigation of Staphylococcal infections.

Most infections are treated on an empirical basis; chemotherapy may be guided by predictable sensitivities or fixed antibiograms for commonly occurring bacterial pathogens. It saves time, allow treatment to begin, and reduce the amount of unnecessary work carried out in the laboratory.

Fixed antibiograms for some common bacterial pathogens are as follows:

Streptococci	– Penicillin, erythromycin, vancomycin
Staphylococci	– Flucloxacillin, clindamycin, fusidic acid, Gentamycin, vancomycin.
Anaerobic cocci	– Penicillin, erythromycin, metronidazole
Enterococci	– Ampicillin, vancomycin
E. coli and *Proteus*	– Gentamycin, trimethoprim, ciprofloxacin, co-trimoxazole.
Pseudomonas	– Gentamycin, ceftazidime, azlocillin, ciprofloxacin.
Hemophilus	– Amoxycillin, co-trimoxazole, tetracycline chloramphenicol, erythromycin
Bacteroides	– Metronidazole, co-trimoxazole,
Salmonella typhi, *S. paratyphi B*	– Chloramphenicol Ampicillin, co-trimoxazole, Amoxycillin.

The use of predictable antibiograms must be qualified by possible differences in the occurrence of resistant strains, particularly in certain areas. For example, for chemotherapy against *Shigella*, *Salmonella* (other than *S.typhi* and *S. paratyphi* B), antibiotic sensitivity must be determined.

ASSAY OF ANTIBIOTICS

Determination of the antibiotic content of a microbial culture, a patient's blood sample or other body fluids, an antibiotic tablet or similar specimens can be done by two methods.

1. Chemical assay. 2. Biological assay.

Chemical Assay

If an antibiotic occurs as part of a solid specimen, such as a powder or tablet, its concentration can be determined by a chemical assay method and expressed in micrograms of the antibiotic per milligram of the specimen.

Chemical assay methods are generally more accurate and require less time than biological methods, but they are less sensitive. Moreover, they may not always be reliable, since antibiotics may degrade into biologically inactive forms that the chemical assay cannot distinguish from the active form.

Microbiological Assay

In biological assay, living microorganisms are used to measure the amount of antimicrobial activity present in an antibiotic-containing specimen. It is based upon comparing the antimicrobial activity of the specimen with that of a standard preparation of the antibiotic under standard conditions.

The biological assay of antibiotics is performed by using either the tube dilution or disc plate technique. In tube dilution technique, two series of tubes are prepared: a standard set using tubes of media containing known (measured) amounts of the antibiotic, and a test sample set using tubes of media containing unknown amounts of the same antibiotic. The tubes are inoculated with a test bacterium, incubated and then observed for growth. By comparing the end points of growth of the known and the unknown, the antibiotic content of the sample can be determined.

The unit of measurement for antibiotics is arbitrary or established by International agreement. For example, the international unit (IU) of penicillin is defined as that amount of penicillin that has antimicrobial activity equal to that present in 0.5988 microgram of an International standard preparation of penicillin. This standard consists of a sample of pure penicillin G that contains 1667 units of activity per milligram.

NON MEDICAL USES OF ANTIBIOTICS

Antibiotics are used mainly for treatment of human and animal infections. But apart from this, antibiotics have several non-medical uses.

1. Some antibiotics are effective against plant pathogens and may be used for treatment of plant diseases.

2. Antibiotics are used as growth stimulants or supplement in animal feeds. *e.g.*, The addition of tetracycline or penicillin to poultry or swine feed at the rate of 5 to 20 gms per ton of feed increases the rate of growth of young animals by at least 10 per cent and some times much more.

3. Antibiotics are used in tissue cultures and embryonated chicken eggs to prevent bacterial growth.

4. Antibiotics are used to prepare selective culture media. *e.g.*, Thayer-Martin medium, a selective medium for the isolation of gonococci, contains antibiotics vancomycin, colistin and nystatin, which do not inhibit the growth of gonococci, but prevent the growth of other bacteria and fungi.

PHAGE THERAPY

Phage therapy involves the use of specific viruses that can infect and lyse pathogenic bacteria. Since, antibiotic-resistance is widely increasing among bacteria, bacteriophages offer a promising field as natural, self-replicating and self-limiting antibiotics. Clinical trials are conducted to use phages against multiple-drug resistant Staphylococcus and Enterococcus. The most powerful and cost-effective application of phage therapy is in the treatment of diseases such as cholera and dysentery.

Phage therapy has agricultural applications to eradicate *Salmonella* from chickens to prevent human infections and to treat diarrhoeal diseases of live-stock such as cattle and fish infections, plant pathogens all of which will reduce the environmental impact of over used chemical antibiotics as well as treat important diseases.

Phage therapy has advantages over antibiotic therapy.

1. Phages can be given in a single dose, since the phages can replicate themselves and are not diluted out by body fluids.

2. Phage-resistant bacterial mutants that develop are much less virulent than the parent wild types.

3. Phage can target bacterial pathogens specifically.

4. In cases of intestinal infection, phages eliminated along with the feces will prevent the spread of infection, if feces contaminates food or water.

BACTERIOCINS

Many gram negative bacteria produce antibiotic-like bactericidal substances active against some other strains of the same or closely related specie. They are called bacteriocins.

The bacteriocins produced by coliform bacilli such as *E. coli* are called colicins, Pseudomonads produce pyocines (aeruginocines) *Bacillus megaterium* produce megacins, *Corynebacterium diphtheriae* produce diphthericins, *Yersinia pestis* produces pesticins and so on.

Bacteriocins are proteins, and when seen under electron microscope, appear like tail structures of phages. They also resemble phages in their ability to adsorb on specific receptor sites on susceptible bacterial cells; some of the receptor sites may be same for both phages and bacteriocins.

The production of bacteriocins is determined by the presence in bacteria of plasmids (colicinogenic factors or col factors), known as bacteriocinogen, that are transmitted from cell to cell by conjugation, transduction. Certain physical (UV rays) and chemical agents (nitrogen mustard) may induce bacteriocin production by the bacteria possessing plasmids.

Bacteriocin typing may be used as a tool for epidemiological studies. Bacteriocin typing is based on the ability of bacteriocins produced by the test strain to kill standard indicator strains of bacteria.

QUESTIONS

Essay Type Questions

1. Define antibiotic. Write in brief the mode of action of antibiotics. List the various methods of antibiotic susceptibility testing

Short Notes

1. Chemotherapeutic test.
2. MIC.
3. Disc diffusion test.
4. Kirby-Bauer method.
5. Explain the different methods of antibiotic sensitivity testing.
6. Bacteriocins.
7. Tube dilution method of antibiotic susceptibility testing.
8. Stokes method.
9. E-test.
10. Assay of antibiotics.
11. Non-medical uses of antibiotics.
12. Antibiogram.

16

Microbial Genetics

- *Introduction*
- *Definitions*
- *Structure of DNA*
- *Structure of RNA*
- *Ribozymes*
- *Differences between DNA and RNA*
- *Central dogma of molecular biology*
- *Replication of DNA*
- *Genetic code*
- *Gene expression/protein synthesis*
- *Regulation (control) of gene expression*
- *Variability in microorganisms*
  - *Genotypic*
  - *Phenotypic*
- *Mutations*
  - *Definitions*
  - *Spontaneous mutations*
  - *Induced mutations*
  - *Mutagens*
  - *Biochemical mutations*
  - *Conditional mutations*
  - *Point mutations*
  - *Frame-shift mutations*
  - *Base-pair mutations*
  - *Reversion mutations*
  - *Inversion*
  - *Drug resistance mutations*
  - *Detection of mutations (selection of mutants)*
- *Mechanisms of gene transfer (genetic recombination)*
  - *Transformation*
  - *Conjugation*
  - *Sexduction*
  - *Transduction*
  - *Lysogeny*
  - *Transposition*
- *Biotechnology*
- *Genetic engineering/Gene cloning/DNA recombinant technology*
- *Applications of genetic engineering*
- *Restriction endonucleases*
- *DNA fingerprinting*
- *Restriction fragment length polymorphism (RFLP)*
- *Polymerase chain reaction (PCR)*
- *Transposable elements (Jumping genes)*
- *Blotting techniques*
  - *Southern blotting*
  - *Northern blotting*
  - *Western blotting*
  - *Eastern blotting*
- *Plasmids episomes*
  - *Functions encoded by plasmids*
  - *Conjugative (transmissible) plasmids*
  - *Nonconjugative plasmids*
  - *F-factor*
  - *R-factor*
  - *Col factor*
  - *Dissimilation plasmids*
  - *Inc plasmids*
  - *Plasmids as cloning vectors*
- *Cosmids*
- *DNA probes*

INTRODUCTION

Genetics is the study of heredity and variation, seeking to understand the similarities and differences between parents and their daughter cells.

Microbial genetics comprises the following aspects:

1. Structure and organization of genome.
2. Replication and expression of genetic material.
3. Mechanisms by which genetic information is changed and exchanged among bacteria.

In all living organisms, the hereditary information resides or is encoded in nucleic acids – DNA and RNA. Nucleic acids are called "life molecules", because they are store house of genetic information. The genetic information in bacteria, as in all cells, is contained in the specific sequence of nucleotides in the cell's Deoxyribonucleic acid (DNA). Thus, DNA is the store house of genetic information required for protein synthesis

GENE or CISTRON. A segment of DNA or a specific nucleotide sequence that specifies the production of a particular polypeptide (protein) chain is called "gene". The unit of heredity is gene.

Genome. The total complement of genes in a cell is known as the cell's genome. In other words, all genes taken together within an organism comprise that organism's genome.

The size of a gene and genome is usually expressed in the number of base pairs (bp) present *e.g.*, kilobases and megabases.

Chromosome. The genome is organised into discrete elements known as "chromosomes". The set of genes within a chromosome are arranged in a linear fashion, but the number of genes per chromosome is variable.

Karyotype. Representation of entire chromosomal complement of a cell or an organism or species, their number and morphology is called karyotype.

Idiogram. A diagrammatic representation of karyotype based on size and morphology of chromosomes is called idiogram.

Gene locus. The position of a gene along chromosome.

Gene pool. It is a term used to describe all the genes at a given locus in the population. The size of the pool is related to the genetic diversity in the population.

Gene mapping. Determination of the relative position of genes on a DNA molecule (chromosome or plasmid) and of the distance, in linkage units or physical units, between them.

Exon. The protein coding DNA sequence of a gene.

Intron. A noncoding DNA sequence within a gene that is initially transcribed into mRNA but is later snipped out.

Sequencing. Determination of the order of nucleotide bases arranged within a DNA molecule and decoding of the genetic information contained therein (amino acid sequence of the corresponding proteins or structure of control regions).

Pedigree. A diagram mapping the genetic history of a particular family.

Eugenics. The improvement of humanity by altering its genetic composition by encouraging breeding of those presumed to have desirable genes.

Genomics. A study of how genes and genetic information are organized within the genome, and how this organization determines their function.

This science was given an impetus by the "human genome project", which led to the development of efficient sequencing techniques. A number of microbial genomes have already been sequenced.

Genomic library. A collection of all the DNA in a species genome, broken into random DNA fragments, inserted into DNA.

Replicon. It is a unit of the genome in which DNA is replicated, contains an origin for initiation of replication.

Regulatory gene. A segment of gene which regulates the switching on (expression) of the gene or not (repression).

Inducer. A small molecule that triggers gene transcription by binding to a regulatory protein.

Operator. A prokaryotic regulatory element that interacts with a repressor to control the transcription of adjacent structural genes.

Promoter is a region of DNA involved in binding of RNA polymerase to initiate transcription.

Template. Single stranded DNA or RNA molecule upon which a complementary nucleotide strand is synthesized.

Repression. It is the ability of bacteria to prevent synthesis of certain enzymes when their products are present; more generally, refers to inhibition of transcription (or translation) by binding of repressor protein to a specific site on DNA or mRNA.

Trait. A character difference associated with a particular gene.

RNA polymerase. It is an enzyme that synthesizes RNA using DNA template. It is also called as "DNA-dependent RNA polymerase".

DNA polymerase. It is an enzyme that catalyzes the synthesis of a daughter strand(s) of DNA (under direction from a DNA template). It is also involved in repair and replication. These enzymes are of three types — DNA polymerase I, DNA polymerase II and DNA polymerase III.

DNA polymerase III is the major enzyme involved in replication. DNA polymerase I is responsible for the repair of damaged DNA and also possesses exonuclease activity in $3' \rightarrow 5'$ direction. The role of DNA polymerase II is unclear but it is believed to be involved in repair of damaged DNA.

BACTERIAL NUCLEUS.

Bacteria possess a prokaryotic nucleus, consisting of a single circular chromosome, made up of a single molecule of double-stranded DNA, of about 1000 to 1300 μ length. Some viruses may possess RNA genome.

STRUCTURE OF DNA

DNA possesses a double-helix structure (Watson and Crick - 1953). The DNA molecule consists of two helically twisted strands, connected together in the form of a double helix. Each strand consists a back bone of deoxyribose (a pentose sugar) and phosphate groups, linked covalently by phosphodiester bonds. The purine and pyrimidine nitrogenous bases are covalently connected to deoxyribose sugar molecules. Purine bases are adenine (A) and guanine (G) and the pyrimidines thymine (T) and cytosine (C).

The double stranded nature of the molecule is stabilised by hydrogen bonding between the bases on the opposite strands in such a manner that adenine base of one strand always binds, via two hydrogen bonds, to the thymine base of the other strand, or vice versa, (A = T). Likewise, the guanine base of one strand always binds by three hydrogen bonds to the cytosine base of the other strand, or vice versa

(G ≡ C). Thus, adenine and thymine form a complementary base pair, and guanine and cytosine form another. A molecule of DNA will, therefore contain as many units of adenine as thymine, and of guanine as cytosine, but the ratio of each pair of bases $\frac{(A + T)}{(G + C)} = 1$, though constant for each species, varies widely from one bacterial species to another.

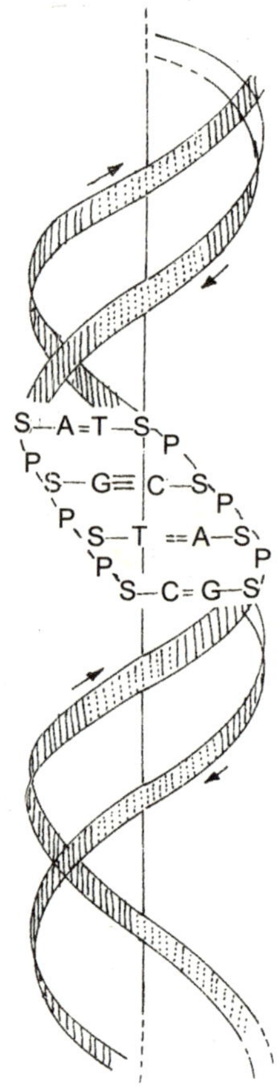

Fig. 16.1. DNA double hellix.

Each strand has a 5´ and a 3´ hydroxyl terminus. Both the strands of DNA run antiparallel, with the 5´ terminus of one strand opposed to the 3´ terminus of the other.

The DNA molecule is a polynucleotide, a polymer consisting of several nucleotides. Each **"nucleotide"** consists of pentose sugar deoxyribose, a phosphate group and a nitrogenous base (purine or pyrimidine).

Deoxyribose sugar and a nitrogenous base together called as **"nucleoside".**

A nucleoside and phosphate together called as **nucleotide.**

The strand completes a turn each 34Å; each nucleotide occupies 3.4Å; thus, there are ten nucleotides per turn.

The order of nitrogenous bases along a DNA or RNA strand is known as the "base sequence". Genetic information is stored in the DNA as a **"code or codon",** consisting of a sequence of 3 bases, *i.e.*, the code is **"triplet".** Each codon specifies for a single amino acid, but more than one codon may exist for the same amino acid. *e.g.*, the codons (triplets) AGA, AGG, CGC, CGU, CGA and CGG code for the same amino acid arginine.

Three codons UAA, UAG, and UGA do not code for any amino acid and are called **"non-sense codons".** They act as punctuation marks (stop codons), terminating the message for the synthesis of a polypeptide. A segment of DNA carrying codons specifying for a particular polypeptide is called a **"gene"** or **"cistron".** A DNA molecule consists of large number of genes, each of which contains thousands of nucleotides.

STRUCTURE OF RNA

RNA is a polymer of ribonucleotides, frequently occurs in single stranded form. It is found in cytoplasm and ribosomes.

RNA is structurally similar to DNA, except for two major differences. It contains the sugar ribose (instead of deoxyribose in DNA) and the base uracil (instead of thymine in DNA). Thymine is absent in RNA.

On the basis of structure and function, three distinct types of RNA can be distinguished.

1. *Messenger RNA (m-RNA).* DNA acts as a template for the synthesis of mRNA, and therefore, the bases will be complementary to each other. The m-RNA is formed on DNA template by transcription and carries message-specific sequence of nucleotides in triplet codons, passes from nucleus to cytoplasm to convey message to ribosomes for the synthesis of protein molecule.

2. *Ribosomal RNA (r-RNA).* It is present in ribosomes, where messages of mRNA are translated into amino acid structure of proteins.

3. *Transfer RNA (tRNA)* or *soluble RNA (sRNA).* It is present mainly in cytoplasm. They are relatively small, single stranded, globular molecules, consisting about 75–100 nucleotides.

Each single stranded tRNA remains folded to form a clover-leaf structure, containing four main arms or loops. The anticodon loop helps to recognize triplet codon on mRNA.

Amino acids in cytoplasm are linked to tRNA molecules, which carry them to the ribosomes.

RIBOZYMES

A few RNA molecules have been shown to function as catalytic enzymes, known as ribozymes. They are found in both prokaryotes and eukaryotes, ribozymes are short RNAs which have as few as 19 bases and are involved in several important cellular reactions. They play a key role as self-splicing introns, and remove themselves from RNA molecules.

It has been proposed that they are the vestigeal remains of a simpler form of life, "RNA life", which may have predated the era of proteins as cell's major catalysts.

DIFFERENCES BETWEEN DNA AND RNA

Table 16.1

DNA	*RNA*
1. DNA is the usual genetic material	1. RNA is the genetic material in some viruses
2. DNA is usually double-stranded (may be single stranded in some viruses)	2. Mostly single stranded (some viruses may have double-stranded RNA *e.g.,* Reo virus)
3. The pentose sugar is deoxyribose	3. The pentose sugar is ribose
4. Nitrogenous bases are adenine, thymine guanine, cytosine	4. Nitrogenous bases are adenine, guanine, cytosine and uracil
5. Adenine pairs with thymine and guanine with cytosine	5. Adenine pairs with uracil and guanine with cytosine
6. Most of the DNA is found in chromosomes in the nucleus. Some DNA may be found in the cytoplasm	6. mRNA is formed on the chromosomes and is found in the nucleolus and cytoplasm. t-RNA and rRNA are found in cytoplasm.
7. DNA on replication forms DNA, and on transcription forms RNA	7. Usually RNA does not replicate or transcribe
8. Genetic messages are encoded in DNA	8. The usual function of RNA is translating messages encoded in DNA into proteins
9. DNA consists large number of nucleotides, up to 4.3 million	9. RNA consists of fewer nucleotides, up to 12,000
10. Purine and pyrimidine bases are almost equal	10. Not equal

CENTRAL DOGMA OF MOLECULAR BIOLOGY

Living organisms from man to viruses, must perform several actions in order to carry out normal life processes. The important action among them is biosynthesis of nucleic acid and protein. Nucleic acid (DNA) is the genetic material in all living systems, the duplication of which is necessary for the passage of genetic information during cell division to yield identical daughter cells.

The duplication of DNA (replication of DNA) is the biosynthesis of an exact copy of parental DNA molecules from the monomeric deoxyribonucleotides. The genetic information is preserved by duplicating the nucleotide sequence of parent DNA. The expression of genetic information of genes in DNA involves the processes of transcription and translation. In transcription, the genetic information stored in the base sequence of DNA is copied in the form of an RNA molecule (mRNA). In the process of translation, the genetic information, now present in the mRNA (transcript) is utilized to direct the synthesis of proteins. The flow of information from DNA to proteins (DNA $\rightarrow$ RNA $\rightarrow$ Polypeptides) is called the "central dogma of molecular biology".

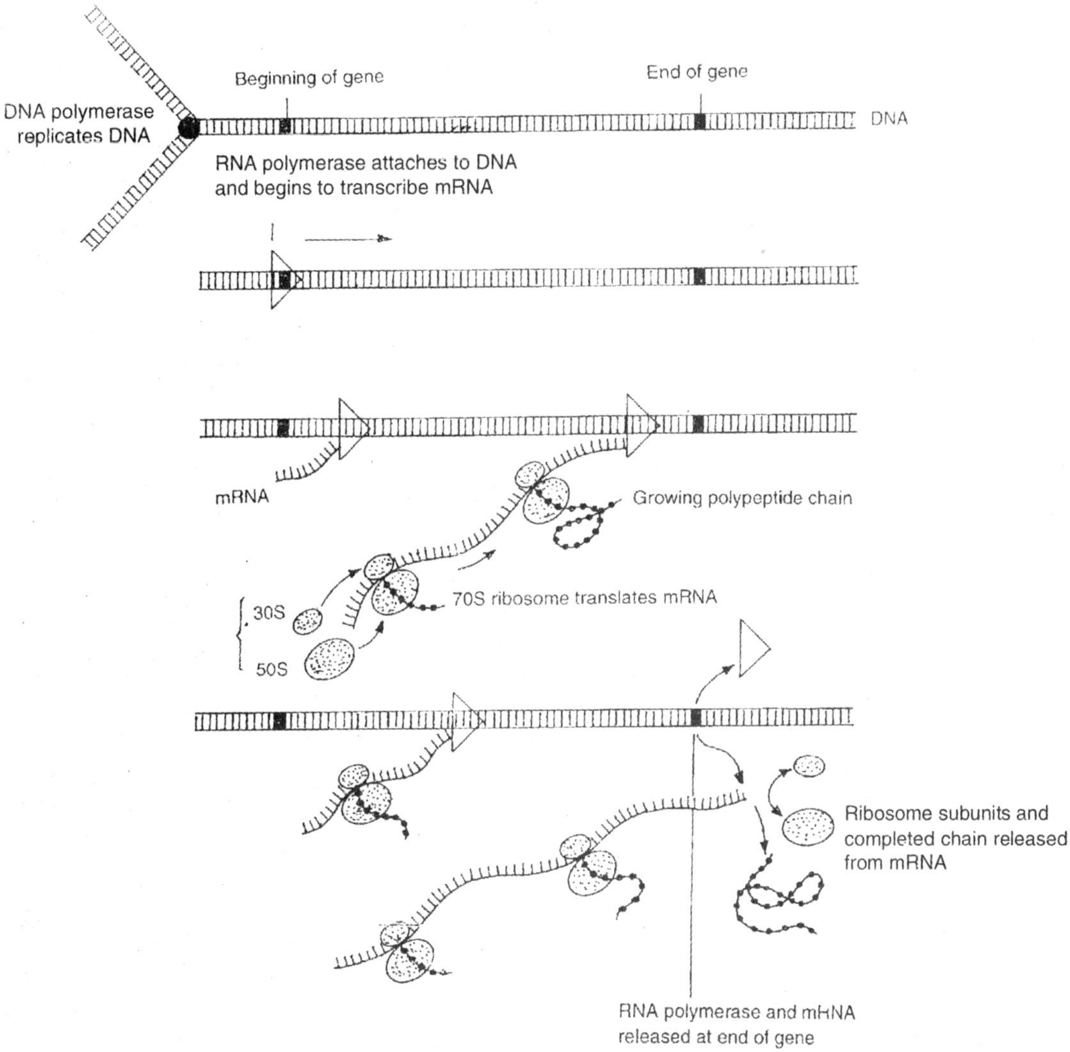

Fig. 16.2. Central dogma of molecular biology.

REPLICATION OF DNA (SEMICONSERVATIVE MECHANISM)

DNA can make exact copies of itself, known as replication and is the very basis of life. DNA replication is the process that copies the nucleotide sequence of a double-stranded parent DNA molecule into two double-stranded daughter DNA molecules-each of which will enter into daughter cell, during cell division.

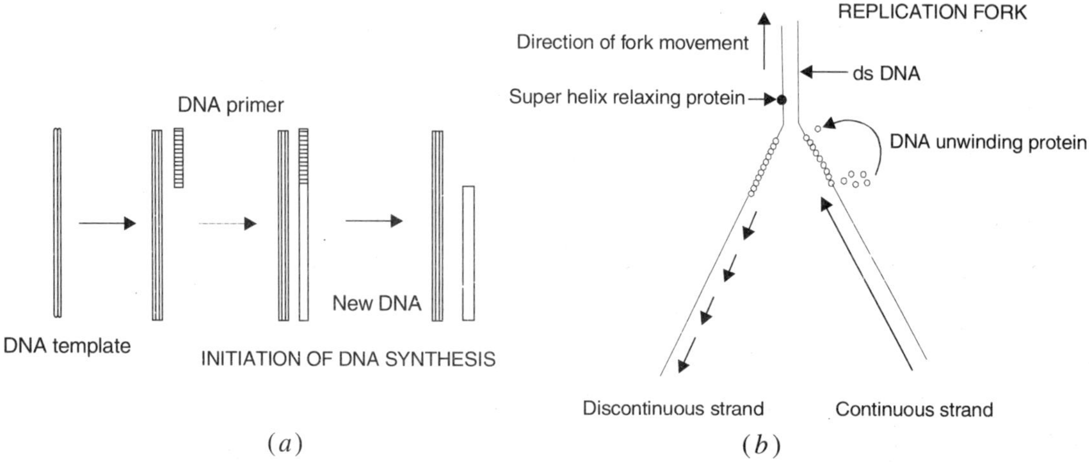

Fig. 16.3. Replication of DNA.

Bacteria replicate, usually by semiconservative method, which means, each daughter DNA molecules contains one strand from the parent DNA molecule (*i.e.,* one old or conserved strand) and one newly synthesized strand.

Replication starts at a unique, specific point called the "origin" on the chromosome. In some, replication starts with a "**nick**" or "**incision**" made by an incision enzyme, known as endonucleases (Fig. 16.3).

The two strands of the DNA double helix unwind with the help of a DNA unwinding protein or DNA binding protein known as "**DNA gyrase**", forming two 'Y' shaped "**replication forks**". The unwinding of the strands imposes strain, which is relieved by the action of a "superhelix relaxing protein" or "swiveling protein". As two parental strands separate, each strand serves as a "template", which acts as a "master copy", in the synthesis of a new strand with complementary base pairing. Each replication fork moves through the parent DNA molecule in opposite directions, so that replication is a bidirectional process. When one strand replicates at 3′ end, the other strand replicates at 5′ end. One strand replicates continuously, known as continuous strand, another strand replicates discontinuously, known as discontinuous strand. DNA polymerase adds nucleotides to the new strand at 3′ end, in a sequence that is complementary to the base sequence in template strand to form a continuous strand.

In discontinuous replication of other strand, near replication fork, a short, complementary RNA molecule, known as "**RNA primer**" is formed by the action of RNA polymerase. Then DNA polymerase adds deoxyribonucleotides to its 3′ end and forms many complementary short segments, known as "**okazaki fragments**", which are joined to form a continuous strand by "**DNA ligase**". Then DNA polymerase removes the RNA primer and catalyzes the synthesis of short DNA fragment in its place, which joins the main strand. The direction of synthesis of okazaki fragments is opposite to that of the movement of replication fork.

Termination of replication occurs when the two replication forks meet, resulting in two complete chromosomes, each containing two complementary strands, one of parental origin and one newly synthesized daughter strand.

GENETIC CODE

The genetic message carried by mRNA are written in a chemical language called genetic code. Genetic code describes relationship between DNA sequence and protein it specifies or codes. Genetic code is a 64-codon dictionary known as genetic codon dictionary. Each codon is a triplet, made up of three nitrogenous bases formed from four letter life – AGCT(U), which is organised in different combinations (4^3) to form 64 three letter codons, sufficient to code for twenty amino acids.

Thus, genetic code particularly refers to codons of mRNA that specifies number, sequence, and type of amino acids in proteins.

Genetic code is degenerate, non-overlapping, commaless, non-ambiguous, universal read in particular frame. It contains three termination codons UAA, UAG, UGA.

GENE EXPRESSION OR PROTEIN SYNTHESIS

Gene acts by protein synthesis, which takes place in two steps : 1. transcription, and 2. translation. The processes of transcription and translation leading to protein synthesis are termed "central dogma of molecular biology". DNA carries genetic information, which is transcribed on to ribonucleic acid (RNA) and then translated as the particular polypeptide.

$$\text{DNA} \longrightarrow \text{RNA} \longrightarrow \text{Polypeptide}$$

1. Transcription or RNA biosynthesis

The synthesis of mRNA on DNA template is called "transcription". The "coding" strand is called "sense" strand and the opposite strand is called "antisense" strand. Transcription takes place by three stages

1. DNA-dependent RNA polymerase first binds to a special sequence of DNA nucleotides, called "promoter" region, whereupon the two DNA strands separate and RNA polymerase begins to move forward in $5' \rightarrow 3'$ direction and synthesize a complementary mRNA strand.

2. mRNA chain elongation takes place by the addition of ribonucleotides in $5' \rightarrow 3'$ direction based on complementary base pairing.

3. Termination of transcription occurs when RNA polymerase stops; as it reaches the end of genetic message indicated by "termination sequence" on the gene or by 'rho' cofactor, which can disrupt mRNA – RNA polymerase – DNA template complex.

II. Translation.

The synthesis of polypeptide chain from amino acids on ribosomes using coded information in m-RNA is called "Translation". It takes place in 4 steps.

1. Amino acids are activated (energized) with the energy of ATP and then linked to tRNA molecules.

2. m-RNA binds to small risbosomal unit and polypeptide synthesis is initiated by initiator codon AUG, sometimes GUG. It requires GTP as energy source and some initiating factors.

3. Polypeptide chain elongation takes place, after the tRNA carry (transport) activated amino acids to ribosomes, which links amino acids together by formation of a peptide bond to form protein.

There is specific tRNA for each of the 20 amino acids. tRNA consists an anticodon loop, with three unpaired bases, which can recognize a complementary codon in mRNA. mRNA and tRNA come together on the surface of the ribosomes. Specific alignment of tRNA anticodons with their complementary mRNA codons allows amino acids to be assembled in correct sequence on ribosomes.

4. Termination of polypeptide chain synthesis stops when the ribosome finally reaches nonsense codons (UAA, UAG or UGA).

REGULATION OR CONTROL OF GENE EXPRESSION

The study of control of gene expression is important because all genes in the organism would not function at all times. Every cell has regulatory mechanisms that depending upon the current environment, allow some genes to be transcribed, while preventing others. Thus, particular genes act at particular time in an organism. Based on the nature of gene expression, two types of genes are known.

1. *Constitutive genes.* An enzyme or protein is always produced by the cell, whether or not the substrate present. This means that the gene for that enzyme or protein is always transcribed. They are known as constitutive genes *e.g.,* glycolysis enzymes. They are not regulated and they are not under the control of inducers or repressors.

2. *Inducible genes* or *regulated genes.* An enzyme or protein is produced by the cell only when needed and only in the presence of a particular substrate. The substance that initiates enzyme induction is called "inducer", the substance that represses enzyme production is called a "co-reprocessor". *e.g.,* β-galactosidase, which splits lactose, is produced by *E.coli*, only when the substrate lactose is present. If lactose is absent, the enzyme is not synthesized. This phenomenon is called "**enzyme induction**" and "**enzyme repression**". This strategy avoids waste and overproduction of products that are already present.

In bacteria, the genes that code for the enzymes of a metabolic pathway are usually arranged in a consecutive manner to form a functional unit called an "**operon**". In bacteria the process of gene expression is mainly regulated at transcriptional level.

Enzyme induction. *Esch.coli* can utilize lactose as a source of energy. The enzyme β-galactosidase is produced only in the presence of lactose and its production is switched off when not required. Lactose (substrate) is called "inducer" and β-galactosidase is called "inducible enzyme".

Operon. The genes associated with fermentation of lactose in *E.coli* are present in "**lac operon**", which contains following structural genes, involved in a common regulatory system.

lac Y gene – codes for a permease required for active transport of lactose into cells.

lac Z gene – codes for the synthesis of β-galactosidase which splits lactose into glucose and galactose.

lac A gene – codes for a transacetylase enzyme that reduces the toxicity of some galactosides by transferring acetyl groups.

lac I gene – codes for the repressor, a regulatory protein.

When the substrate (inducer) is absent, the lac operon can be switched off by the attachment of a repressor molecule to a specific region of the DNA, known as the "operator", which lies between the promotor and the lac Z gene. When the inducer is present, the repressor is released from the operator, and transcription takes place.

The repressor is an allosteric molecule with two active sites. One recognizes operator of the lac operon and binds to it to prevent transcription. The other recognizes inducer (lactose) and binds to it and gets released from operator, so that transcription can resume.

Enzyme Repression (End-Product Repression)

In *E.coli,* a promotor, an operator, and five genes that code for tryptophan synthesizing enzymes form the "**trp operon**". A trp regulator gene codes for the synthesis of inactive repressor protein, which cannot bind to the trp operator, if tryptophan is absent; so that RNA polymerase can transcribe the trp operon, for enzyme synthesis. However, if tryptophan is present, the repressor binds to tryptophan and is activated, which binds to the operator to prevent transcription and subsequent enzyme synthesis.

Thus, trp operon is regulated by end product (tryptophan), hence called "end-product repression" and the operons are called "repressible operons". Operons of arginine, histidine and tryptophan are examples of this type.

VARIABILITY IN MICROORGANISMS

Genetic information is transmitted from parents to progeny with great accuracy, carrying specific traits from generation to generation. However, genetic variability is also necessary for a biological species. Living organisms maintain a proper balance between these two properties *i.e.,* variability and constancy. Variability is associated with two properties of an organism, its genotype and phenotype.

Genotype

The sum total of genes that make up the genetic apparatus or genetic constitution of a cell is known as its genotype.

It is stable, permanent and hereditary, that is transmitted to its progeny.

The genotype includes inheritable complete genetic potential of the cell, all of which may or may not be expressed at a time, in a given environmental situation.

In a bacterial cell, genotype includes the chromosomal DNA plus any plasmid DNA that may be present; In an eukaryotic cell, it includes the chromosomal DNA plus the DNA of the mitochondrion; in algal or plant cell, chromosomal DNA plus mitochondrial DNA plus the DNA of the chloroplasts.

Phenotype

The phenotype is the physical expression of a genotype in a given set of environmental conditions. A cell may exhibit different phenotypic appearances in different situations. *e.g.,*

1. color or size of bacterial colony
2. ability of microbes to utilize specific chemicals as energy sources
3. presence or absence of bacterial flagellae
4. presence or absence of bacterial capsules.

Genotypic variations. Genotypic changes are due to alterations in genome or genotype.

Genotypic variations are stable, permanent, heritable and not influenced by the environment. They may occur by, 1. mutations, 2. one of the methods of genetic exchange or gene transfer or genetic recombination. They are:

(*i*) Transformation (*ii*) Conjugation
(*iii*) Sexduction (*iv*) Transduction
(*v*) Lysogency (*vi*) Transposition

Phenotypic variations. Both the genotype and environment influence the phenotype of an organism.

Phenotypic variations are temporary, not heritable, limited in range by the genotype, influenced by the environment. Phenotypic changes caused by changes in the environment, will return back to original phenotype, if the original environmental conditions are restored. *e.g.,*

1. *Salmonella typhi* is normally flagellated but when grown in phenol agar, the flagellae are not synthesized. When it is subcultured on to medium without phenol, the flagellae are resynthesized.

2. *E.coli* produces β-galactosidase enzyme for lactose fermentation, only when lactose is present whereas the enzyme is not produced when lactose is not available.

3. *Azomonas* bacterium forms large, gummy colonies when grown in presence of sucrose; and smaller, non-gummy colonies in the absence of sucrose.

MUTATIONS

Definitiions

The term "mutation" was first coined by Huge Devries and is derived from the latin word "mutate" meaning "to change".

Mutation is defined as a random, undirected, heritable variation caused by an alteration in the nucleotide sequence at some point of the DNA of the cell.

Any gene can undergo mutation. Mutated gene will have an altered nucleotide sequence, and the protein coded by it may have an altered amino acid sequence. Hence, mutations may produce changes in morphology, enzyme activity, nutritional requirements, biochemical reactions, antigenic structure, host range and susceptibility to antibiotics and phages.

The importance of mutations lies in the field of drug resistance and the development of live attenuated vaccines.

Mutant strain. A cell of an organism carrying a mutated gene (with altered nucleotide sequence) is called a mutant.

Wild strain. The organism or cell with a normal, nonmutated gene is called wild type.

Mutagenesis. The process of mutation is called mutagenesis.

Mutagen. Any agent physical or chemical, which increases the frequency of mutations is called mutagen.

Mutations can be classified into various types as described here below:

Spontaneous Mutations

Mutations which occur under natural conditions are called "spontaneous mutations".

Mutation is a natural event, taking place all the time at its particular frequency in all dividing forms of life. Each gene undergoes mutation with a fixed frequency. Mutation rates of individual genes in bacteria range from 10^{-2} to 10^{-10} per bacterium per division.

Spontaneous mutations usually arise due to errors in DNA replication or tautomerism or damage to DNA spontaneous mutations are usually rare and may be dominant or recessive. Recessive mutations are more frequent.

Induced Mutations

Though mutations occur spontaneously, its frequency can be increased by several physical and chemical agents, called mutagens; and mutations induced by mutagens are called induced mutations.

Induced mutations differ from spontaneous mutations only in frequency, not in kind.

Many mutagens are also carcinogens.

Physical mutagens. Physical mutagens include radiations such as

Non-ionizing – UV rays or over exposure to sunlight.

Ionizing – X-rays, gamma rays, beta rays, alpha rays.

UV rays causes the formation of thymine dimers, in which two adjacent pyrimidines on a DNA strand become bonded together; this bonding distorts the normal conformation of the DNA.

UV radiation also causes addition of water molecules (hydration) to pyrimidines in both DNA and RNA resulting in the formation of hydrated pyrimidines.

X-rays bring about mutations by breaking the phosphodiester linkages at one or more points in DNA. When X-rays pass through a cell, they can remove electrons from molecules, forming ions. These ions can directly or indirectly cause alterations in the structure of purine and pyrimidine bases.

Chemical mutagens. They can be classified according to the way in which they bring about mutations.

(*i*) ***Base analogues.*** Chemical substances resembling bases are called base analogues. A base analogue may be incorporated into newly synthesized DNA, instead of a normal base *e.g.,* 5-Bromouracil, 2-amino purine, 2, 6 diaminopurine, 5-bromodeoxyuridine and nitrogen mustard.

(*ii*) ***Agents that modify purines and pyrimidines.***

e.g.,	Deaminating agents	– nitrous oxide, hydroxyl amine
	Alkylating agents	– dimethyl sulphate, ethyl methane sulphonate, ethyl ethane sulphonate, nitrosoguanidine.

(*iii*) ***Intercalating substances.*** They produce distortion in DNA. *e.g.,* fluorescent acridine dyes such as proflavine, acridine orange.

(*iv*) ***Chemicals in cigarette smoke.*** Polycyclic aromatic hydrocarbons such as benzopyrene in smoke induce cancer.

Biological mutagens. Transposons–small, mobile pieces of DNA, contain genetic information and insert themselves into chromosomes at numerous locations, randomly. They cause mutations by interrupting the nucleotide sequence of the genes into which they are inserted.

Biochemical Mutations

In some mutations, the organism loses the ability to synthesize an essential metabolite, and unable to grow in a medium that does not contain this essential metabolite and therefore require this nutrients. These mutants are called "**auxotrophs**". Thus, an auxotroph is a microbial cell that, through mutation has lost the ability to synthesize an essential metabolite, and gained a growth requirement for this metabolite, which must be supplied in the medium for its growth; whereas the wild type strains capable of growing on minimal media are known as "**prototrophs**".

Conditional Mutations

They are expressed only under certain environmental conditions. For example, temperature sensitive (ts) mutant of *E.coli,* which behaves normally below 34°C and as a mutant above 39°C. It is known "conditional mutant". Temperature sensitive mutation creates a gene product that is functional at low temperature but inactive at high temperature. The reverse relationship is called cold-sensitive.

Point Mutations

They are produced when a single base is substituted for another in a gene. They are of several types.

(*i*) ***Silent mutations or neutral mutations.*** The altered nucleotide sequence continues to code for the same amino acid as before, hence there will be no change in phenotypic expression.

(*ii*) ***Non-sense mutation.*** The nucleotide substitution produces a nonsense codons such as UAA, UAG and UGA, resulting in premature polypeptide chain termination.

(*iii*) ***Missense mutations.*** One base of a codon may be substituted by another base. The changed codon may code for another amino acid. As a result, there is a simple change of one amino acid in polypeptide chain.

A good example of missense mutation in humans is the disease sickle cell anemia. A single base substitution in the codon for the sixth amino acid of normal hemoglobin A changes this amino acid from glutamic acid (codon GAG) to valine (codon GUG). The result is the abnormal hemoglobin, hemoglobin S, that characterizes sickle cell anemia. At low oxygen concentrations in the blood, the hemoglobin S molecules become stacked into crystals, distorting RBC into sickle shapes.

Frame Shift Mutations

A mutation in which there is deletion or addition of one or a few nucleotides is called a frame shift mutation. The name is derived from the fact that there is a shift in the reading frame either backwards or forwards by one or two nucleotides. This usually leads to the formation of a nonfunctional protein.

(*i*) ***Addition or insertion mutations.*** Addition of one or few bases to a nucleotide chain.

(*ii*) ***Deletion nucleotides.*** Removal of one or a few bases from a nucleotides chain.

Base Pair Substitutions

They occur due to incorporation of wrong bases during replication of DNA due to tautomerism.

All the four common bases of DNA have usual tautomeric forms. They are normally present in "keto" form due to tautomerism they may be transformed into "enol" form.

Base pair substitutions are categorised into two major types.

(*i*) ***Transitions.*** They are the most common type of substitutions where a purine base is replaced by another purine base and a pyrimidine by another pyrimidine.

(*ii*) ***Transversion.*** They are substitutions where a purine base is substituted by a pyrimidine base or vice versa. This type of substitution is very rare.

Reversion Mutations

The effect of a mutation on the phenotype can be reversed, so that the original phenotype is brought back. This reversal may be due to true reversion or suppression.

(*i*) ***True reversion or back mutations.*** True reversion is restoration at the site of mutation. In true reversion, there is a reversal of original genetic exchange. Such a mutation is called "back mutation".

(*ii*) ***Suppression.*** A change at a site different from the mutation, causes suppression of mutation resulting in phenotypic restoration of gene function.

Suppressor mutations are of two types:

(*a*) ***Intragenic suppression.*** A mutation in a gene is suppressed by another mutation in the same gene.

(*b*) ***Extragenic or intergenic suppression.*** A mutation in a gene is overcome by a mutation in another gene.

Inversion

If a segment of DNA is removed and reinserted in a reverse direction, it results in an inversion mutation.

Based on the extent of base pair alterations, mutations can be divided into two groups.

(*i*) ***Microlesions.*** Also known as point mutations, usually a single base pair may alter. They may be base pair substitutions or frame shift mutations.

(*ii*) ***Macrolesions.*** Alterations of large number of base pairs in DNA may be due to additions, deletions, inversions and duplications.

Drug Resistance Mutations/Mutational Drug Resistance

Mutations may offer survival advantage on bacteria by the development of drug resistance.

For many antibiotics, a particular mutation produces only a slight increase in resistance; but a series of consecutive mutations can produce a step-wise increase in resistance, usually seen with penicillin.

Resistance to streptomycin arises quite readily by a "single large-step mutation" in many bacteria, which is a serious problem in clinical practice *e.g.,* in the treatment of tuberculosis. The mutants may vary widely in the degree of resistance, some exhibiting low resistance, while others may be highly resistant, and some mutants may become streptomycin dependent for growth.

Detection of Mutations or Selection of Mutants

There are several experiments to detect mutants. The most important are:

1. Replica plating technique.
2. Penicillin enrichment technique.
3. Fluctuation tests.
4. Ames test.

Highly automated techniques have been developed for the detection and isolation of mutant cells.

1. ***Replica plating technique.*** Nutritional mutants (auxotrophs) can be detected by the technique of replica plating. A nutritional mutant that has developed a requirement for a growth factor is called an "**auxotroph**" and the wild type parent from which the auxotroph was derived is called a "**prototroph**".

The technique involves imprinting of colonies from a master plate on to an agar plate lacking the nutrient, using a sterile velvet cloth covered on a cylinder, called velvet disk replicator. Here the colonies of the parental type will grow normally, whereas those of the mutant will not. Thus, the inability of a colony to grow on the replica plate will be a signal that it is a mutant. The colony on the master plate corresponding to the vacant spot on the replica plate can then be picked, purified and characterized.

2. ***Penicillin enrichment technique.*** The mutagen-treated culture is inoculated into a liquid medium lacking the nutrient needed by the mutant (auxotroph). After a short incubation for 15 – 20 minutes, penicillin is added to the culture. This antibiotic kills only cells that are reproducing. Thus, the wild type cells are killed, whereas the mutant cells are not killed, because they are not growing due to the lack of limiting nutrient.

The enzyme penicillinase is added to destroy penicillin or the cells can be centrifuged out and plated on to an agar medium containing the nutrient required by mutants. The auxotrophs multiply and form colonies, which can be picked up and characterized.

3. ***Fluctuation tests.*** It is first devised by Luria and Delbruk (1943). This test is used to demonstrate the occurrence of spontaneous mutations. The experiment is based on the observation that, in a population of cells sensitive to a particular phage, there are a few resistant cells. When equal volumes of broth culture, each containing approximately 10^9 *E.coli,* were spread on plates seeded with the bacteriophage the number of colonies arising from resistant cells showed a small fluctuation from plate to plate.

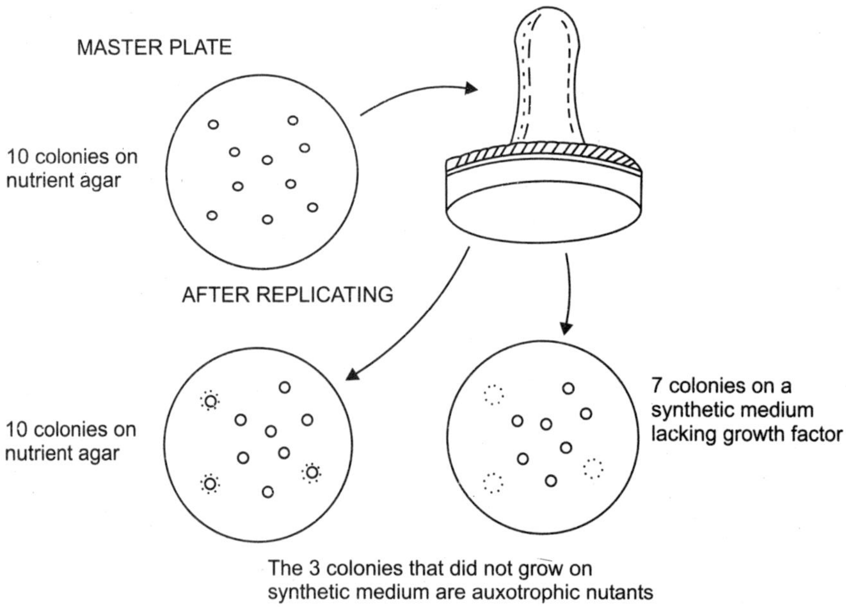

Fig. 16.4. Replica plating to detect auxotrophic mutants.

Small inocula of the same culture is inoculated to produce a series of 50 separate broth cultures. When similar volumes (10^9 bacteria) are spread on agar seeded with bacteriophage, large fluctuations were seen in the number of colonies obtained per plate.

These results indicate the randomly occurring spontaneous mutations, arising at different times during development in each culture.

4. ***Ames test or the Salmonella test or reverse mutation test.*** The most widely used short term test to detect whether a substance can induce mutations or not is developed by Bruce Ames et al (1971), and known as Ames test.

The test uses normally seven specially constructed strains of *Salmonella typhimurium*, that lack the "his" gene (his^-) and consequently lost the ability to synthesize histidine amino acid. Thus, the bacteria that are already mutants are treated with test compound (mutagen) to determine whether the test compound can induce a second mutation either frameshift or base pair substitution or reverse mutation which directly reverses or suppresses the original mutation, so that the strains acquire his gene (his^+) and consequently the capacity to synthesize histidine amino acid.

MECHANISMS OF GENE TRANSFER OR GENETIC EXCHANGE OR GENETIC RECOMBINATION IN BACTERIA

In bacteria, gene transfer that can lead to genetic recombination, may occur by any one of following methods.

1. Transformation or Griffith phenomenon.
2. Conjugation.
3. Sexduction.
4. Transduction.
5. Lysogeny.
6. Transposition.

Transformation or Griffith Phenomenon

Some bacteria can take up or acquire DNA fragments or genes from surroundings, that is released into the environment due to bacterial death or lysis.

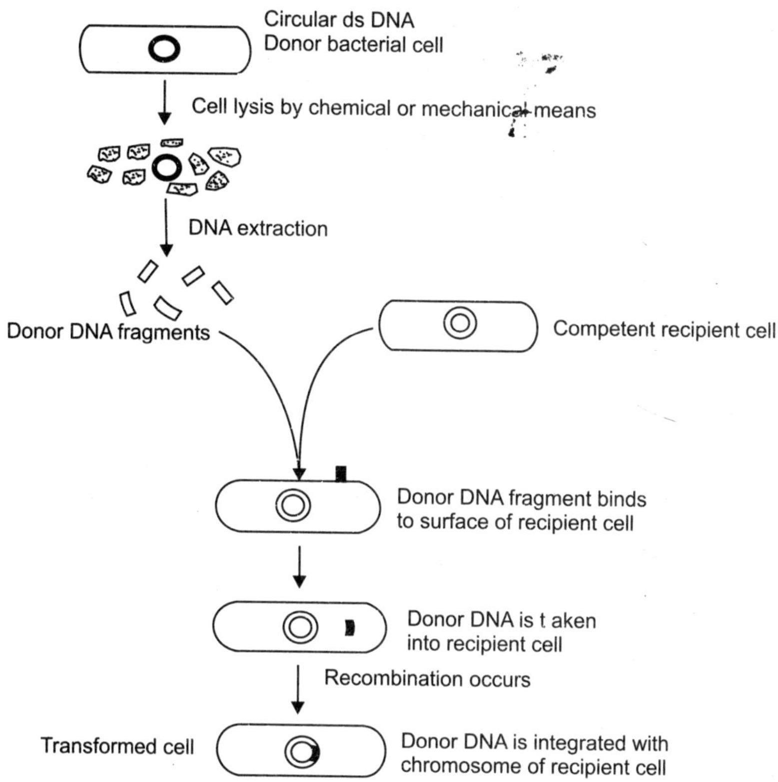

Fig. 16.5. Transformation.

It is found in both Gram positive and Gram negative bacteria. Transformation has been studied mainly in pneumococci, *Bacillus* species and *Hemophilus influenzae*. Any character may be transferred by transformation. The fragments of DNA involved in transformation may carry about 10 to 50 genes.

It is first discovered by Griffith (1928) hence known as Griffith phenomenon. Griffith found that mice died when injected with a mixture of live noncapsulated (Rough or R) pneumococci and heat killed capsulated (Smooth or S) pneumococci, neither of which proved fatal when injected separately. From blood cultures of dead mice, the live capsulated (S) pneumococci was isolated, which shows that some factor from heat-killed capsulated pneumococci (S) had transferred the genetic information for capsule synthesis to the live noncapsulated (R) pneumococci.

Cells that are able to take up DNA from their environment and incorporate it into the genome are said to be "competent". Although chromosomal DNA can be readily transferred to competent recipient bacteria, plasmid DNA is not easily transferred by ordinary transformation procedures. In genetic engineering, to accomplish transformation with plasmid DNA, the recipient cells (*e.g., E.coli*) are treated with $CaCl_2$ under cold temperatures (0 – 4°C) and then heat shock (to 42°C for 2 – 5 min.).

Transformation can be used as a genetic tool for gene mapping and the quantitative determination of gene dosages.

Transfection. It is a process where bacteria can be transformed with DNA released from a bacterial virus (phage) rather than from another bacterial cell. Transfection is used as a tool for studying the mechanism of transformation and recombination.

Conjugation

It was first discovered by Lederberg and Tatum (1946) in *E.coli* K12 strain, for which they were awarded Noble prize, since it opened up the era of molecular genetics.

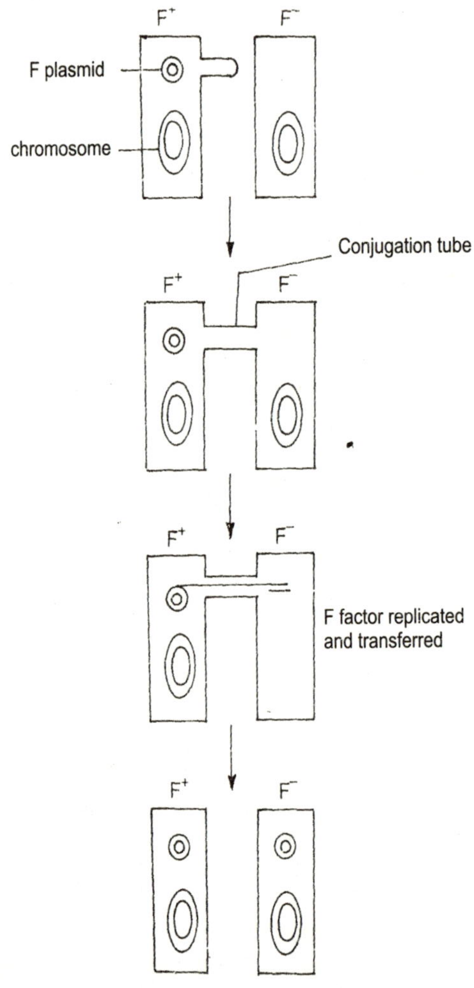

Fig. 16.6. Bacterial conjugation.

Conjugation is a process whereby DNA is transferred by cell to cell physical contact, from one bacterium to another. This may be regarded as a primitive means of sexual reproduction. Conjugation takes place between a "male cell" or "donor cell" or "+ strain" and a "female cell" or "recipient cell" or "– strain". The donor status or maleness of a cell is determined by the presence in it of a plasmid which codes for special fimbriae, called "sex pili". This plasmid is called fertility factor (F factor) or sex factor or transfer factor. It contains genetic information necessary for the synthesis of sex pilus or F pilus. Cells carrying F factor are called F^+ cells and cells without F factor are called F^- cells.

When F^+ and F^- cells are mixed together ($F^+ \times F^-$ cross), the end of the F^+ sex pilus binds to a nearby F^- cell and then retracts, pulling the F^- and F^+ cells into close contact. A conjugation tube is formed between two cells by sex pilus. The plasmid DNA (F factor) replicates and a copy of it passes from the F^+ cell into F^- cell, through conjugation tube. As a result, the recipient acquires donor status and can in turn conjugate with other female (– strain) cells. In this way, the conjugation process can continue until all the F^- cells in the culture are converted. In an $F^+ \times F^-$ cross, it is usually only the donor's F plasmid that moves to the F^- cell, and do not transfer any chromosomal genes.

Genetic mapping by interrupted mating is one of the most powerful genetic tools of conjugation. It is the most common mode of spread of drug resistance among Gram negative bacilli.

Sexduction

In conjugation F^+ cells can transmit only F factor to F^+ cells and do not transmit any chromosomal genes. However, there are exceptions. Certain F^+ cells can transfer chromosomal genes to F^- cells at rates atleast 1000 times greater than normal F^+ cells. These special donor cells are called "High-frequency recombination (Hfr) cells". They are F^+ cells in which the F plasmid has become integrated into the bacterial chromosome and replicates synchronously with it.

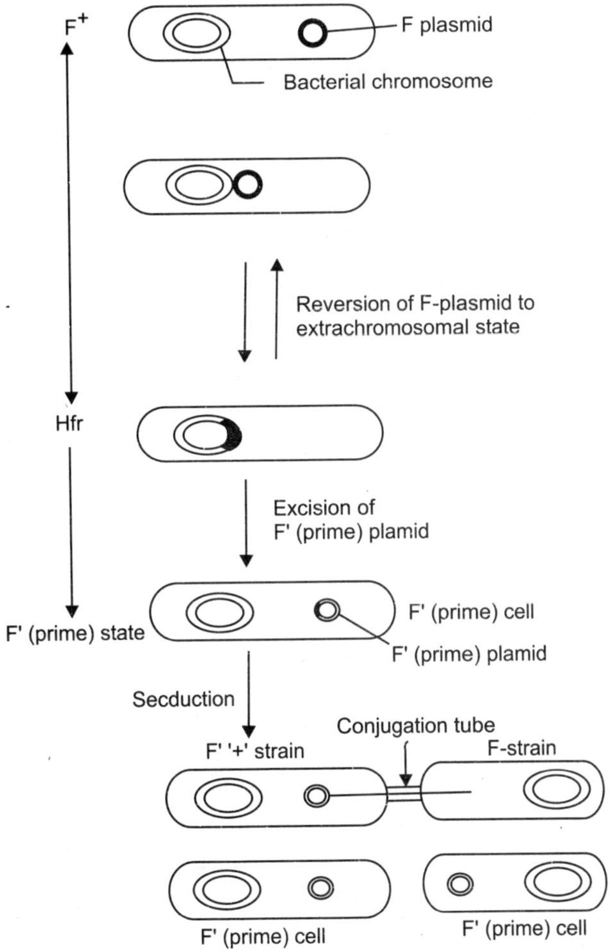

Fig. 16.7. F^+ to Hfr interconversion and sexduction.

F factor usually exists in free independent state in F^+ cells. But in some F^+ cells it is also able to exist in the "integrated state" or "inserted" into the bacterial chromosome. Such cells are able to transfer chromosomal genes with high frequency and are known as "Hfr cells". In Hfr × F^- cross, a single strand of Hfr chromosome is transferred to recipient cell in a linear fashion, sequentially like beads on a string. It takes about 100 minutes to complete strand transfer. However, conjugation may be interrupted by accident before transfer is complete. The donor strand transferred to the recipient cell becomes incorporated into the recipient's chromosome by recombination.

Thus in Hfr × F^- cross, the frequency of gene recombination is high, but the transfer of F plasmid itself low; and most recipient cells remain F^- cells after conjugation with Hfr cells.

The conversion of F^+ cell into Hfr state is reversible. When the F plasmid reverts from the integrated to the free state, it may sometimes carry with it some chromosomal genes from the bacterial chromosome. Such F factor possessing some chromosomal genes is called "F prime factor" of "F′ factor" and the cells are "F prime cells" or "F′ cell".

When F′ cell mates with a recipient, it transfers, alongwith the F plasmid, the host chromosomal genes incorporated with it. This process of transfer of host genes through the F factor, resembles transduction, and has, therefore, been called "sexduction".

Transduction

Transduction is a process where DNA is transferred from cell to cell through the agency of bacteriophages. In other words, it is a method of gene transfer in which a virus (phage) acts as a vehicle for carrying DNA from a donor bacterium to recipient bacterium.

Viruses that attach (infect) bacteria are called bacteriophages or simply phages. A phage consists of a nucleic acid, usually DNA, surrounded by a protein coat to form a head and a tail that helps the phage to attach to the surface of a susceptible host bacterium. After the phage injects its DNA into the host cell, the phage DNA is replicated rapidly, which then directs the synthesis of new phage proteins. The DNA and proteins, then assemble to form daughter phages, which are released due to the lysis of host bacterium.

During the assembly of phage progeny inside the bacterial cell, "packaging errors" may occur; a fragment of bacterial DNA may be incorporated into daughter phage head instead of the phage DNA. Any phage carrying such bacterial DNA is called "transducing phage", because, if it infects another bacterium, it injects the bacterial DNA fragment into the new host. Because the transducing phages do not contain all the viral DNA, they do not kill the new host cell. The DNA fragment can then undergo recombination with the new host's chromosome. Thus, the second bacterial host acquires one or more genes from the first host. Besides chromosomal genes, plasmids can also be transferred to recipient cells via phages. The plasmids coding for the synthesis of penicillinase (β-lactamase), that provide drug resistance to penicillin in Staphylococci are transferred from cell to cell by transduction.

Transduction is the most wide spread mechanism of gene transfer among prokaryotes and provides an excellent tool for the genetic mapping of bacteria. Transduction is especially useful for determining the order and location of genes that are closely linked, since interrupted mating (conjugation) experiments do not permit separation of genes that are very close together. Transduction has been proposed as a method of genetic engineering in the treatment of some inborn errors of metabolism. The metabolic defects in fibroblasts from galactosaemic patients can be corrected by transduction using the lambda phage carrying the "gal" gene. Transduction may be seen occasionally in eukaryotes also. Transduction may be generalised or specialized.

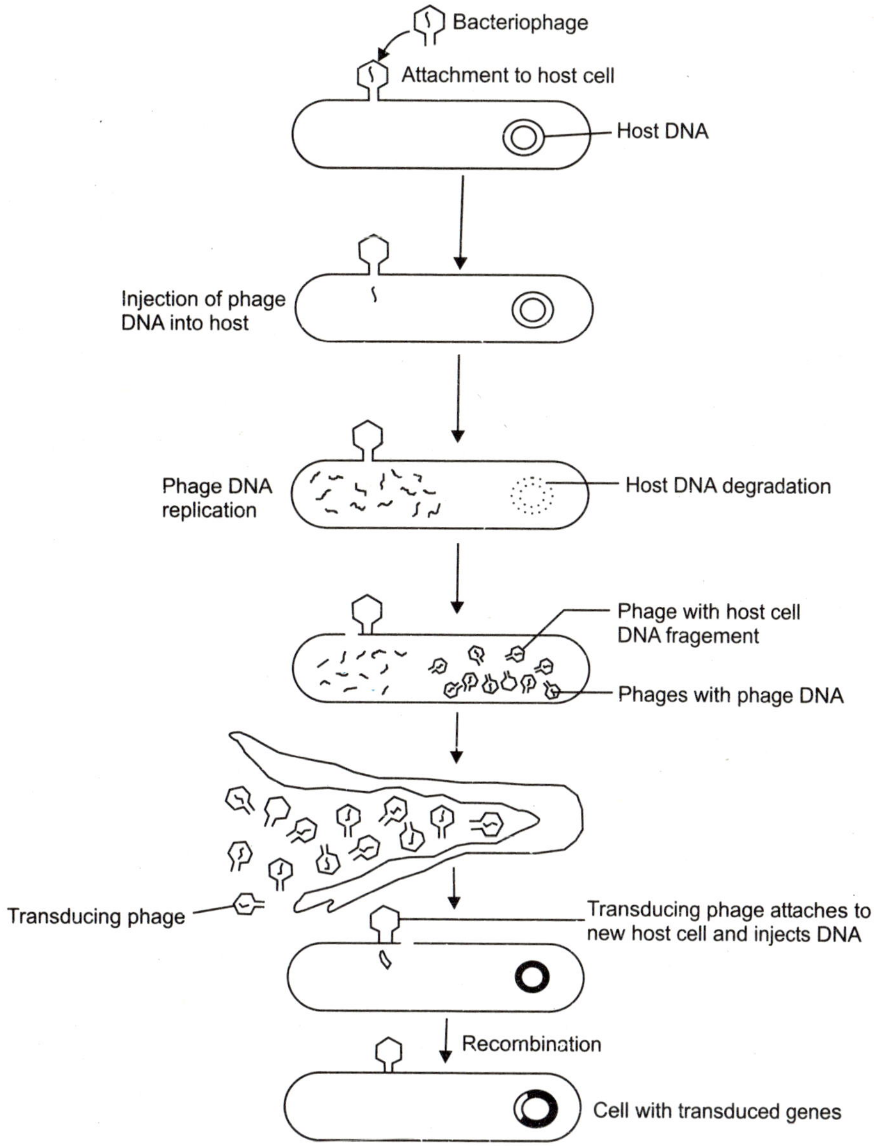

Fig. 16.8. Transduction.

Generalised transduction. Phage particle can transduce any fragment of the host DNA randomly. Generalized transducing bacteriophages can transduce chromosomal genes as well as plasmids. *e.g.,* penicillinase gene in *Staphylococci* is located on a plasmid and may be transferred to other Staphylococcal cells by generalised transduction.

Specialized or restricted transduction. When a specific bacteriophage transduces only a particular genetic trait. Specialized transduction is generally limited to genes near the attachment site of temperate phages. *e.g.,* transduction of the gal gene or bio gene by the temperate lambda (λ) phage of *E.coli*. The phage DNA is inserted at a certain position in *E.coli* chromosome between the "gal" gene (for galactose utilization) and "bio" gene (for biotin synthesis). During excision, the prophage can carry alongwith it, the adjacent host chromosomal genes, either 'gal' or 'bio' and transfer these genes to other bacterial cells. This phenomenon is called restricted or specialized transduction.

Abortive transduction. The transduced DNA fragment may present in a circular form in the cytoplasm, extrachromosomally. It may be protected from nucleases by host protein cover. It can not replicate and is, therefore, segregated to one daughter cell at each division. This state is known as abortive transduction; this state can persist for several generations.

Lysogeny or Lysogenic Conversion or Phage Conversion

Bacteriophages exhibit two types of life cycle.

1. ***Virulent or lytic cycle*** – large number of progeny phages are built up inside the host bacterium, which ruptures to release them.

2. ***Temperate or nonlytic cycle*** –The host bacterium is unharmed. The phage DNA becomes integrated with the bacterial chromosome, known as "prophage", which multiplies synchronously with the host DNA and is transferred to daughter cells. This process is called "lysogeny" and bacteria harbouring prophages are called lysogenic bacteria.

Lysogeny is extremely frequent in nature. In lysogenic bacteria, the prophage behaves as an additional fragment of the bacterial chromosome, coding for new characters. This process by which the prophage confers genetic information to a bacterium is called "lysogenic conversion" or "phage conversion". *e.g.,* diphtheria bacilli acquire toxigenicity on lysogenic conversion with beta phage. Elimination of the phage, renders it nontoxigenic.

Lysogeny is same as specialized transduction.

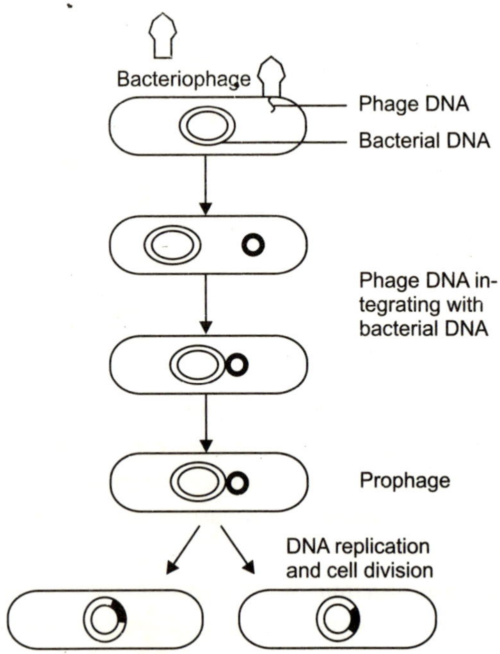

Fig. 16.9. Lysogeny.

The lambda phage DNA is inserted at a certain position in *E.coli* chromosome between the "gal" gene (for galactose utilization) and " bio" gene (for biotin synthesis). During excision, the prophage can carry alongwith it the adjacent host chromosomal genes, either 'gal' or 'bio' and transfer these genes to other bacterial cells. This phenomenon is called restricted or specialized transduction as the transducing phage can transfer only specific genes adjacent to its site of attachment in the host DNA.

A lysogenized bacterial cell can be cured of its prophage by superinfection with a heteroimmune phage which results in the excision of the prophage.

Transposition

Transposable elements are pieces of specific sequences of DNA that move from one genetic element to another, from one plasmid to other or within the chromosome or plasmid to chromosome or vice versa. Because of the ability of transposable elements to insert into a large number of sites both on the chromosome and on plasmids, they are popularly called "jumping genes", and this phenomenon is known as transposition.

When a transposable element is inserted into target DNA, base sequences in target DNA are altered that leads to mutations; or during transposition genes may be carried from one genetic element to other. Thus transposition is a mode of gene transfer, which may confer drug resistance.

BIOTECHNOLOGY

The term biotechnology is schematically explained underneath –

Biological sciences + Chemical sciences = Biochemistry

Biological sciences + Engineering = Bioengineering

Chemical sciences + Engineering = Chemical engineering

Biochemistry + Bioengineering + Chemical engineering = Biotechnology.

Biotechnology is defined as "application of scientific and engineering principles to the processing of materials by biological agents to provide goods and services".

In this definition we refer to "scientific and engineering principles" means, it covers wide range of subjects like biology, biochemistry, chemistry, engineering sciences. Similarly biological agents refer to microbes, enzymes, plants and animal cells. The concept of "materials" include organic and inorganic materials. "Goods and services" means products like medicines, antibiotics, vaccines, antibodies, proteins, hormones etc., and services include medicine, diagnostics, agriculture, veterinary, waste treatments, pollution control, leaching of minerals etc.

There are several methods in biotechnology. Among them the following three are important.

1. Genetic engineering or gene cloning or recombinant DNA technology.
2. Cell culture or tissue culture and organ culture.
3. DNA (Genetic) finger printing.

GENETIC ENGINEERING *OR* GENE CLONING *OR* RECOMBINANT DNA TECHNOLOGY

The basic steps in producing a genetically engineered bacterium are as follows:

1. Isolation of genes from donor DNA by

(*a*) Shotgun method – by using restriction endonucleases

(*b*) Obtaining from mRNA by hybridization method or reverse transcriptase method.

(*c*) Making an artificial gene. An artificial insulin gene was already made in this manner.

2. Plasmid DNA is isolated to serve as the "carrier" or "vector" for the particular gene. Bacteriophages (*e.g.*, Lambda phage) can also be used as vectors.

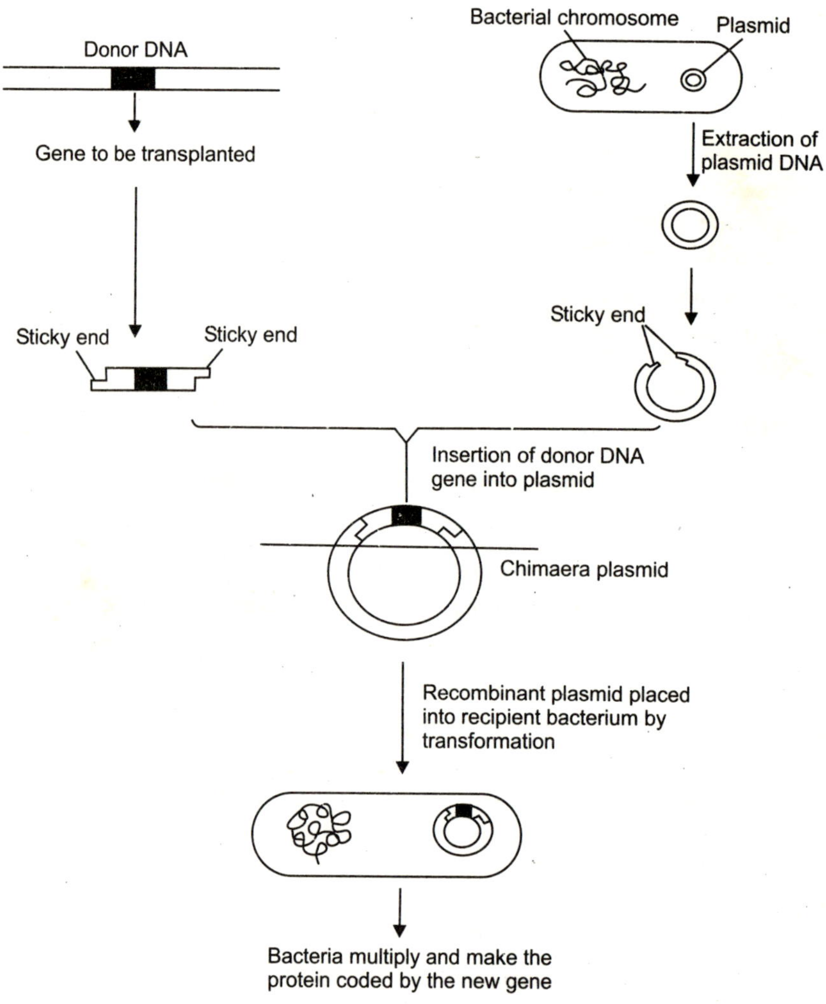

Fig. 16.10. General scheme of genetic engineering

In isolating plasmid DNA, the outer membrane of host bacterium is first dissolved by detergent so that DNA is released. The plasmids are separated from chromosomal DNA by placing in cesium chloride and ethidium bromide by using "density gradient centrifugation" in an ultra centrifuge.

3. Plasmid DNA is subjected to the action of same restriction enzymes. Since both donor DNA and plasmid DNA are treated with the same enzyme, a "restriction endonuclease", that cleaves or cuts the DNA in such a way as to form complementary single-stranded ends ("sticky ends"). These ends are capable of joining to other fragments of DNA having the same complementary single-stranded ends.

4. Foreign DNA or isolated genes from donor are mixed with plasmid DNA (vector) fragments. The sticky ends of the donor DNA joins with sticky ends of plasmid DNA by hydrogen bonding, thus

forming a modified plasmid which now carries the donor DNA fragment, known as "chimaera plasmids" or "recombinant DNA".

Although the sticky ends can join, the structure is fragile, because the breaks in the sugar-phosphate backbone still remain. Another enzyme called "**DNA ligase**" together with ATP forms covalent bonds between sugar-phosphate linkages.

5. The recombinant chimaera plasmids are placed or inserted into recipient bacteria, usually by transformation. *E.coli* is the most important bacterium used as cloning organism in genetic engineering. Yeasts are safer than *E.coli* for recombinant DNA studies, because they do not live in humans and are not pathogenic to man. But, most bacteria do not readily take up plasmid DNA. However, $CaCl_2$ transformation is very effective.

The recipient cells are treated with $CaCl_2$ under cold temperature 0–4°C for *E.coli*, adding chimaera plasmids, and then heating the recipient cells (to 42°C for 2 – 5 min. for *E.coli*), suddenly, in order to heat-shock them. This alters bacterial permeability, allowing the recombinant DNA to enter the cells. Electric shock treatment also makes the cells to take up the plasmid DNA.

6. To identify the recipient bacteria that have acquired the chimaera plasmid, antibiotics are used. Genes for resistance to antibiotics such as tetracycline and ampicillin are often present in a plasmid. If the recipient bacteria are initially sensitive to those antibiotics, then only those cells that have acquired chimaera plasmids will become antibiotic-resistant.

When the mixture of plasmid containing and plasmid lacking bacteria is spread on to agar media containing the antibiotics, only the bacteria that contain the chimaera plasmid will be able to form colonies.

7. Once colonies of plasmid containing bacteria that either have the gene or can make the product of the transplanted gene are identified; cells are inoculated on agar medium and upon incubation form colonies, which contain large population of identical cells, called a "clone", in which the new gene is present in every cell. Thus, the new gene is inherited, called a "cloned gene". Since, a plasmid is the vehicle, by which the new gene is placed into recipient bacterial cell, the plasmid is called a "cloning vector". Some times bacteriophages are used as "cloning vectors", when yeast cells are used as recipients.

For certain plasmids, exposure to low levels of antibiotic chloramphenicol results in uncontrolled plasmid replication so that many copies of recombinant plasmid DNA can be made per bacterial cell. Such abnormal enhanced replication of plasmids is called "amplification". The result is that larger amounts of the product of a cloned gene can be made per bacterial cell.

8. Finally, it is essential to identify the recipient bacteria that express the gene to make a particular gene product. For example, if the gene of interest is the one for human insulin; a small amount of the same is injected into a rabbit to produce antibodies. These antibodies can be purified from the rabbit's serum and labelled with radioactive isotope. They can be used to identify the colonies of bacteria, as they bind to insulin produced by bacteria and can be detected by an instrument that measures radioactivity.

APPLICATIONS OF GENETIC ENGINEERING

Genetic engineering has a wide range of applications for the welfare of mankind.

I. Medical Applications

Recombinant DNA technology is useful in the production of

1. Hormones – *e.g.*, Human insulin, growth hormone, thymosin alpha–1 (effective against brain and lung cancer) and beta endorphin (pain killer produced by the brain).
2. Vaccines – *e.g.*, Hepatitis B vaccine, rabies vaccine, foot and mouth disease vaccine.

3. Enzymes – *e.g.*, Streptokinase or urokinase (used to dissolve blood clots).
4. Monoclonal antibodies by the production of hybridomas.
5. Biologically active substances such as interferon, interleukin-II, tumor necrosis factor, clotting factor VIII, erythropoietin.
6. **Gene therapy** – It aims at inserting one or few genes into target tissues such as bone marrow or chromosomes by using plasmids or Retroviruses as vectors. Many genetic disorders like hemophilia, phenyl ketonuria, sickle cell anemia, thalassemia, alkaptoneuria, galactosemia etc., which are due to defective genes can be cured by replacing with correct genes.
7. Beer for diabetics.

II. Environmental Applications

Genetically modified microorganisms can be used for degradation of wastes in sewage, biological waste treatment processes and pollution control industries. They can be used in leaching minerals such as copper from low grade ores in mining and also in the exploration and recovery of oil and petroleum products.

A strain of *Pseudomonas* sp. is produced by genetic engineering by placing several plasmids into it. This "multiplasmid organism" can eat crude oil and can be used as oil spill scavanger.

III. Industrial Applications

Microorganisms can be modified by gene cloning for increased production of enzymes, vitamin C (ascorbic acid), ethylene oxide (for making plastics), ethylene glycol (antifreeze), organic acids, alcohol etc.

IV. Agricultural Applications

Genetic engineering techniques are used in agriculture

1. to increase soil fertility by cloning nitrogen fixation genes (Nif genes) into soil microbes or plants.

2. to protect fruits against frost damage.

3. to control plant diseases by developing plants with resistance to insects, pests and microbial pathogens.

4. to develop biopesticides and biofertilizers.

V. Food Processing

Genetically modified microorganisms are used for the production of single cell protein (SCP) from algae and yeasts, that are rich in proteins.

Different varieties of yeast *Saccharomyces* have been improved to produce calorie beer for diabetics.

VI. Fundamental Understanding of Biological Processes

Genetic engineering techniques have been used for acquiring basic knowledge about biological processes like gene structure, gene regulation, gene expression, gene mapping, cell differentiation and integration of viral genomes. This could lead to the better understanding of genetics of microbes, humans, animals and plants.

The human cell contains thousands of genes. At present, the exact location and function of vast majority of the genes is not known. Human genes can be introduced into *E.coli*, one at a time and the bacterium could be made to reproduce on large scale. This will provide millions of copies of individual genes and enable a detailed analysis of their structure and function.

Many of the genes of Drosophila have been isolated and identified by this method.

VII. Biological Warfare

Recombinant DNA methods offer horrible new possibilities for efficient creation and widespread use of biological weapons. Bacterial toxins such as botulinum toxin or highly virulent forms of existing diseases (anthrax, cholera, plague, small pox etc.) can be produced to use on enemy countries.

RESTRICTION ENDONUCLEASES (Molecular scissors)

Restriction endonucleases are enzymes produced by bacteria, that identify and destroy foreign DNA, that might enter a cell, particularly bacteriophages. These enzymes are sometimes known as "gene shears".

Restriction enzymes produced by bacteria, do not act on the DNA of their own cell, because some parallel enzymes produced by the cell, keep on adding methyl groups to specific adenine or cytosine residues to recognize self-DNA. This process is known as "DNA-modification".

Restriction enzymes are broadly of three types. The type I and type III enzymes recognize and bind to specific base sequences and cut the DNA at a site away from the point of attachment, the distance of break being either definite (type III) or unpredictable (type I).

Type II enzymes are most useful in genetic engineering experiments. They recognize certain sites of DNA, consisting short, specific nucleotide sequences of 4 to 6 base pairs with palindromic sequences *i.e.,* a sequence of nucleotide bases that can be read same in both the 3′ to 5′ and 5′ to 3′ direction; and makes a cut in deoxyribose-phosphate back bones of both DNA strands, like a pair of scissors cutting a piece of tape. Hence, these restriction enzymes are represented as "scissors" in diagrams.

Restriction endonucleases recognize and cleave at specific sites on DNA. This cleavage positions may be "even" or "staggered".

In "even cleavage" the cuts on the two strands at the same position, exactly opposite each other, resulting in DNA fragments with blunt ends or non-sticky ends.

In "staggered cleavage", the cuts on each strand are in a different position or the cuts are staggered so that the cleaved DNA molecule has two single-stranded ends, known as sticky ends or cohesive ends. Such DNA is called "sticky-ended DNA" and these complementary single-stranded ends can join by hydrogen bonds, but the resulting structure is fragile, because the breaks in the sugar-phosphate back bone still remain. Another enzyme, called "DNA ligase", together with ATP as an energy source, connects or ligates these broken sugar-phosphate linkages.

Restriction endonucleases are important tools in molecular biology, particularly in genetic engineering. *e.g.,* Eco RI, Hin d-III, Hae-III.

DNA FINGERPRINTING

This technique is now widely used in research and a variety of legal situations to help identify individuals

1. to identify criminals in forensic science.
2. to determine paternity.
3. to study genetic variations among populations.

4. to diagnose various hereditary and infectious diseases.

DNA fingerprinting can be done with minute quantities of DNA; for example, from a single strand of hair, a drop of semen, a spot of blood, saliva residue on cigarette butts; from these specimens, DNA can be amplified by PCR and used in DNA fingerprinting.

In each person, certain DNA segments contain base sequences that are repeated several times. Both the number of repeat copies in one region and the number of regions subject to repeat are different from one person to another. Except for identical twins, the chance that two people would have the same DNA fingerprint is about 1 in 10 billion.

In DNA fingerprinting a technique called "Restriction Fragment Length Polymorphism (RFLP)" is used. The technology includes following steps:

1. Extraction of DNA (from blood, amniotic fluid, hair, semen etc.).

2. The DNA is cut into fragments by using restriction endonucleases.

3. The DNA fragments are then separated by gel electrophoresis.

4. Then specific base sequences in DNA fragments are identified by using radioactive isotope labelled DNA probes of known base sequence.

5. DNA probes pair with complementary base sequences. These are then subjected to autoradiography to set band like pattern called DNA fingerprints.

6. Such DNA fingerprints are compared to identify criminals or to solve disputed paternity etc.

RESTRICTION FRAGMENT LENGTH POLYMORPHISM (RFLP)

Refers to inherited differences in sites for restriction enzymes (for example, caused by base changes in the target site) that result in differences in the lengths of the fragments produced by cleavage with the relevant restriction enzyme. RFLPs are used for genetic mapping to link the genome directly to a conventional genetic marker. It is widely used in DNA fingerprinting to solve paternity dispute.

POLYMERASE CHAIN REACTION (PCR)

PCR is an invitro DNA amplification method for producing large amounts of DNA (unlimited number of copies of DNA) from very tiny initial quantities of DNA, impossible to detect by routine methods. The PCR technique involves a repeated cycling process composed of 3 stages.

1. Denaturation – Double-stranded DNA is heated at 90 – 95°C for 60 seconds to form two single stranded DNAs.

2. Annealing – Specific oligonucleotide primers (15 – 22 bases) are added by reducing temperature to 40 – 50°C. They are allowed to react for 60 – 120 seconds so that they bind (hybridize) to their complementary bases on single stranded DNA.

Oligonucleotide primers used in PCR are chemically; synthesized sequences of polynucleotides, complementary to DNA sequences to be amplified.

3. Extension of annealed primers at 72°C for 60 – 180 seconds by sequential addition of nucleotides at 3′ end by DNA polymerase. Usually Taq polymerase, a heat stable DNA polymerase is used. It is produced by a thermophilic bacterium, *Thermus aquaticus* found in hot springs that produce enzymes resistant to high temperature.

These three steps constitute one cycle and generally 25 to 50 cycles are performed, using an automated thermal device which is usually completed within 3 to 4 hours. The product of first cycle becomes template for next cycle. By the third cycle double stranded DNA molecules, whose ends are defined by the two oligonucleotides, begin to appear and accumulate exponentially. By the twenty-fifth cycle, millions of copies are formed.

Large amounts of DNA can be produced from minute amounts present in water, food, blood, hair, semen, saliva and clinical samples taken from patients.

PCR has several applications in basic research. Forensic (legal) medicine, clinical diagnosis, immunology and in molecular biology and human genetics

1. to study the structure of genome and DNA sequencing

2. to detect mutations, polymorphisms, gene defects, tumor cell markers.

3. in the early diagnosis of infectious diseases to detect and identify viral and bacterial pathogens, genetic disorders and cancer.

4. to obtain large amounts of DNA for subsequent analysis, as in forensic science.

5. to obtain genetic mapping of genes.

6. in immunology widely used to characterize HLA, T-cell receptors, antibody diversity and quantification of lymphokines.

7. used in epidemiological, phylogenetic and developmental studies.

TRANSPOSABLE ELEMENTS *OR* JUMPING GENES *OR* GENES WITH MOBILITY

Transposable elements are pieces (specific sequences) of DNA that move from one genetic element to another, from one plasmid to other or within the chromosome or plasmid to chromosome or vice versa. They do not exist as separate entities within the bacterial cell because do not contain information for self replication and depend on chromosomal or plasmid DNA. Thus they must either be incorporated into a plasmid or the chromosome. Transposable elements were first discovered by Barbara McClintock (1930) in Maize. They are found widely in bacteria.

Transposable elements are of two types : 1. Insertion sequences (IS), 2. Transposons. They differ in size and gene content.

Insertion sequences. They are small (1–2 Kb) consisting a central coding sequence and flanking short, inverted repeat sequences at either end. They contain genes that encode for information required for movement among plasmids and chromosomes and for replicative recombination. Usually they do not alter phenotype of the cell.

Transposon. They are larger (4 – 25 Kb) composite elements contain genes for movement as well as genes that encode for various functions such as drug resistance and toxin production. They can alter the phenotype of the cell. Transposons contain one or more genes in the centre, and the two ends carrying very long "inverted repeat" sequences of nucleotides, *i.e.,* nucleotide sequences complementary to each other but in the reverse order. Because of this, transposons can form a single stranded loop carrying the gene, and a double-stranded stem formed by hydrogen bonds between the terminal inverted repeat sequences.

Bacteriophage mu is a large transposable element and inserts in many sites on *E.coli* chromosome. Because of the ability of transposable elements to insert into a large number of sites both on the chromosome and on plasmids, they are popularly called "jumping genes", and this phenomenon is known as **"transposition".**

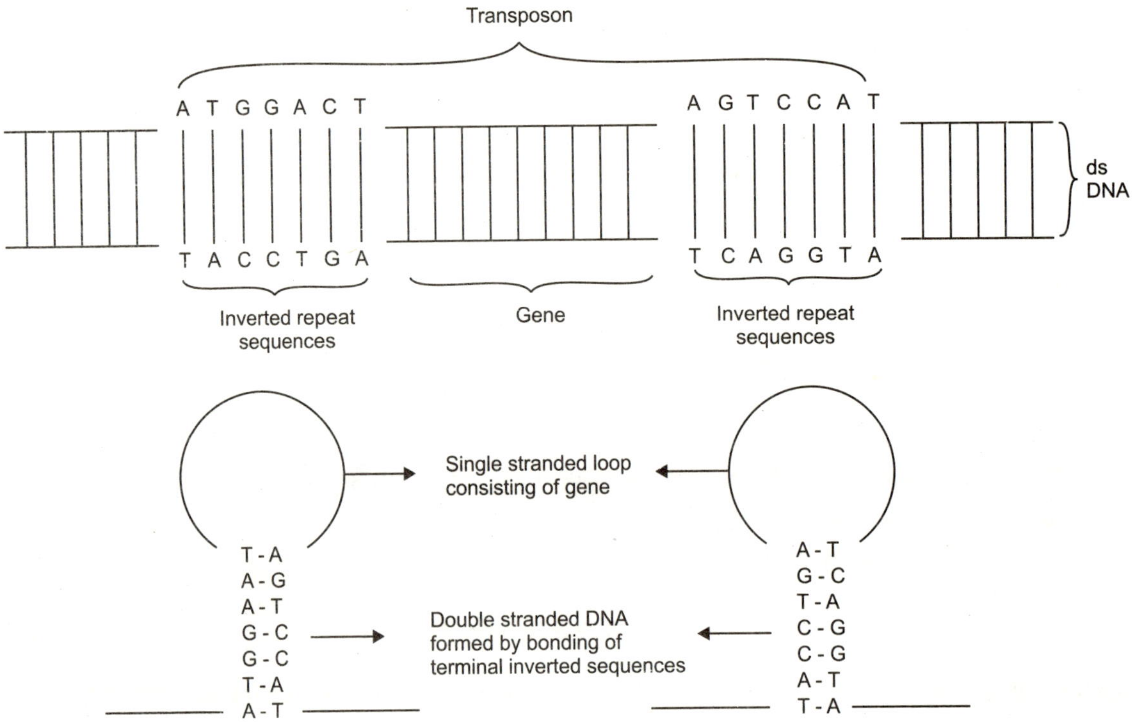

Fig. 16.11. Transposon.

There are two distinct mechanisms of transposition-conservative and replicative. In conservative transposition the transposable element is excised from one location in the chromosome and becomes reinserted at a second location in the same chromosome. The copy number therefore remains unchanged. In replicative transposition, the transposable element is duplicated and inserted at another location in the chromosome. Thus one copy of transposing element remains at the original site and another copy is found at the new site.

Transposition requires an enzyme "transposase" which is coded by IS and transposons and may also be coded by the chromosome, plasmid or phage to which transposable element is inserted.

When a transposable element is inserted into target DNA, base sequences in target DNA are altered that leads to polar mutations, due to deletion, duplication, inversion and other alterations besides disturbance in chromosomal DNA.

BLOTTING TECHNIQUES

Blotting techniques are very sensitive and specific and have become important tools in both molecular biology and clinical research. The tests are based on nucleic acid hybridization and are used to identify DNA, RNA and proteins.

Three main blotting techniques are developed and one more under development

1. Southern blotting to identify DNA.
2. Northern blotting to identify RNA.
3. Western blotting to identify proteins.
4. Eastern blotting to identify lipids and fats.

Southern Blotting Technique

It is named after E.M. Southern, who first discovered it. It has a wide application in DNA analysis. It is a DNA–DNA hybridisation technique used to identify DNA fragments by hybridisation with DNA probes. In other words, it can be used to identify the location of a single gene on chromosomal DNA. The technique consists of following steps.

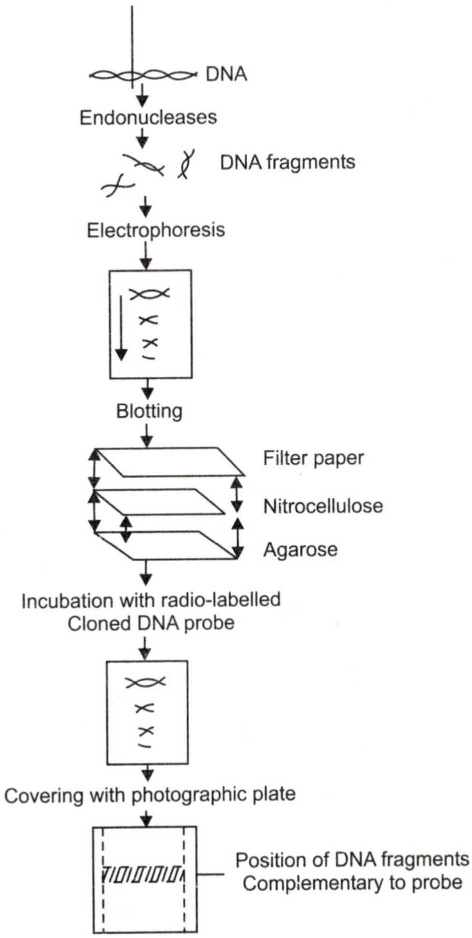

Fig. 16.12. Southern blotting.

1. Fragments of DNA are produced from chromosomes by using restriction endonucleases, which cleave DNA at specific sites.

2. The DNA fragments are subjected to electrophoresis on agarose gel, so that they are separated based on their size; the smaller DNA fragments migrate farthest.

3. The DNA bands in the gel are denatured into single strands by using alkaline solution.

4. The electrophersis gel is then covered with a sheet of nitrocellulose or nylon membrane, on to which DNA fragments are transferred and immobilised or blotted.

5. This nitrocellulose membrane with absorbed DNA fragments is treated and incubated with radioactive isotope labelled single stranded DNA probe. These will hybridise with homologous DNA to form radioactive double-stranded DNA probes, which can be detected by autoradiography.

Zooblot. It is a technique which uses southern blotting to test the ability of a DNA probe from one species to hybridize with the DNA from the genomes of a variety of other species.

Northern Blotting Technique

It is used to identify RNA (messenger RNA) by hybridisation with labelled DNA or RNA probes. With this method the transcripts of specific genes can be studied and measured.

Since, it is an analogous procedure for the analysis of RNA, and patterned after southern blot it has been called "northern blotting" as opposite to southern blotting.

Here the RNA (mRNA) mixture is separated, according to size by gel electrophoresis and then transferred and immobilized or blotted on nitrocellulose membrane or on a chemically reactive paper prepared by diazotization with aminobenzyloxymethyl paper. RNA fragments that bind to this membrane or paper can be hybridized with radiolabelled DNA, which can be detected by autoradiography.

Western Blotting Technique

This technique is used to identify proteins (antigens) by using specific antibodies as analytical probes. Thus, nucleic acid probes are not used in this method. The sources of antibody probes may be serum from patients with known infections or purified polyclonal antibody preparations or monoclonal antibodies.

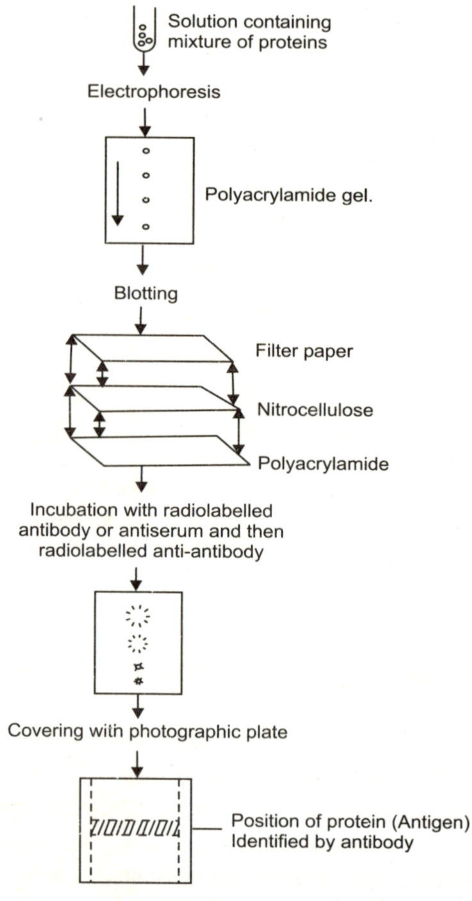

Fig. 16.13. Western blotting.

Since this test is used for the identification of protein antigens, it is known as "immunoblotting" or "western blotting" in conformity with other blotting techniques.

Protein antigen mixture is first separated into its components by polyacrylamide gel electrophoresis, and then blotted on to nitrocellulose membrane. It is then incubated with specific antibody. This primary antibody binds to its target protein antigen and is immobilised on the nitrocellulose blotting support.

This antigen-antibody complex can then be identified with radioactive or enzyme labelled antibodies (anti-antibody) to primary antibodies, and can then be visualised by autoradiography. If required the labelled anti-antibody can be removed and the protein antigens can be studied further.

Western blot test is very popular as a confirmatory test for AIDS.

Eastern Blotting Test

It is used for the identification of lipids and fats. The technique is under development.

PLASMIDS *OR* EPISOMES *OR* EXTRA CHROMOSOMAL GENETIC ELEMENTS

Plasmids are small, circular, covalently closed, double-stranded DNA molecules found in cytoplasm. They are self-replicating extrachromosomal genetic elements, that reproduce themselves and are thus conserved, apart from chromosome, through successive cell divisions, and segregate into daughter cells.

Some plasmids are capable of replicating autonomously as well as integrating into the chromosome. They are known as episomes *e.g.,* F-factor.

Plasmids can be detected and isolated by gel electrophoresis and electron microscope. Plasmids can be extracted from bacterial cells by treating them with certain chemicals or dyes such as sodium dodecyl sulphate and acridine orange or with high temperature. Cells thus treated are said to be "cured". For example, *E.coli* can be cured by using the dye acridine orange. Quinolones are also used to cure plasmids.

Plasmids are widely distributed among various species of bacteria and in some yeasts. They are not essential for the normal life of the bacteria, but confer on it certain survival advantages such as toxigenicity, drug resistance etc.

Functions Encoded by Plasmids

By all plasmids

1. Self-replication

By some plasmids

2. Self-transfer
3. Resistance to antimicrobial agents
   (*a*) Antibiotics *e.g.,* Penicillin, streptomycin, kanamycin, neomycin, tetracycline, chloramphenicol.
   (*b*) Synthetic chemotherapeutic agents *e.g.,* sulfa drugs and trimethoprim.
   (*c*) Heavy metals *e.g.,* Mercury, silver, cadmium.
4. Toxin production
5. Enterotoxin production
6. Pigment production
7. Antibiotic production
8. Bacteriocin production

9. H_2S production
10. Urease production
11. Catabolic functions *e.g.*, degradation of lactose, octane, xylene, camphor, toluene, naphthalene etc.
12. Phage sensitivity and resistance
13. Nitrogen fixation
14. Induction of plant tumors
15. Host controlled restriction and modification.

Plasmids are divided into two broad categories.

Conjugative Plasmids or Transmissible Plasmids

Plasmids containing information for self-transfer to another cell by conjugation are called conjugative or transmissible plasmids. They are usually large (about 60–120 Kb) and undergo stringent multiplication so that they are maintained at one or two copies per cell. In addition to self-transfer, these plasmids encode genes for autonomous replication as well as a variety of other properties such as toxin production, bacteriocin production, drug resistance etc.

Examples of conjugative plasmids include F-factor, R-factor, Col-factor etc. They are commonly found in Gram negative bacilli such as *E.coli, Klebsiella, Shigella, Salmonella, Proteus* etc.

Non-Conjugative Plasmids or Non-Transmissible Plasmids

They are usually small (1.5 to 15 Kb), undergo relaxed multiplication, so that, multiple copies (10–20 per cell) are maintained per cell. They lack the functions of self-transfer by conjugation; although they may be transferred by co-operative action of conjugative plasmids. They may be transmitted from one cell to another by transformation or transduction through the agency of bacteriophages. All Staphylococcal plasmids are non-transmissible and non-conjugative. The plasmid for penicillinase (β-lactamase) is transmitted from cell to cell by transduction.

F-factor or Sex factor or Transfer factor or F-plasmid

F-factors were the first plasmids to be discovered by Hayes. F-factor is a transfer factor that contains the basic genetic information for extrachromosomal existence, self-transfer by conjugation and for the synthesis of sex pilus (F-pilus), but does not contain other genetic markers such as drug resistance gene.

Cells that contain F-factor are called F^+ cells. F-factor codes for the synthesis of sex pilus, which mates with F^- cell by forming a conjugation tube and promotes transfer of plasmid DNA from one bacterium to another, quickly converting F^- population into F^+.

High-frequency recombination (Hfr) strains are bacterial cultures in which the F-factor is stably integrated into the chromosome. Recombinations occur with high frequency in Hfr matings than in F^+ matings.

F prime factors (F′ factor) are rare. F factors excised from Hfr chromosomes alongwith a small segment of the chromosome. These F′ factors transfer chromosomal genes from one cell to another through a process called “sexduction”.

R-factors or R-plasmids or Resistance factors or Resistance transfer factor (RTF)

R-plasmids carry genes (determinants) for resistance to various antibiotics. They are numerous among intestinal Gram negative bacilli and responsible for the spread of multiple drug resistance among them. They are also found in a variety of other organisms. Each antibiotic resistance gene in these R-plasmids codes for an enzyme that destroys or inactivates a particular antibiotic.

Conjugative R-plasmid can confer simultaneous resistance to several antibiotics particularly to frequently used antibiotics such as ampicillin, chloramphenicol, tetracycline, kanamycin and streptomycin; makes it difficult to treat infections successfully.

Indiscriminate use of antibiotics can increase the incidence of antibiotic-resistant bacteria. Transfer of multiple drug resistance was demonstrated between *E.coli* and *Shigella* strains both *in vitro* and *in vivo*. This resistance is plasmid mediated and is transferred by conjugation. This mechanism of drug resistance is known as "infectious or transferable or episomal drug resistance". Bacteria carrying R-factors can be transmitted from animals to man. Hence, indiscriminate use of antibiotics in veterinary practice or in animal feeds can also lead to an increase of multiple drug resistance in the community. Transferable drug resistance is now universal in distribution and involves all antibiotics in common use. Its incidence is directly proportional to the frequency of use of antibiotics in the area.

R-plasmid consists of two components – 1. the resistance transfer factor (RTF), which is responsible for conjugational transfer, and 2. the resistance determinant (r-det) for each of several drugs. Both of them together (RTF + r-det) constitute the whole R-plasmid. R-factor can have several r-determinants, and resistance to as many as eight or more drugs can be transferred simultaneously. Some times, the RTF may dissociate from the r-determinants, and the two components can exist as separate plasmids. In such cases, though the host bacterium remains drug resistant, the resistance is not transferable. The RTF can have determinants other than drug resistance, coding for the synthesis of enterotoxin, hemolysins in some enteropathogenic *E.coli* (EPEC).

Frequently, the drug resistant genes are carried on highly mobile transposons. Transposons are discrete genetic and physical entities able to move (jump) from one position to another or to a new genome. They assort randomly to produce a wide variety of R-factors.

Col-Factor or Colicinogenic Factors or Bacteriocinogenic Plasmids

Bacteriocinogenic plasmids contain a gene that directs the host bacterium to synthesize a bacteriocin-antibiotic like substance which specifically and selectively lethal to other bacteria. A bacterium that forms a particular bacteriocin is not killed by that bacteriocin, although it may be killed by other bacteriocins. Chemically, bacteriocins may be proteins or lipoprotein-polysaccharide complexes or particles resembling a defective phage.

The bacteriocins produced by coliform bacilli are called colicins and the bacteriocinogenic plasmids are called colicinogenic plasmids or col-factors. Similarly, bacteriocins produced by *Pseudomonas pyocyanea* are called pyocins; *Corynebacterium diphtheriae* are called diphthericins; and *Serratia marcescens* are known as marscesins.

Col-factor contains genes that promote self-transfer by conjugation, self-replication and capable of transferring chromosomal segments.

The specificity of bacteriocin action is utilized in intraspecies classification of certain organisms such as *Shigella sonnei* and *Pseudomonas aeruginosa*.

Dissimilation plasmids

Plasmids that code for important degradative or dissimilatory enzymes are called dissimilation plasmids. These plasmids are responsible for certain *Pseudomonas* species to breakdown industrial solvents such as toluene and xylene which are otherwise difficult to degrade.

Bacterial plasmids can also convert harmless mercury compounds in industrial wastes to harmful neurotoxic organomercurial (methyl mercury) compounds.

By genetic engineering, a combination of several plasmids were cloned into *Pseudomonas* sp., so that it can breakdown complex hydrocarbons such as camphor, naphthalene, xylene present in crude oil. These bacteria have potential use for treatment of environments contaminated by oil spills.

Mercury Resistance Plasmids

Plasmids-coded resistance to mercury has been found in *Pseudomonas* and resistance to nickel, cobalt, mercury and arsenate in *E.coli* and *Salmonella*.

Incompatible Plasmids or Inc. Plasmids

Certain pairs of plasmids, for example, F-plasmid and F′-plasmid, cannot be stably replicated in the same bacterial cell. Two such plasmids are said to be "incompatible" and a collection of incompatible plasmids constitute an "incompatibility group", designated as Inc. The plasmids of same incompatibility group are closely related, so this property is used as a system of classification. Some plasmids can replicate only in a few species of closely related, while others have a much broader host range. It is a cause of plasmid immunity.

Cryptic plasmids or silent plasmids are those for which a function has not yet been identified. They confer no phenotype on their host.

Plasmids as Cloning Vectors (Vehicles)

Plasmids are widely employed as vectors or vehicles in cloning genes in recombinant DNA technology, because of the following features.

1. They can be readily isolated from bacterial cells by physical means, because they exist as super coiled circles less readily broken by shearing forces.

2. Possess a single restriction site for one or more restriction enzymes.

3. Insertion of a linear molecule of gene (DNA) at one of these sites does not alter its replication properties.

4. It can be reintroduced into a bacterial cell (recipient) conveniently by transformation and the recipient cells by harbouring recombinant plasmids can be easily selected or identified.

5. They do not occur in nature but are found only in bacterial cells.

PBR 322 is the most widely used plasmid in genetic engineering techniques.

COSMIDS

Cosmids are hybrid vectors derived from the plasmids which contain 'cos' site of lambda phage. Cosmids are constructed from plasmids containing cloned DNA by ligating the lambda phage "cos" (cohesive ends) region to the plasmid DNA. The modified plasmid can then be packaged into lambda phages *in vitro*. Cosmids lack genes for encoding viral proteins.

The advantages of cosmids over plasmids in genetic engineering is that they can be used for cloning large fragments of DNA and phages are more stable than plasmids so that recombinant DNA can be preserved for a long time in gene bank or gene library.

Phasmids. When plasmids are inserted into the genome of lambda phage (λ phage) they are said to be phasmids. They can be used as cloning vectors.

DNA PROBES

Each species will have a unique DNA base sequence, that differentiates it from every other species. If this sequence can be identified and isolated, a chemical label (such as radioactive isotopes) can be attached to it so that this labelled DNA sequence can be used as a probe to detect. Complementary DNA sequences present in a given sample by hybridization reactions.

Hybridization is a process in which two single strands of nucleic acid with complementary base sequences bind together to form a stable double-stranded molecules.

Labelled DNA probes that are specific for particular pathogens can be used to detect and identify pathogen specific DNA present in clinical samples, directly; even without any isolation of pathogen.

DNA probes have already been used to identify a wide variety of pathogens such as viruses, bacteria and parasites. Commercial kits using DNA kits for diagnostic use are available. DNA probes have also been developed to detect and identify specific antibiotic resistance genes, so that antimicrobial sensitivity of an organism can be determined directly from clinical sample, without primary isolation and growth.

QUESTIONS

Essay Type Questions

1. Describe the mechanisms of genetic exchange or gene transfer among bacteria.
2. Describe mutations and their importance in clinical microbiology.

Short Notes

1. Genome.
2. Genomics.
3. Karyotype and idiotype.
4. DNA polymerase.
5. Gene or cistron.
6. Genetic code.
7. Differences between DNA and RNA.
8. Central dogma of molecular biology.
9. Replication of DNA.
10. Gene expression.
11. Regulation or control of gene expression.
12. Operon.
13. Genotype.
14. Phenotype and phenotypic variations.

15. Mutations.
16. Mutagens.
17. Wild strain.
18. Replica plate technique.
19. Penicillin technique.
20. Fluctuation tests.
21. Ames test or the *Salmonella* test or reverse mutation.
22. Transformation or Griffith phenomenon.
23. Bacterial conjugation.
24. Transduction.
25. Specialized transduction.
26. Lysogenic conversion.
27. Transfection.
28. Biotechnology.
29. Describe the principles of genetic engineering or gene cloning or recombinant DNA technology.
30. Applications of genetic engineering.
31. Restriction endonucleases.
32. DNA finger printing.
33. RFLP.
34. Auxotroph.
35. PCR.
36. Transposons or transposable elements or jumping genes or insertion sequences or transposition.
37. Blotting techniques.
38. Southern blotting.
39. Northern blotting.
40. Western blotting.
41. Plasmids or episomes or extrachromosomal genetic elements.
42. R-plasmids.
43. RTF.
44. F-factor.
45. Hfr.
46. Sexduction.
47. F′ cell.
48. Why plasmids are preferred as cloning vectors ?
49. DNA probes.
50. Col factor.

17

Drug Resistance

INTRODUCTION

Strains of microorganisms differ in their degree of susceptibility to antibiotics and chemotherapeutic agents. The susceptibility of an organism to any particular drug may change with time. An organism that had once been highly susceptible to a drug may develop resistance, over time.

BIOLOGICAL RESISTANCE

It refers to changes that result in the organism being less susceptible to a particular drug than has been previously observed.

Biological development of drug resistance is an ongoing process, which may not be detected by laboratory procedures. Microorganisms may undergo marked changes in their levels of biological resistance without notice.

CLINICAL RESISTANCE

When antimicrobial susceptibility has been lost to such an extent that the drug is no longer effective for clinical use; the organism is said to be achieved clinical resistance. Most of the laboratory methods used to detect resistance are meant to detect clinical resistance.

CROSS-RESISTANCE

Microorganisms resistant to a certain drug may also be resistant to other drugs. It is commonly seen among drugs that are closely related chemically.

e.g., Polymyxin-B and colistin, erythromycin and oleandomycin, neomycin and kanamycin.

Cross-resistance may be seen between unrelated chemicals such as erythromycin and lincomycin.

ENVIRONMENTALLY MEDIATED DRUG RESISTANCE

It is defined as resistance that directly results from physical or chemical characteristics of the environment that either directly alter the drug or alter the microorganism's normal physiologic response to the drug.

Environmental factors that mediate resistance include pH, anaerobic atmosphere, cations such as Mg^{++} and Ca^{++}, thymine-thymidine content etc.

Examples. 1. Antimicrobial activity of erythromycin and aminoglycosides diminish with decreasing pH, whereas the activity of tetracycline decreases with increasing pH. Thus, several antibiotics are affected by pH.

2. Inhibition of bacterial protein synthesis by aminoglycosides requires intracellular uptake through cell membrane, driven by oxidative process, so that in the absence of oxygen (anaerobic atmosphere), uptake and hence activity is diminished.

3. Aminoglycoside activity is also affected by the concentration of cations, such as Mg^{++} and Ca^{++}, in the environment. It is most commonly seen with *Pseudomonas aeruginosa.* Aminoglycoside molecules have a net positive charge and most Gram negative bacilli have a net negative charge. The Ca^{++} and Mg^{++} ions found in bacterial environment compete with aminoglycoside molecules for the negatively charged receptor sites on bacterial surface, so that less drug will be taken up and antimicrobial activity diminishes.

Information regarding environmentally mediated resistance is used to standardize testing methods that minimize the impact of environmental factors so that microorganism mediated resistance is more accurately determined.

BIOCHEMICAL MECHANISMS OF DRUG RESISTANCE

There are different mechanisms by which microorganisms exhibit resistance to drugs.

1. Microorganisms may produce enzymes that destroy the active drug. *e.g.,* Staphylococci resistant to penicillin G produce penicillinase (β-lactamase) that destroys the active drug. similarly, Gram negative bacilli resistant to chloramphenicol produce chloramphenicol acetyl transferase enzyme.

2. Microorganisms may change their permeability to the drugs. Microbes may cease active uptake of certain drugs *e.g.,* resistance to tetracyclines and polymyxins. Streptococci have a natural permeability barrier to aminoglycosides. Resistance to amikacin and to some other aminoglycosides may depend on a lack of permeability to the drugs, due to changes in outer membrane that impairs active transport into the cell.

3. Microorganisms develop an altered structural target for the drug. Microbial drug receptor sites may undergo change resulting in decreased antibiotic binding and action *e.g.,* erythromycin-resistant organisms have an altered receptor on the 50S subunit of the ribosome, resulting from methylation of a

23S ribosomal RNA. Chromosomal resistance to aminoglycosides is associated with the loss or alternation of a specific protein in the 30S subunit of the bacterial ribosome that serves as a binding site in susceptible organisms. Resistance to some penicillins may be a function of the loss or alteration of PBPs.

4. Microorganisms develop an altered metabolic pathway that bypasses the reaction inhibited by the drug. *e.g.*, some bacteria have developed resistance to sulphonamides by acquiring the ability to synthesize PABA by utilizing preformed folic acid.

5. Microorganisms develop an altered enzyme that can still perform its metabolic function but is much less affected by the drug than the enzyme in the susceptible organism. *e.g.*, in some sulphonamide-susceptible bacteria, the tetrahydropteroic acid synthetase has a much higher affinity for sulphonamides than for PABA. In sulphonamide resistant bacteria, the tetrahydropteroic acid synthetase has high affinity for PABA than for sulphonamide.

MICROORGANISM MEDIATED DRUG RESISTANCE

Microorganism mediated drug resistance can be divided into two categories

1. Intrinsic or inherent or natural resistance.
2. Acquired resistance.

Intrinsic resistance

Drug resistance resulting from the normal genetic, structural or physiologic state of microorganism is referred to as "Intrinsic resistance". It is natural, inherited characteristic that is usually associated with a species or genus or a group of strains. Therefore, this is a predictable resistance of a particular organism.

Intrinsic resistance profiles are useful 1. as markers in the identification of certain bacteria, 2. to determine which drug should be tested against a particular organism.

Table 17.1 Examples of intrinsic resistance

Natural (Intrinsic) resistance	***Mechanism***
Anaerobic bacteria versus aminoglycosides	Lack of oxidative metabolism to drive uptake of aminoglycosides
Gram positive bacteria versus aztreonam (β-lactam)	Lack of penicillin binding proteins (PBPs)
Gram negative bacteria versus vancomycin	Lack of uptake due to inability of vancomycin to penetrate outer membrane
Pseudomonas aeruginosa versus sulphonamides, trimethoprim, tetracycline, chloramphenicol	Lack of uptake due to inability of antibiotics to achieve effective intracellular concentrations
Klebsiella sp. versus ampicillin (β-lactam)	Production of β-lactamases that destroy the drug
Aerobic bacteria versus metronidazole	Inability to anaerobically reduce drug to its active form.

Acquired resistance

Drug resistance that results from altered cellular physiology and structure caused by changes in a microorganism's genetic makeup is known as acquired resistance. It is a character associated with only some strains and unpredictable and that's why laboratory methods to detect resistance are necessary.

Acquired resistance mechanisms are all genetically encoded and may be acquired by

1. Mutations.

2. Mechanisms of genetic exchange such as transformation, transduction, lysogeny, conjugation and transposition.

ORIGIN OF DRUG RESISTANCE

The origin of drug resistance may be genetic or nongenetic.

Nongenetic Origin of Drug Resistance

1. Antibiotics can act and kill bacteria that are in log phase and actively multiplying. Microorganisms, which are metabolically inactive and dormant are usually resistant to antibiotics. *e.g.*,

Mycobacterium tuberculosis can survive in tissues without multiplying for many years and may be resistant to antibiotic action.

2. Microorganisms may lose the specific target structure for a drug for several generations and becomes resistant to drugs. *e.g.*,

Penicillin-susceptible organisms (Staphylococci) may change to cell wall deficient L-forms, when penicillin is administered; and thus becomes resistant to penicillins, cephalosporins which act by inhibition of cell wall synthesis. When these L-forms revert to their parent form, become susceptible to penicillin.

3. Microorganisms may infect the host at sites where antibiotics are excluded or are not active *e.g.*, aminoglycosides such as gentamycin are not effective in treating enteric fever, because the *Salmonella* are intracellular and the aminoglycosides do not enter the cells.

Genetic Origin of Drug Resistance

Microorganisms may develop drug resistance due to genetic changes mediated by either chromosomal or extrachromosomal genetic elements.

Chromosome Mediated Drug Resistance or Mutational Drug Resistance

It is mainly due to spontaneous mutations in a gene locus that determines susceptibility to a drug.

Mutations confer resistance to only one drug at a time. Development of multiple drug resistance would require multiple mutations, which is very rare. Mutational drug resistance can be overcome by high dosage of drug as the degree of resistance is usually low. It can be prevented by treatment with a combination of drugs as in tuberculosis. Resistant mutants may be metabolically defective and their virulence may be low (live attenuated vaccines).

For many antibiotics, a particular mutation produces only a slight increase in resistance; but a series of consecutive mutations can produce a step-wise increase in resistance, usually seen with penicillin mutation can result in the loss of penicillin-binding proteins (PBPs) making such mutants resistant to β-lactam drugs.

Resistance to streptomycin arises quite readily be a "single large-step mutation" in many bacteria, posing a serious problem in clinical practice, as in the treatment of tuberculosis, the mutants may vary widely in the degree of resistance, some exhibiting low resistance, while others may be highly resistant, and some mutants may become streptomycin-dependent for growth.

Spontaneous mutations occurs with a frequency of 10^{-12} to 10^{-7}, but for rifampin, streptomycin, novobiocin drug, the development of drug resistant mutants can occur with a high frequency, and, once resistant mutants appear, they become selected, and grow replacing susceptible organisms. When, for example, streptomycin is used alone to treat tuberculosis or *E.coli* urinary tract infection, initially a few mutants appear resistant to streptomycin and within a few day replace and the whole population becomes resistant as susceptible (non-mutants) die out in the presence of drug. A high degree of resistance can appear due to mutations in bacterial DNA so that the bacterial ribosome is altered so that streptomycin cannot bind and act. Due to the selective growth of chromosomal-resistant mutants in tuberculosis, multiple drugs are used for therapy.

Extrachromosomal Resistance or Infectious Drug Resistance or Transmissible Drug Resistance

Bacteria contain extrachromosomal genetic elements called plasmids. R-plasmids are a class of plasmids that carry genes (determinants) for resistance to various antibiotics and heavy metals. They are numerous among intestinal Gram negative bacilli and responsible for the spread of multiple drug resistance among them. They are also found in a variety of other organisms. Each antibiotic resistance gene in the R-factors codes for and enzyme that destroys or inactivates a particular antibiotic. *e.g.,*

1. Plasmids carrying genes for the formation of β-lactamases confer resistance to penicillin and cephalosporins.

2. Plasmids carrying genes for the production of acetyl transferase, confer resistance to chloramphenicol.

3. Plasmids carry various genes for enzymes that inactivate aminoglycosides.

4. Plasmids carry genes for enzymes that determine the active transport of tetracyclines across the cell membranes.

R-plasmids can confer simultaneous resistance to several antibiotics particularly to frequently used antibiotics such as ampicillin, chloramphenicol, tetracycline, kanamycin and streptomycin; makes it difficult to treat infections successfully. Transfer of multiple drug resistance was demonstrated between different genera of bacteria. For example, between *Shigella* and *E.coli.* This mechanism of drug resistance is known as "infectious drug resistance" or "transferable drug resistance". The degree of resistance is usually high and cannot be prevented by a combination of drugs.

Bacteria carrying R-factors can be transmitted from animals to man. Hence, indiscriminate use of antibiotics in veterinary practice or in animal feeds can also lead to an increase of multiple drug resistance in the community. Transferable drug resistance is now universal in distribution and involves all antibiotics in common use. Its incidence is directly proportional to the frequency of use of antibiotics in the common area.

R-plasmid consists of two components – 1. the resistance transfer factor (RTF), and 2. the resistance determinant (r-det) for each of several drugs. Both of them together (RTF + r-det) constitute the whole R-plasmid. R factor can have several r-determinants, and resistance to as many as eight or more drugs can be transferred simultaneously. Sometimes, the RTF may dissociate from the r-determinants, and the two components can exist as separate plasmids. In such cases, though the host bacterium remains drug resistant, the resistance is not transferable.

Transferable drug resistance can be transferred between different bacteria by the transfer of plasmids and genetic material through following mechanisms:

1. Conjugation
2. Sexduction
3. Transduction
4. Lysogeny
5. Transformation
6. Transposition.

1. *Conjugation.* Conjugation is a process whereby genetic material is transferred unilaterally between bacteria of the same or different genera by mating (physical contact). Conjugation takes place between '+' strain or donor strain and '–' strain or recipient. The donor status is conferred by F-factor, that codes for sex pili, which forms a conjugation tube and establishes physical contact with recipient, through which plasmid or other DNA is transferred. This is the commonest method by which R-factors and consequently multidrug resistance spreads among different genera of Gram negative bacteria. Transfer of R-plasmids also occurs among some Gram positive cocci.

2. *Sexduction.* Sometimes F-factor may integrate with bacterial chromosomes. Such cells can transfer genes with a high frequency, and are called "High frequency cells (Hfr). When the F-plasmid reverts from the integrated state to free state, it may sometimes carry some chromosomal genes and is called F prime factor (F′ factor) and the cells are F prime cells (F′ cells). When F′ cell mates with a recipient, it transfers alongwith F plasmid, the chromosomal genes incorporated with it. This process of transfer of host chromosomal genes through the F factor resembles transduction, and has therefore been called sexduction.

3. *Transduction.* Transduction is a process where plasmid DNA is enclosed in a phage and transferred from cell to cell of the same species, through the agency of bacteriophages. In other words, it is a method of DNA transfer in which a virus (phage) acts as a vehicle for carrying genes from one bacterial cell to another.

e.g., Plasmids carrying genes for the production of β-lactamases in Staphylococci are transferred by transduction, by a phage. Similar transduction occurs in *Salmonella.*

4. *Lysogeny.* The phage DNA, sometimes, becomes integrated into the bacterial chromosome, known as "prophage", multiplies synchronously with host chromosomal DNA and is transferred to daughter cells. This process is called "lysogeny" and bacteria harbouring prophages are called "lysogenic bacteria". The presence of phage DNA confers new properties such as toxigenicity, drug resistance etc. a phenomenon, known as "lysogenic conversion" or "phage conversion".

5. *Transformation.* Free DNA or naked DNA passes from one cell of a species to another cell, altering its genetic structure. This can occur either spontaneously or in laboratory manipulation as in recombinant DNA technology.

6. *Transposition.* Transfer of short DNA sequences, called transposons or transposable elements occurs between one plasmid and another or between a plasmid and a portion of bacterial chromosome within a bacterial cell, causing alterations in base sequences.

Table 17.2 Differences between mutational and transferable drug resistance.

Mutational drug resistance	*Infectious (transferable) drug resistance*
1. Mutations confer resistance usually to one drug at a time	Mediated by plasmids, may confer resistance to multiple drugs or all drugs used in treatment, simultaneously
2. Degree of drug resistance is low	Degree of drug resistance is usually high
3. It can be overcome by administering high dose of drug	It cannot be overcome by high drug dosages
4. It can be prevented by treatment with a combination of drugs (multidrug therapy)	It cannot be prevented by a combination of drugs
5. Mutational drug resistance does not spread from cell to cell	Transferable drug resistance spreads to other cell of same or different species by various methods of gene transfer such as conjugation, transduction, transformation, transposition etc.
6. Resistant mutants are usually metabolically defective	Drug resistant strains are metabolically normal
7. The virulence of resistant mutants may be decreased	Virulence is not decreased

DRUG DEPENDENCE

Certain organisms not only develop resistance to a drug but require it and depend on it for growth. This has been best demonstrated with streptomycin, When streptomycin is used for treatment of tuberculosis, the tubercle bacilli develop resistance by mutations, with varying degrees some of which may become drug dependent. This phenomenon may also be seen with meningococci.

EPIDEMIOLOGY OF DRUG RESISTANCE

With the introduction of antibiotics, bacteria have adopted resistance mechanisms as a part of their survival strategy. There are several factors which influence the emergence of drug resistant strains.

1. Overuse and abuse of antibiotics in hospitals and in general population contributed to the development and spread of drug resistance.
2. The occurrence and spread of plasmids and transposons, which carry drug resistant genes.
3. Indiscriminate use of antibiotics in veterinary practice and in animal feeds.
4. The degree of cross-infection with drug-resistant strains of bacteria.

Because of overuse and abuse of antibiotics, indiscriminately led to selective pressure on bacterial strains; so that bacteria have developed new genes *e.g.,* methicillin-resistant Staphylococci, vancomycin-resistant Enterococci; or there is a movement of old genes into new bacterial hosts *e.g.,* penicillin resistant gonococci; or mutations of old genes resulting in more potent resistance *e.g.,* beta-lactamase mediated resistance to advanced cephalosporins in *E.coli* and *Klebsiella* sp.

CLINICAL IMPLICATIONS OF DRUG RESISTANCE

Emergence of drug-resistant organisms and their selection by wide spread use of antibiotics can be explained by following examples:

1. Gonococci were initially highly susceptible to penicillin. In the 1970s, β-lactamase producing strains appeared first in philippines and West Africa and spread to other parts of the world. Thereafter, spectinomycin came into use for treatment of gonorrhoeae. Resistance to spectinomycin is now appearing.
2. Meningococci were susceptible to sulphonamides until 1962; and developed resistance thereafter; then penicillins came into use for therapy, and rifampin for prophylaxis. However, meningococci now developed resistance to rifampin and penicillin.
3. In 1944, most Staphylococci were sensitive to penicillin. But in 1948, Staphylococci acquired the capacity to form β-lactamases which inactivate penicillins. Then β-lactamases-resistant penicillins such as methicillin came into use. But now methicillin-resistant *Staphylococcus aureus* (MRSA) strains have emerged.
4. Pneumococci were sensitive to penicillin-G until 1963. But, thereafter penicillin resistant strains emerged in various parts of the world, due to altered penicillin binding proteins.
5. Drug resistance among Gram negative bacilli spread through R-plasmids. Several strains of *Shigella* are now resistant to multiple drugs. Similarly, *Salmonella* also developed resistance, particularly to those incorporated into animal feeds *e.g.,* tetracyclines. The indiscriminate and abundant use of antibiotics among patients leads to the emergence and spread of drug resistance among Gram negative bacilli such as *Klebsiella, Proteus, Enterobacter, Serratia* and *Pseudomonas.*

PREVENTION OF DRUG RESISTANCE

The emergence of drug resistance can be prevented by following ways.

1. Indiscriminate use of antibiotics must be avoided.
2. It is essential to use the correct dosage and schedule (complete course) of the antibiotic to overcome the infection early.
3. Maintain sufficiently high levels of the drug in the tissues to inhibit both the original population and first step mutants.
4. Use a mixture of drugs that have different modes of action so that the organism cannot quickly undero adaptation. Multi-drug therapy may prevent the emergence of mutants *e.g.*, rifampin and isoniazid in the treatment of tuberculosis.
5. Antibiotics used in veterinary practice can lead to emergence of drug resistant strains, that may be transferred to humans.
6. Incorporation of antibiotics in animal feeds may cause animals to grow more rapidly, but associated with increase of drug resistant strains in farm workers. Hence, use of antibiotics in animal feeds must be controlled.
7. The drug of choice has to be replaced at the first sign of resistance by the organism.
8. Antibiotics should only be used in situations where a bacterial infection is either proven or strongly suspected.
9. The drug chosen should be targeted for the specific organism to be eradicated rather than opting for a more broad-spectrum drug.

QUESTIONS

Essay Type Questions

1. Describe the genetic mechanisms of drug resistance with examples.
2. Describe various mechanisms of drug resistance in bacteria.

Short Notes

1. Drug resistance.
2. Transferable drug resistance or infectious drug resistance.
3. Mutational drug resistance.
4. Control of drug resistance.
5. Environmentally mediated drug resistance.
6. Clinical implications of drug resistance.

18

Infection and Host-Parasite Interactions

- *Definitions*
- *Infection and Infestation*
- *Types of infections*
- *Sources of infections*
  - *Endogenous (autogenous) infections*
  - *Exogenous infections*
    - *Human patients*
    - *Human carriers*
    - *Animals*
    - *Insects*
      - *Mechanical vectors*
      - *Biological vectors*
  - *Water*
  - *Food*
  - *Soil*
- *Portals of entry (Mode of transmission)*
  - *Direct contact*
  - *Indirect contact*
  - *Inhalation/Air-borne transmission*
  - *Ingestion/food and water borne transmission*
  - *Venereal transmission*
  - *Vertical transmission*
  - *Congenital infections*
  - *Perinatal infections*
  - *Inoculation/percutaneous transmission*
  - *Zoonotic transmission*
  - *Insects*
  - *Iatrogenic transmission*
  - *Laboratory infections*

DEFINITIONS

Saprophyte

(Sapros = decayed ; phyton = plant) – Any microorganism (or plant) living on dead or decaying organic matter is known as saprophyte. They are free living in soil and water and carry out biodegradation of organic matter in nature. They cannot invade living tissues, and only on very rare occasions enter into parasitic relationship with man.

Parasite

Parasite is an organism living in or on another living organism (host) for food and shelter, benefitting at the expense of the host.

By convention, when the word "parasite" is used, it refers specifically to a protozoan or helminthic organism.

Obligatory parasites are those which can only live as parasites and cannot live or multiply outside the host *e.g.,* gonococci, meningococci.

Facultative parasites are those which can lead a parasitic life, but may also live outside the host body *e.g.,* Staphylococci.

Ectoparasite is an organism, which lives on the surface of its host *e.g.,* lice, ticks, mites and leeches.

Endoparasite is an organism, which lives inside the body of the host; in the tissues, blood, body cavity, digestive tract and other organs.

Commensal

(Com = with ; Mensa = table ; living together) Commensals live in complete symbiosis (friendship) with the host, without causing any damage or lesion or invasion. They derive nutrition from secretions, food residues, debris, excretory products etc. They constitute the normal flora of the body *e.g., Staphylococcus epidermidis* (*albus*). They are normally non-pathogenic, hence known as "non-pathogens". But some commensals are capable of causing infections, when transferred to an abnormal site for example, *Escherichia coli* is normally a harmless commensal in the gut, but causes infection in a wound or urinary tract. *Streptococcus viridans*, a normal mouth commensal, can cause subacute bacterial endocarditis, when it enters blood stream, after a tooth extraction. *Clostridium welchii*, a normal intestinal commensal can cause gangrene in locally damaged tissues.

Pathogen

(Patho = disease; gen = to produce) – A microorganism capable of causing a disease is called a pathogen. An organism is said to be pathogenic, when it satisfies the Koch's postulates.

Opportunistic Pathogen/Facultative Pathogen

An opportunistic pathogen or facultative pathogen is one which is normally non-pathogenic (a commensal) but can invade healthy tissues and produce disease, when the host resistance is impaired, that is, when the host is immunocompromised.

Host

Host is a person or animal including birds and arthropods that provide lodgement and nourishment to an infectious agent under natural conditions.

Etiologic agent

It is a microorganism responsible for causing infection or infectious disease. "Etiology" is the science dealing with causes of disease.

INFECTIONS

The entry, lodgement and multiplication of an infectious agent in the body of man and animals is called infection. The term "infection" also implies that the body responds in some way to defend itself against the infectious agent either in the form of an immune response or disease. An infection may or may not lead to a disease state.

Multiplication of normal flora of the body is generally not considered an infection. Whereas, multiplication of pathogenic bacteria is considered an infection, even if the person is asymptomatic.

INFESTATION

It is defined as the lodgement, development and reproduction of parasites (particularly helminthes) in the host or parasitic invasion of the organs and tissues.

It is also defined as the lodgement, development, and reproduction of arthropods (insects such as lice, ticks and mites) on the skin of the body or in the clothing of humans.

Invasion. The process whereby microorganisms enter host cells or tissues and spread in the body is called invasion.

Contamination. The presence of an infectious agent on a body surface and also on or in clothes, bedding, surgical instruments or surgical dressings etc. or substances including water, milk and food. Contamination on body surface does not imply a carrier state.

Infectious disease. A clinically manifested disease of man or animals resulting from an infection.

Contagious disease. An infectious disease that is transmitted by direct contact. *e.g.,* sexually transmitted diseases.

Communicable disease. It is a disease due to an infectious agent or its toxic products capable of being transmitted directly or indirectly from man to man, animal to animal or from the environment to man.

Primary infection. It is an initial (or first) infection caused by a microorganism.

Reinfection. When the same (or a single) microorganism cause infections repeatedly, subsequent infections are termed reinfections.

Secondary infections. When a new microorganism sets up an infection in a host whose resistance is lowered by a pre-existing disease, it is termed secondary infection.

Opportunistic infections. When the host resistance is impaired, as in immunocompromised patients, a non-pathogenic organism may set up infection, which is known as opportunistic infection. For example, opportunistic infections are very common in AIDS due to immunodeficiency.

Superinfection. An infection superimposed on an already existing infection or occurring after the primary pathogen is under control.

Vertical infection. Infections transmitted from one generation to another either congenitally (transplacentally) or perinatally (just before or during birth) are known an vertical infections. *e.g.,* syphilis, AIDS, rubella, CMV, toxoplasmosis.

Systemic infection. Systemic infection is one which affects the body as a whole. A systemic disease can spread throughout the body.

Mixed infection. When more than one microorganism infects a host simultaneously it is called a mixed infection.

Focal infection. It refers to localised or circumscribed chronic infection or sepsis in the body; in areas like gums of teeth, tonsils, nasal sinuses, appendix etc.

Cross infection. When a patient is suffering from a disease, a new infection is set up from another host or exogenous source, termed as cross infection. In other words, it is an infection transmitted between hosts infected with different organisms.

Nosocomial/hospital-acquired infection. Cross infections in hospitals are called hospital-acquired infections; developing in hospitalized patients, which were not present or in incubation at the time of their admission; originating from patient (endogenous) himself or external source (exogenous). In other words, it is an infection in which etiological agent is acquired in hospital.

Iatrogenic infection. It is a physician induced infection resulting from diagnostic, preventive (immunization) or therapeutic (drug therapy) procedures.

Subclinical/inapparent infection. It is an infection, where clinical effects are not apparent. In other words, there will be no overt symptoms.

Covert infections. They are subclinical, without symptoms.

Overt infections. They are symptomatic infections.

Atypical infection. Atypical infection is one in which the typical or characteristic clinical manifestations of the particular infectious disease are not present.

Exogenous infection. It is an infection caused by the entry of organism from an external source such as food, water, air, fomites or other persons.

Endogenous infection. It is an infection caused by a microorganism, derived from the host's body itself; and is often due to lowering of resistance of the host. It is often an opportunistic infection caused by commensals. *e.g., E .coli* derived from bowel may cause urinary tract infection; *Staphylococcus aureus* from nostrils may cause a boil in the skin or infection of wound; pneumococci from nasopharynx may cause bronchitis and bronchopneumonia.

Latent infection. It is an infection in which infecting organism is quiescent, but may reactivate. Some microorganisms following infection, may remain in the tissues for long periods, without producing any symptoms, in a latent or hidden form proliferating and producing clinical disease, when the host resistance is lowered. This is termed latent infection.

e.g., Herpes simplex virus (HSV) infections, Brill-Zinsser disease, slow virus infections.

Fulminating infection. Fulminating infections are those where infectious agent multiplies with great intensity.

Generalized infection. Generalized infections are those that affect many parts of the body. *e.g.,* streptococcal infections.

Localized infection. Localized infections are those which are restricted to a limited region or to one or more anatomical areas. *e.g.,* Staphylococcal abscess.

Pyogenic/suppurative infection. Pyogenic or suppurative infections are those which result in the formation of pus.

Terminal infection. Terminal infections are those which occurs near the end of a disease and frequently causes death.

Abscess. A localized infection with a collection of pus surrounded by an inflamed area.

Acute infection. Acute infections are those with short course but severe symptoms.

Chronic infection. Chronic infections are those which persists over a long time.

Bacteremia. Presence or circulation of viable bacteria in the blood stream is called bacteremia. Transient bacteremia occurs in healthy persons during chewing, brushing of teeth and while straining during excretion of feces.

Septicemia (Sepsis). A systemic disease or blood poisoning in which microorganisms multiply in the blood stream, form toxic products, producing clinical signs and symptoms such as fever.

Sepsis may occur as a complication of intravenous catheterisation or child birth (puerperal).

Pyemia. Pyemia is a condition where pyogenic bacteria produce septicemia with multiple abscesses in the internal organs of the body.

Toxaemia. Toxaemia is a condition arising from toxins in the blood.

Epidemiology. Epidemiology is defined as the study of the nature, distribution, causation, mode of transfer, prevention and control of disease. It has also been regarded as "the natural history of disease" or as "the human face of ecology".

Surveillance. Any type of epidemiological investigation that involves data collection and evaluation of data for characterizing conditions or factors related to the incidence or prevalence of a particular disease or infection, is called surveillance. It is useful for control and prevention of infectious diseases.

Morbidity. The state of disease and its associated effects on the host is called morbidity and the incidence of a particular disease state is called morbidity rate.

Mortality. Mortality is defined as death resulting from disease. The incidence in which a disease results in death is known as mortality rate.

Vector. A living entity (insect, animal or plant), that transmits the pathogen is called vector.

Vehicle. A non-living entity that is contaminated with the pathogen and acts as a mode of transmission. *e.g.,* surgical instruments, bedding, eating utensils.

In epidemiology, these common vehicles are called **"fomites".** Food (*Salmonella* food poisoning) and water (cholera) are common vehicles for many human diseases.

Outbreak. A larger than normal number of diseased or infected individuals that occurs over a relatively short period is known as an outbreak of a disease.

Sporadic. The word sporadic means scattered about. The cases occur irregularly, haphazardly from time to time and infrequently. The cases are few and separated widely in space and time. Many zoonotic diseases are characterized by sporadic transmission to man. Some times, a sporadic disease may be the starting point of an epidemic.

Epidemic (epi = upon ; demos = population). It refers to increased occurrence of disease and a larger number of diseased or infecting individuals in a particular location; spreads rapidly involving many persons at the same time in an area. *e.g.,* influenza.

Epizootic. An epidemic that occurs in animals is called epizootic. *e.g.,* plague in rats.

Endemic. A disease constantly or persistently present at some rate of occurrence in a defined population or geographical area. *e.g.,* typhoid fever.

Enzootic. An endemic occurring in animals is called enzootic. *e.g.,* plague in rats, brucellosis in cattle.

Pandemic. An epidemic that spans the world is called pandemic disease; spreading through many areas of the world involving very large numbers of people within a short period.

e.g., influenza, cholera, plague, enteroviral conjunctivitis.

Prosodemic. A disease which passes directly from one person to another; they evolve more slowly and produce smouldering epidemics. *e.g,,* meningitis.

Exotic. Diseases which are imported into a country, where they do not occur are known as exotic diseases.

SOURCES OF INFECTION

The term "source of infection" refers to the location (*e.g.,* man, animals, fomites etc.) from which the pathogen is disseminated to the host.

The "Reservoir" is the natural habitat of the infectious agent, in which it lives, multiplies and infects the host. *e.g.,* water, food, soil, insects, fomites, animals or humans.

The sources of infection to a man can be endogenous or exogenous.

Endogenous (Autogenous) Infections

When the source of infection is from one's own normal flora within the body, it is said to be endogenous infection. *e.g.,*

E.coli, which lives as a harmless commensal in the intestine, may cause acute infections in the urinary tract.

Staphylococcus aureus from nostrils may cause a boil in the skin or infection in a wound.

Pneumococci from the nasopharynx may cause bronchitis and bronchopneumonia.

Streptococcus viridans, a normal mouth commensal may cause subacute bacterial endocarditis, following tooth extraction.

Table 18.1 Source of infection

I. Endogenous (Autogenous) infections	
II. Exogenous infections	
1. Human patients	
2. Human carriers	
3. Animals (zoonoses)	– Reservoir hosts, Amplifier hosts
4. Insects (vectors)	– Mechanical vectors, Biological vectors
5. Water	– Due to the presence of pathogen
	– Due to the presence of an aquatic host.
6. Food	– Food poisoning – Microbial, Toxic
7. Soil	

Exogenous Infections

When the source of infection is from outside the body, the infection is said to be exogenous. The exogenous sources are – 1. human patients, 2. human carriers, 3. animals, 4. insects, 5. Water, 6. food, 7. soil.

Human Patients

Infections due to some microorganisms are acquired mainly or exclusively from patients with active infection. *e.g.,* pulmonary tuberculosis, leprosy, whooping cough, syphilis, gonorrhoea, measles, small pox, mumps and influenza.

Human Carriers

Carrier is defined as an infected person, who harbours the pathogen, without any clinical disease (asymptomatic infection), and acts as a potential source of infection for others.

Carriers play an important role in the epidemiology of the disease. *e.g.,* Marry Mallon ("Typhoid Mary"), a New York cook, who over a period of 15 years, caused atleast seven outbreaks affecting over 200 persons. Carriers are of several types:

Healthy carrier is an individual who harbours the pathogen but is not ill. *e.g.,* salmonellosis, cholera, dysentery, diptheria, meningitis, staphylococcal, streptococcal and pneumococcal infections, poliomyelitis.

Incubatory carrier is an individual who is incubating the pathogen in large numbers, during the incubation period of an illness, but is not yet ill. *e.g.,* pertussis, influenza, measles, mumps.

Convalescent carrier is an individual who has recovered from the infectious disease, but continues to harbour large numbers of the pathogen. *e.g.,* typhoid fever, dysentery, cholera, diphtheria and pertussis.

Temporary carriers harbour the pathogen for less than 6 months. Healthy, incubatory and convalescent carriers may harbour the pathogen for only a brief period – hours, days or weeks and then are called **casual, acute,** or **transient** carriers.

Chronic carriers harbour the pathogen for long periods – months, years or life.

Contact carrier is one who acquires the pathogen from a patient.

Paradoxical carrier is one who acquires the pathogen from another carrier.

According to portal of exit, carriers may be classified as urinary carriers, intestinal carriers, respiratory carriers and others.

Table 18.2 Classification of carriers

Type	Healthy carriers Incubatory carriers Convalescent carriers
Duration	Temporary carriers (casual, acute or transient carriers) Chronic carriers
Portal of entry	Contact carriers Paradoxical carriers
Portal of exit	Urinary carriers Intestinal carriers Respiratory carriers Others (open wound infections, skin eruptions)

Animals

Some pathogens that are primarily parasites of different animals, may spread from the infected animal to man and called "**zoonoses**". In these infections man is generally an "end-host". Many animals serve to maintain the parasite in nature by acting as "**Reservoir hosts**" or "**Amplifying hosts**". Some diseases are endemic among animals, known as "**enzootic**", whereas epidemics that occur in animals are known as "**epozootic**". Animals which live in close association with man are the greatest danger. From wild animals, diseases may spread to man by insects.

Various bacterial, viral, parasitic and fungal zoonoses are listed here below.

Table 18.3 Bacterial zoonoses

Disease	*Etiologic agent*	*Animal host*	*Mode of transmission*
1. Anthrax	*Bacillus anthracis*	Cattle, sheep, goats, horses, swine	Inhalation or ingestion of spores; direct contact
2. Plague (Bubonic)	*Yerisinia pestis*	Domestic rats, wild rodents	Rat flea bite
3. Brucellosis (undulant fever)	*Brucella melitensis* *Brucella abortus* *Brucella suis*	Cattle, goats, sheep, swine, dogs, pigs	Milk; direct or indirect contact
4. Salmonellosis (*Salmonella* food poisoning/gastroenteritis)	*Salmonella* sp. (except *S. typhi*)	Fowl, sheep, cattle, horses, dogs, cats, rodents, reptiles	Direct contact; food
5. Tuberculosis	*Mycobacterium bovis*	Cattle, horses, dogs, cats	Milk; direct contact
6. Leptospirosis (Weil's disease)	*Leptospira interrogans*	Rats, wild animals	Direct contact with urine infected tissue, and contaminated water
7. Rat-bite fever	Spirillum minus	Rats, mice, cats,	Rat bit
8. Q. fever	*Streptobacillus moniliformis*	Rats, mice, squirrels	Rat bite; contaminated food, water
		Cattle, sheep, goats	Inhalation of contaminated dust, soil
9. Lyme disease	*Borrelia burgdorferi*	Ticks	Tick bite
10. Tularemia	*Francisella tularensis*	Rabbits, other rodents	Direct contact with infected carcass; tick bite; biting flies
11. Campylobacteriosis	*Campylobacter jejuni*	*Cattle, sheep, poultry, birds*	Raw milk; contaminated water and food
12. Pasteurellosis	*Pasteurella multocida*	Fowl, cattle, sheep, swine, goats, mice, rabbits, rats, dogs, cats	Animal bite (dog or cat bite)
13. Relapsing fever (Borreliosis)	*Borrelia* sp.	Rodents, ticks, lice	Tick bite; lice bite
14. Listeriosis	*Listeria monocytogenes*	Sheep, goats, cattle, guinea pigs, chickens, horses	Contact, inhalation or ingestion
15. Glanders	*Pseudomonas mallei*	Horses	Contact, inhalation
16. Melioidosis	*Pseudomonas pseudomallei*	Rats, mice, rabbits, dogs, cats	Arthropod Vectors
17. Boutonneuse fever African tick typhus	*Rickettsia conorii*	Dogs	Tick bite
18. Rickettsial pox	*Rickettsia akari*	Mice	Mice bite
19. Rocky mountain spotted fever	*Rickettsia rickettsii*	Rabbits, squirrels, rats, mice	Tick bite
20. Scrub typhus	*Rickettsia tsutsugamushi*	Wild rodents, rats	Mice bite
21. Cat scratch fever	*Rochalimaea* sp.	Cats, dogs	Cat of dog scratch
22. Psittacosis	*Chlamydia psittaci*	Psittascine birds	Direct contact; Respiratory aerosols

Table 18.4 Viral zoonoses

Disease	*Etiologic agent*	*Animal host*	*Mode of transmission*
Colorado tick fever	Arbovirus	Squirrels, mice	Tick bite
Cow pox	Cow pox virus	Cattle, horses	Skin abrasions
Encephalitis			
St. Louis	Arbovirus	Birds	Mosquito
California	Arbovirus	Rats, squirrels, horses, deer, cows	Mosquito
Eastern equine	Arbovirus	Birds, ducks, fowl, horses	
Venezuelan equine	Arbovirus	Rodents, horses	Mosquito
Western equine	Arbovirus	Birds, snakes, squirrels, horses	Mosquito
Herpes B viral encephalitis	Herpes virus simiae	Monkeys	Monkey bite; contact
Lymphocytic choriomeningitis	Arbovirus	Mice, rats, dogs, monkeys, guinea pigs	Inhalation of contaminated dust; Ingestion of contaminated food
Orf (contagious ecthyma)	Virus	Sheep, goats	Skin abrasions
Rabies	Rabies virus	Dogs, bats, opposums, skunks, foxes, cats	Bite of rabid animal
Vesicular stomatitis	Virus (Rhabdovirus group)	Cattle, swine, horses	Direct contact
Yellow fever (jungle)	Yellow fever virus	Monkeys, marmosets mosquitoes	Mosquito

Table 18.5 Parasitic zoonoses

Babesiosis	*Babesia sp.*	*Ticks*	*Tick bite*
Cryptosporidiosis	*Cryptosporidium* sp	Calves	Contact
Giardiasis	*Giardia lamblia*	Rodents, deer, cattle, dogs, cats	Contaminated water
Leishmaniasis			
Visceral	*Leishmania donovani*	Dogs	Sandfly bite
Cutaneous (Oriental sore)	*Leishmania tropica*	Dogs	Sandfly bite
Espundia	*Leishmania brasiliensis*	Rodents	Sandfly bite
Hydatid disease	*Echinococcus granulosus*	Dogs	Ingestion

Table 18.6 Fungal zoonoses

Disease	*Etiologic agent*	*Animal host*	*Mode of transmission*
Dermatophytosis	Zoophilic dermatophytes	Cats, dogs	Direct contact
Histoplasmosis	*Histoplasma capsulatum*	Birds	Inhalation

Insects

Insects such as mosquitoes, flies, lice, ticks, mites and fleas that transmit infections are called vectors. Blood sucking insects may transmit pathogens to humans. These diseases are called "Arthropod-borne" diseases. Vectors are classified into two types based on mode of transmission and propagation of pathogens, mechanical and biological.

(*i*) ***Mechanical vectors.*** They transmit the pathogen mechanically, through soiling of its legs or probascis; sometimes the pathogen may be ingested by insect vector and get excreted passively. There is no development or multiplication of the pathogen on or within the vector *e.g.,* transmission of dysentery bacilli or typhoid bacilli by domestic fly.

(*ii*) ***Biological vector.*** The pathogen undergoes development or multiplication or both in vector and requires an incubation period before transmission. *e.g.,*

Female anopheles mosquito – malaria
Aedes aegypti mosquito – yellow fever
Culex mosquito – filariasis, Japanese B encephalitis
Rat flea – plague
Louse – epidemic typhus
Tick – spotted fevers, relapsing fever
Mite – scrub typhus
Tsetsefly – African sleeping sickness (Trypanosomiasis)
Sandfly – Leishmaniasis

Table 18.7 Bacterial diseases transmitted by biological vectors

Disease	*Causative agent*	*Biological vector*	*Animal reservoir*	*Insect-pathogen-human interrelationship*
Epidemic relapsing fever	*Borrelia recurrentis* (a spirochete)	Human body louse (*Pediculus humanus*)	None	Pathogen multiplies in tissues of louse; humans inoculated by crushing louse on skin
Endemic relapsing fever	*Borrelia hermgii* and other borrelia	Ticks (*ornithodoros* sp)	Ticks, wild rodents and other small animals	Pathogen multiplies throughout body of tick; transovarian passage occurs; humans are inoculated by tick salvia or tick feces.
Epidemic typhus	*Rickettsia prowazekii*	Human body louse (pediculus humanus)	Usually none. It is found in flying squirrels in the south eastern United States	Pathogen multiplies in tissues of louse; the louse excretes the Rickettsiae in its feces; humans are inoculated by rubbing the louse feces into bite.

Scrub typhus	Rickettsia tsutsugamushi	Red mites (trombicula sp.)	Wild rodents	Pathogen multiplies in gut of mite; transovarian passage occurs; humans infected through bite of larval mite.
Murine typhus	*Rickettsia typhi* (*R. mooseri*)	Rat flea (*Xenopsylla cheopis*)	Rats and mice	Pathogen multiplies in lining of the flea's midgut; humans infected through bite.
Rickettsial pox	*Rickettsia akari*	Mouse mite (*Allodermanyssus sanguineus*)	House mice	Pathogen multiplies in gut of mite; humans infected through bite.
Trench fever	*Bartonella quintana*	Human body louse (*Pediculus humans*)	None	Pathogen multiplies in mid gut of louse; humans inoculated by louse feces or by crushing louse on skin.

Table 18.8 Virus diseases transmitted by biological insect vectors

Causative agent	*Geographical distribution*	*Disease*	*Vector*	*Animal reservoir*
Alphavirus	Eastern North America	Eastern equine encephalitis	Mosquitoes (*Culex melanura* and *Aedes* sp.)	Wild birds
	Western North America	Western equine encephalitis	Mosquitoes (*Culex tarsalis*)	Wild birds
	Central and South America and Southern USA	Venezuelan equine encephalitis	Several kinds of mosquitoes	Horses, rodents
	Australia	Murray valley encephalitis	Mosquitoes (*Culex annulirostris*)	Birds
Flavivirus	Tropical and subtropical regions of the world	Dengue fever	Mosquitoes (*Aedes aegypti, A. albopictus*)	Other *Aedes* sp. maintain a sylvatic cycle in monkeys similar to that of yellow fever.
	USA	St. Louis encephalitis	Mosquitoes (*Culex pipiens* and other *Culex* sp.)	Wild birds
	Russia and Northern Europe	Tick-brone encephalitis	Ticks (*Ixodes ricinus* and others	Small wild mammals and birds
	Africa, Europe, Middle Esat	West Nile fever	Mosquitoes (*Culex* sp.)	Birds
Bunyavirus	Central Asia	Crimean-Congo haemorrhagic fever	Ticks (*Hyalomma marginatum*)	Many mammals
Orbivirus	Western United States	Colorado tick fever	Ticks (*Dermacentor andersonii*)	Small mammals

Table 18.9 Protozoan diseases transmitted by biological insects

Causative	*Geographical distribution*	*Disease*	*Biological Vector*	*Animal reservoir*	*Insect-pathogen-human inter relationship*
Leishmania donovani	China, India, Africa, Mediterranean area, Latin America	Kala-azar	Sand flies (*Phlebotomus* sp.)	Wild rodents, other wild animals; dogs	Pathogen multiplies in mid-guts and reaches mouth-parts of fly; humans infected through bites
Leishmania tropica	Mediterranean area to Western India	Oriental sore	Sand flies (*Phlebotomus* sp.)	— do —	— do —
Leishmania	Mexico to Northern Argentina	Espundia	— do —	— do —	— do —
Trypanosoma Sub sp. *gambiense* Sub sp. *rhodesiense*	West and Central Africa East and Central Africa	African trypanosomiasis (sleeping sickness)	Tsetse flies (Glossina sp.)	Antelops and other wild game animal in Africa	Pathogen multiplies in mid gut and passes to salivary glands; human are infected by bite
Trypanosoma cruzi	Latin America	Chaga's disease	Reduviid bugs (*Triatoma* sp. *Panstrongylus* sp.)	Armadillos, opossums, dogs, and other animals	Pathogen multiplies in hind gut of bug; humans infected by rubbing bug's feces into the bite
Plasmodium (Malarial parasite)	World wide	Malaria	Female anopheles mosquito (*Anopheles gambia*)		Pathogen multiplies in the gut of mosquito and passes to salivary glands; humans are infected by bite

Table 18.10 Helminthic (Filariases) transmitted by biological vectors

Causative agent	*Geographical distribution*	*Disease*	*Biological vector*
Wuchereria bancrofti	Tropical and subtropical regions throughout the world	Bancroft's filariasis (Wuchereriasis)	Mosquitoes (*Aedes* sp, *Culex* sp, *Anopheles* sp)
Brugia malayi	South East Asia	Brugian filariasis	Mosquitoes (*Anopheles* sp, *Mansonia* sp)
Brugiya timori	Indonesia	Brugian filariasis	Mosquitoes (*Anopheles barbirbostris*)
Loa loa	Africa	Loasis	Horse or deerflies (*Chrysops* sp)
Onchocerca volvulus	Africa, Central and South America	Onchocerirasis	Black flies (*Simulium* sp)

Causative agent	*Geographical distribution*	*Disease*	*Biological vector*
Tetrapetalonema perstans	Africa, South America	Tetrapetalonemiasis	Midges (*Culicoides* sp)
T. Streptocera	Africa	Tetrapetalonemiasis	Midges (*Culicoides* sp)
Mansonella ozzardi	Central and South America	Ozzard's filariasis	Midges (*Culicoides* sp)

Biological transmission is of three types:

(*i*) ***Propagative.*** The pathogen merely multiplies in vector, but no change in form. *e.g.,* plague bacilli in rat fleas.

(*ii*) ***Cyclopropagative.*** The pathogen changes in form and number. *e.g.,* malarial parasites in female *Anopheles* mosquitoes.

(*iii*) ***Cyclodevelopmental.*** The pathogen undergoes only development but no multiplication. *e.g.,* microfilaria in *Culex* mosquito.

The interval of time required for the biological vector to become infective, beginning from the time of entry of pathogen into it, is termed the extrinsic incubation period.

Some insects may act as reservoir hosts. *e.g.,* ticks in relapsing fever and spotted fevers.

When the pathogen is transmitted vertically from the infected female to her progeny in the vector, it is known as **transovarial transmission.**

Transmission of the pathogen from one stage of the life cycle to another is known as **transstadial transmission.**

Water

Water acts as a source of infection due to contamination with pathogens from humans or animals (usually excreta). Water-borne diseases may be due to the presence of a pathogen or an aquatic host in it.

Water borne diseases

I. Due to the presence of pathogens

1. Bacteria: *Vibrio cholerae, Salmonella* sp, *Shigella, Esch.coli, Vibrio Parahemolyticus, Yersinia enterocolitica, Campylobaer, Leptospira.*
2. Viruses: Hepatitis 'A' virus, Poliovirus (enteroviruses), Rotavirus.
3. Protozoa: *Entamoeba histolytica, Giardia lamblia, Cryptosporidium, Acanthamoeba, Naegleria fowleri.*
4. Helminthes: Round worm, whip worm, pin worm

II. Due to the presence of an aquatic host

1. Cyclops Guinea worm, fish tape worm
2. Snail *Schistosoma*

Food

Many diseases are transmitted by foods contaminated with pathogens or their toxins. Foods may be contaminated by flies mechanically or carriers due to handling or eating utensils infected by handling or washing in contaminated water. "**Bacterial food poisoning**" is due to the growth of the bacteria and the production of enterotoxins in the contaminated food.

e.g., Staphylococcus aureus, Clostridium botulinum, Clostridium welchii (Type A), *Bacillus cereus, Salmonella* species, *Campylobacter jejuni, E.coli, Shigella, Yersinia enterocolitica, Vibrio parachemolyticus, Listeria monocytogenes* etc. may be transmitted by contaminated food. Tape worm infestations may be transmitted by undercooked pork or beef.

Soil

Some infectious diseases of man are caused by saprophytes derived from the soil, vegetation etc. The soil derived infections are not infectious from one man to another.

e.g., Tetanus, gasgangrene, botulism, maduramycosis, sporotrichosis, histoplasmosis, coccidioidomycosis; hook worm and round worm.

Clostridium tetani and *Clostridium welchii* live as commensals in the intestine of animals and humans and enter the soil in fecal droppings.

METHODS/MODES/ROUTES OF TRANSMISSION/PORTALS OF ENTRY

Humans may acquire microorganisms by various routes referred to as the 'modes of transmission". Infections can spread from host to host by a variety of mechanisms:

1. Direct contact
2. Indirect contact
3. Inhalation/Air-borne transmission
4. Ingestion/food and water-borne transmission
5. Venereal transmission
6. Vertical transmission
7. Inoculation/percutaneous transmission
8. Zoonotic transmission
9. Insects
10. Iatrogenic transmission
11. Laboratory infections.

Direct Contact

Direct contact implies an actual physical interaction with the infectious source. This route is frequently called person-to-person contact, which occurs primarily –

(*i*) by touching of bodies as in handshaking,

(*ii*) by kissing

(*iii*) by contact of clothing, *e.g.,* HSV-I, boils, Staphylococcal infections.

Indirect Contact

Indirect contact refers to the transmission of the pathogen from the source to the host via an inanimate objects, known as "Fomites". This mode of transmission is often considered a form of "vehicle" transmission. *Pseudomonas* bacteria are easily transmitted by this route. Pens and pencils shared by school children may act as fomites in the transmission of diphtheria and face towels in trachoma.

Fomites : Surgical instruments, thermometers, eating utensils, spoons, drinking cups, bedding, clothing, pillows, towels, handkerchiefs, doctor's coats, nurses uniform, pens, pencils, toys, pockets, books, door handles, taps, etc.

Inhalation/Air-Borne Transmission

Air-borne infections are transmitted by aerosols and dust, containing pathogens, generated from human or environmental sources.

Aerosols/droplet spray. Microorganisms that cause respiratory infections occur in nasal and oral secretions of individuals. During coughing, sneezing, singing or talking, aerosols may be expelled. The large droplets (10 μ or more in diameter) can be inhaled by people nearby, particularly in over-crowded areas or settle on clothing or inanimate objects, which in turn can infect people. The small droplets (1 to 4 μ in diameter) tends to evaporate quickly, leaving **"droplet nuclei",** a dried residue of solid material containing microorganisms. These droplet nuclei remain suspended in air for hours or days and may be carried long distances. *e.g.,* common cold, influenza, chicken pox, measles, mumps, pneumonia, diphtheria, tuberculosis, meningitis and pertussis.

Aerosols generated from contaminated water of air-conditioners and mist sprays used to keep vegetables fresh, may transmit diseases. *e.g.,* legionnaire's disease.

Mycobacterium intracellulare causes respiratory infection, resembling, tuberculosis, but is not transmitted from person to person. It lives in water and can be ejected into air by air bubbles.

Dust-borne. During sneezing, coughing, singing or talking, large aerosol droplets are expelled and settle on handkerchief, bed clothes, floor, carpets, furniture and other objects, where they evaporate to form a dry residue. Disturbance of these residues by handling a dried handkerchief, by bed making or by sweeping the floor or during dusting the furniture; can generate dust particles that may add pathogens to air. Some microorganisms can survive for relatively longer periods in dust. The diseases carried by infections dust include Staphylococcal and Streptococcal infections, pneumonia, tuberculosis, Q fever, psittacosis. Infectious dust is primarily inhaled, but may settle on food, water and milk. This type of transmission is most common in hospitals causing nosocomial infections.

Some pathogens that inhabit soil may be raised as dust and transmitted through inhalation. *e.g.,* histoplasmosis, coccidioidomycosis.

Air-borne transmission

I. Aerosols

1. From human sources
   - (*a*) droplets
   - (*b*) droplet nuclei

   e.g., common cold, tuberculosis, pneumonia, meningitis, pertussis, diphtheria, influenza, measles, mumps, chicken-pox.
2. From environment — *e.g.,* legionnaire's disease, *Mycobacterium intracellulare*

II. Dust infectious dust

1. From human sources — *e.g.,* Nosocomial infections, Staphylococcal and Streptococcal infections, pneumonia, tuberculosis, psittacosis
2. From environment — *e.g.,* Histoplasmosis, coccidioidomycosis

Ingestion/Food and Water-Borne Transmission

In alimentary tract infections, pathogens are discharged in the feces of infected persons, and are transmitted by fecal-oral routes, leading to their ingestion by the recipient.

Intestinal pathogens such as typhoid and dysentery bacilli may survive for several weeks and spread by moist vehicles such as water or food.

Intestinal infections may be transmitted by following ways:

1. Contamination of water supplies with excreta – water-borne infection.

2. Through contaminated or uncleaned fingers – hand to mouth infection. Nurses may infect their hands in attending patients and in touching bed-pans.

3. Contamination of food – due to a carrier handling the food or mechanically by insects – food-borne infection.

4. Contamination of vegetables and fruits grown fertilised with feces (sewage).

5. Through fomites such as door handles, water taps, lavatory seats contaminated by patients or carriers.

e.g. Cholera, enteric fever (salmonellosis), dysentery, intestinal tuberculosis, Type A hepatitis, enteroviral infections (poliomyelitis), intestinal parasitic infestations.

Venereal Transmission

The diseases that are transmitted by sexual contact are called venereal diseases or sexually transmitted diseases (STD).

e.g. Syphilis, gonorrhoea, chancroid, granuloma inguinale, lymphogranuloma venereum (LGV), AIDS, HSV-2.

Vertical transmission/congenital infections/teratogenic infections/transplacental transmission

The infections that are transmitted from one generation to another, either transplacentally (congenital) or perinatally are known as vertical infections. These infections usually lead to the deformity or malformations in the developing embryo. Hence, they are also called teratogenic infections.

Congenital infections are those diseases, that are acquired by the fetus in utero, through the transplacental route.

e.g. Congenital syphilis, AIDS, congenital toxoplasmosis, congenital rubella syndrome, congenital cytomegalovirus infections.

Congenital infections during first three months of pregnancy may lead to abortion, still birth, miscarriage, premature delivery and a wide range of congenital defects or malformations (teratogenic) such as cardiac defects, blindness, deafness, mental retardation etc.

Perinatal infections are those diseases, that are acquired either during birth or just before birth leading to neonatal complications. *e.g.*, neonatal herpes with HSV-2 and ophthalmia neonatorum by gonococci. Perinatal infections can be prevented by caesarian section, instead of delivering vaginally.

Inoculation/Percutaneous Transmission

Infections may be transmitted by inoculation through the skin or mucus membranes to deeper tissues. *e.g.*, surgery, trauma, injections, dressing of surgical wounds, insect bites etc.

Diseases such as syphilis, AIDS and Type B hepatitis may be introduced by injection of serum, plasma or blood, particularly among intravenous drug addicts. Infection by inoculation may be iatrogenic when it is due to unsterile syringes, surgical instruments and catheters.

In some occasions, the pathogens may be directly implanted or inoculated into the tissues. Inoculation of rabies virus by dog bite, implantation of gas gangrene and tetanus spores in the depth of wounds, and injection of Arboviruses by mosquitoes are examples.

Zoonotic Transmission

See sources of infection.

Insects

See sources of infection.

Iatrogenic Transmission

Infections caused as a result of health care are called iatrogenic or physician induced infections. It refers to adverse consequences resulting due to physician's professional health care activities such as diagnostic, preventive (immunization) and therapeutic procedures. Modern methods of treatment such as exchange transfusion, dialysis and heart and transplant surgery have increased the possibilities for iatrogenic infections.

e.g. Administration of injections, lumbar puncture, aplastic anemia following the use of chloramphenicol, purpura following administration of sedormid, childhood leukemia due to prenatal X-rays, AIDS, hepatitis B following blood transfusion.

Laboratory infections

Technicians, nurses and other paramedical laboratory workers occasionally become infected from cultures or from infectious materials collected from patients or experimental animals. When working with dangerous pathogens such as sputum samples for AFB and blood samples for screening AIDS and Type B hepatitis, special care should be taken to prevent laboratory infections.

QUESTIONS

Essay Type Questions

1. What is an infection ? Describe various types of infections.
2. Describe in detail the sources of infections to humans beings.
3. Describe the portals of entry or routes of transmission or methods of transmission of infections.

Short Notes

1. Define and differentiate primary, secondary, opportunistic and reinfections.
2. Cross infections.
3. Iatrogenic infections.
4. Define epidemic, endemic, pandemic and sporadic.
5. Define bacteremia, septicemia and pyemia.
6. Define exogenous and endogenous infections.
7. Carrier.
8. Zoonoses.

9. Define and mention two zoonotic infections.
10. Name two zoonotic bacterial diseases.
11. Name four parasitic zoonotic diseases.
12. Name four viral zoonotic diseases.
13. Name two fungal zoonotic diseases.
14. Vectors/biological vector/mechanical vector.
15. Name any four water-borne diseases.
16. Fomites.
17. Droplet nuclei/name any four air-borne diseases.
18. Vertical infections/teratogenic infections/congenital infections.
19. Define and differentiate secondary infection and opportunistic infections.

19

Hospital-Acquired Infections Cross-Infections in Hospitals/ Nosocomial Infections/ Hospital Infections

- *Definition*
- *Sources of nosocomial infections*
- *Opportunisitic infections*
- *Transmission of nosocomial infections*
- *Factors contributing to nosocomial infections*
- *Types of nosocomial infections*
- *Causative agents of nosocomial infections*
- *Emergence of drug-resistant microorganisms in hospitals*
- *Lab. diagnosis of Hospital infections*
- *Prevention, control and management of nosocomial infections*
- *Hand washing*
  - **Asepsis**
- **Antisepsis, disinfection and sterilisation**
- **Hospital environmental sanitation**
- **Hospital personnel**
- **Monitoring**
- **Isolation**
- **Universal blood and bodyfluid precautions**
- **Laundry services**
- **Dietetics services**
- **Instrumental procedures**
- **Hospital building and ward design**
- **Antibiotic policy**
- **Surveillance**
- **Infection control program/policy**

DEFINITION

The term "Nosocomial infections" (nosocomeion = hospital) is applied to infections developing in hospitalised patients, after their admission into the hospital which were not present or in incubation at the time of their admission.

Nosocomial infections may be

(1) Infections acquired outside the hospital which become clinically apparent when the patient is in hospital. *e.g.*, Measles.

(2) Infections acquired and developing within hospitals *e.g.*, wound infections, post-operative infections.

(3) Infections acquired in hospital, which become clinically apparent after the discharge of patients from hospital *e.g.,* infections in babies.

SOURCES OF NOSOCOMIAL INFECTIONS

The "**Reservoirs**" of nosocomial infections can be either living organisms (usually humans, animals or insects) that harbor pathogens; or inanimate objects contaminated with infectious microorganisms, known as "**fomites**".

The sources of nosocomial infection in a patient may be exogenous or endogenous.

1. Exogenous Infections

The source of infection is from external sources, such as (*i*) hospital personnel (*ii*) visitors (*iii*) hospital environment– air conditioners floors, bed linen, utensils, water taps, sinks dish mops, food, water, dust, flowers in patient's room, air-borne droplets (*iv*) contaminated medical equipment and fluids, such as – urinary catheters, oral thermometers, intravenous fluids, respiratory equipment, suction apparatus, anesthetic machines such infections are usually Iatrogenic, that may be induced by diagnostic or therapeutic procedures carried out in the hospital.

2. Endogenous Infections

The source of the most nosocomial infections is endogenous, the pathogen being derived from the patient body itself; caused by bacteria found on the skin and mucus membrane surfaces (*e.g., Staphylococcus aureus*), the intestine (*e.g., E.coli, Streptococcus fecalis*) etc.

OPPORTUNISTIC INFECTIONS

Many of the normal flora may act as opportunistic pathogens, which cause infection and disease, when patient's immunity is compromised. The two important sources of opportunistic infections in hospitals are

(*i*) hands of health care personnel

(*ii*) the skin, mucus membranes, saliva, feces and urine of the patient.

TRANSMISSION OF NOSOCOMIAL INFECTIONS

The transmission of infectious microorganisms from one host to another and the subsequent infection of the new host may occur in a number of ways. Pathogens may escape from Reservoir and transmitted to susceptible persons in a variety of ways; as shown below.

RESERVOIR

Growth and reproduction of pathogen

⇓

Escape Routes of Pathogen
From Reservoir

⇓

Respiratory tract – Oral and nasal droplets expelled from mouth and nose during sneezing, coughing or even talking. These droplets may settle on inanimate objects, which then serve as fomites.

- Gastrointestinal tract
- Genitourinary tract
- fluids exuded from lesions in skin and mucosa and wound infections

⇩

MODE OF TRANSMISSION

Direct contact – hand shaking, coughing, sneezing, kissing, rarely infected animals.

Indirect contact – water, food, milk, air currents, insects, contaminated hands, fomites.

⇩

PORTAL OF ENTRY

Respiratory tract – Air-borne diseases

Gatrointestinal tract – Food-borne and water-borne diseases

Genitourinary tract – Sexually transmitted diseases.

Breaks in skin; wounds and burns – wound and skin infections

Parenteral – inner tissues; – Puncture, injections Insect bite – Arthropod-borne diseases

⇩

SUSCEPTIBLE HOSTS

- New born and geriatric patients
- Ill patients
- Surgical patients
- Wounded and burned patients
- Patients undergoing radiation therapy or chemotherapy
- Patients with invasive devices.

FACTORS CONTRIBUTING TO NOSOCOMIAL INFECTIONS OR SUSCEPTIBILITY OF PATIENTS TO INFECTION

Several factors are responsible for frequent occurrence of infections in hospitalized patients.

(1) Many patients, particularly infants and elderly patients may have impaired defense mechanisms due to secondary infections, cancer, surgery, radiation, immuno-suppressive agents or procedures and instruments used on the body; making them more vulnerable to infections.

(2) Major invasive procedures, diagnostic or therapeutic, such as invasive devices, arterial and urinary catheters, implants, carried out in hospitals may lead to infections.

(3) Hospital infections are generally more serious and refractory to treatment as the causative agents are resistant to most antibiotics in common use.

(4) Modern methods of treatment such as organ transplantation, implanted prostheses (*e.g.*, heart valves, pace makers, hip joints), dialysis, exchange transfusion have enhanced the risk of hospital infections.

(5) Hospital environment is heavily laden with a wide variety of pathogens. Patients shed them through their bodies. Hospital personnel spread them through their hands and clothing. Bedding, linen and utensils may act as fomites. Equipment may be contaminated. Pathogens are present in hospital dust and air, and sometimes even in antiseptic lotions and ointments. Contamination of hospital food or water may cause outbreaks of infections.

(6) Patient's susceptibility to microorganisms may be increased by clinical conditions and medical procedures which may allow normal flora to be shifted from their normal habitat to some other area of the patient's body and thereby become opportunistic pathogens for example, *E.coli* from intestine may cause severe infections when transferred to urinary tract. Urinary catheterization can introduce pathogens into the bladder.

Breaking the skin barrier by surgery, biopsy, injection or withdrawal of a blood sample may allow normal skin flora such as *Staphylococcus aureus*, *Staphylococcus epidermidis* to enter tissues and cause infections.

Factors affecting patient's susceptibility to infection

	Factors	*Examples*
1.	Inadequate cell mediated immunity	Infants very old patients
2.	Health status	Malnutrition Diabetes chronic debilitating diseases Hematological disorders Renal diseases Immunodeficiencies, AIDS
3.	Accidents	Severe debilitation Severe burns Shock
4.	Surgery	Size of wound amount of wound drainage Duration of operation; skill of surgeon. Tissue trauma length of hospitalization foreign bodies – sutures, catheters prostheses
5.	Therapy	Antibiotics Radiation Steroids immunosuppressive drugs

TYPES OF NOSOCOMIAL INFECTIONS

1. Surgical or Nonsurgical Wound Infections

Some patients may develop surgical site infections and stitch abscesses after the patient is discharged from the hospital. Causative organisms may be *Staphylococcus aureus*; *Streptococcus pyogenes*; Gram negative bacilli – *E coli, Klebsiella, Pseudomonas*, Nonsporing anaerobes – *Bacteroides fragilis*; clostridial infections.

Non-surgical sites of wound infections include injections, cut-downs, umbilical stumps, ulcers and burns. *Pseudomonas aeruginosa* is most important causative agent of burns infections.

2. Urinary Tract Infections

Majority of hospital-acquired urinary tract infections are caused by Gram negative bacilli such as *E.coli, Klebsiella, Proteus* and *Pseudomonas*. A few urinary tract infections may be caused by *Staphylococcus* aureus, *Candida* species. The predisposing factors to nosocomial urinary tract infections are old age, female gender, catheterization and other serious underlying diseases.

3. Respiratory Infections

The most common pathogens which cause nosocomial Respiratory tract and lung infections (pneumonia) are *Staphylococcus aureus*, *Streptococcus pyogenes*, Gram negative bacilli-*Klebsiella* sp, *Moraxella catarrhalis*.

The risk factors that predispose patients to acquire nosocomial respiratory infections are – coma, old age, chronic pre-existing lung (cardiopulmonary) diseases, chest surgery, intubation (placement of a breathing tube down a patient's throat), attachment to a mechanical ventillator to control breathing, hospitalization in intensive care units, monitoring intracranial pressure in which a catheter inserted through the skill. Sometimes the microorganisms in upper respiratory tract may be coghed up and lodge in lungs instead of being spit out or swallowed.

4. Blood Stream Infections (Bacteremia and Septicemia)

Bacteremia and septicemia may occur as a consequence of the use of intravenous cannulae as in blood transfusion or intravenous rehydration, phlebitis and cut downs in infants and small children.

The causative organisms may be Gram negative bacilli, *Staphylococcus epidermidis, Staphylococcus aureus*, Enterococci, *Candida* sp. etc.

Staphylococcus epidermidis bacteremia is usually associated with implanted artificial heart valves.

The risk factors predisposing to blood stream infections are malnutrition intravenous cannulae, immunosuppressive therapy, severe preexisting diseases, skin lesions–burns, bedsores and prolonged stay in ICU.

5. Gastrointestinal Infections

Out breaks of Diarrhea, cholera, shigellosis, *Salmonella* gastroenteritis, typhoid fever, Hepatitis type A and Amoebic dysentery etc. can occur in hospitals due to contaminated food and water either from hospital personnel or patients or visitors.

CAUSATIVE AGENTS OF NOSOCOMIAL INFECTIONS

Staphylococcus aureus, Pseudomonas and *E.coli* are the most important causative agents of nosocomial infections among bacteria. Most of these strains, that are prevalent in hospital environment are drug resistant.

Viral infections in hospitals are frequently encountered in neonates, infants and immunocompromised patients. Fungal infections are on the rise due to prolonged antibiotic therapy, steroid therapy, immunosuppression, malignancies and Diabetes.

Commonly occurring microorganisms in hospital infections are listed here below.

Urinary tract infections	*E.coli, Klebsiella, Proteus, Serratia, Pseudomonas*, fecal streptococci, *Candida albicans.*
Wound and skin infections	*Staphylococcus aureus, E. coli, Proteus sp., Pseudomonas,* fecal streptococci, Anaerobes–*Bacteroides* *Staphylococcus epidermidis* *Streptococcus pyogenes*
Respiratory infections	*Staphylococcus aureus* *Streptococcus pyogenes* Gram negative bacilli – *Klebsiella* sp, *Pseudomonas.* *Haemophilus influenzae.* *Streptococcus pneumoniae* *Moraxella catarrhalis* Respiratory viruses
Blood stream infections	*Staphylococcus epidermidis* *Staphylococcus aureus* Enterococci Gram negative bacilli *Candida albicans*
Gastrointestinal infections	*Salmonella, Shigella* sp, virus–Rotavirus.

Most of the infections caused by enterococci, other nonhemolytic streptococci, anaerobic cocci, *Bacteroides* and gasgangrene producing clostridia are endogenous and self infectious. Group A streptococcal infection is always exogenous, which spreads from person to person (cross infection). Infections by *Staphylococcus aureus*, Group B streptococci. Enterobacteria (*E.coli, Klebsiella, Proteus* etc.) may be acquired either exogenously or endogenously. Infections with *Clostridium tetani, Flavobacterium, Pseudomonas aeruginosa*, Klebsiellae, *Serratia, Enterobacter* are often acquired from environment sources. HIV and HBV may be acquired from HIV and HBV positive patients by direct inoculation or through contact with broken skin or mucus membrane.

EMERGENCE OF DRUG RESISTANT MICROORGANISMS IN HOSPITALS

The widespread use of antibiotics, chemotherapeutic agents, antiseptics and aseptic techniques in hospitals have produced selective pressures so that sensitive microorganisms die out and those that are resistant multiply, spread and infect patients and become predominant in patients, hospital staff and hospital environment.

In the 1940s and 50s, with the advent of treatment of patients with penicillin and sulfonamides, resistant strains of *Staphylococcus aureus* appeared. Then in the 1970s, treatment of patients with narrow-spectrum cephalosporins and aminoglycosides led to the development and emergence of resistance among Gram negative bacilli – *Klebsiella, Enterobacter, Serratia, Pseudomonas.* During the late 1970s and early 1980s, the use of more potent cephalosporins played a role in the emergence of antibiotic resistant coagulase negative staphylococci, Enterococci, Methicillin–Resistant *Staphylococcus aureus* (MRSA). The 1990s has witnessed the emergence of betalctamase-resistant and vancomycin–resistant enterococci.

After hospitalization, patients normal flora quickly changes and will be replaced by drug-resistant organisms found in hospital environment and spread to other patients, staff and recontaminate hospital environment.

LAB DIAGNOSIS OF HOSPITAL INFECTIONS

For the diagnosis of nosocomial infections the sampling may be done from various possible sources of infection such as – hospital staff. Fomites, water, food, air, equipments, various surfaces, disinfectants, antiseptics, operation theatres, sterilised items (to monitor sterilisation) etc.

Aetiological diagnosis is by routine bacteriological methods like Microscopic examination of stained smear, culture, identification by biochemical tests and antibiotic sensitivity testing. Information about the sensitivity pattern of strains, known as antibiogram is useful as a guide to therapy and may also be used as an epidemiological marker in tracing the source of hospital-acquired infections. Other epidemiological markers used to identify the source of nosocomial infections include biotyping, phage typing, serotyping and bacteriocin typing.

PREVENTION, CONTROL AND MANAGEMENT OF NOSOCOMIAL INFECTIONS

The prevention, control and management of nosocomial infections consists of various measures as described below.

1. Hand Washing

It is a simple procedure where microorganisms are mechanically removed by rubbing soap-lathered hands for atleast ten seconds and rinsing under running water before and after contact with each patient.

All hospital personnel require scrubbing the lower arms and hands with soap and brush for about ten minutes, then rinsing under running water and with an antiseptic. This procedure is called "surgical scrub".

2. Asepsis

Asepsis is the prevention of contact with microorganism to prevent infections.

"**Medical asepsis**" consists of all practices used to keep hospital personnel, hospital environment and patients free from infectious microorganisms *e.g.*, hand washing, sanitation, isolation of patients etc.

"**Surgical asepsis**" is practiced in the operation theatre and in treatment procedures such as wound dressing, catheterization and intravenous therapy. All surgical instruments, gloves and other items that come in contact with patients are sterilized. The operation theater environment is sanitized, fumigated. Operation theatre staff should scrub their hands and arms and put on protective clothing such as sterile caps, gowns, masks and gloves. Antiseptics may be used on patient's skin.

3. Antisepsis, Disinfection and Sterilization

The provision of sterile instruments, dressings and fluids is very important in hospital practice. Sterilisation is done in autoclave and hot air oven in hospital practice.

The use of sterile, pre-packed, single-use disposable items, such as syringes, thermometers, needles, gloves, masks, catheters and drainage bags must be recommended (they are commercially sterilized by gamma radiation or ethylene oxide). This disposed infective waste must be incinerated or autoclaved before disposal in a landfill.

The materials and equipment used for patient care based on the risk of infection during their use into three categories – critical, semicritical and noncritical items.

Critical items *e.g.,* surgical instruments, surgical dressings, catheters, implants and other invasive items; must be sterilized.

Semicritical items such as thermometers must be cleaned and disinfected for reuse.

Noncritical items are those that touch only intact skin, such as bed boards, crutches and other medical accessories. They should be washed with a detergent.

4. Hospital Environmental Sanitation

The general hospital environment can be kept in good order by attention to basic cleaning, waste disposal and laundry. To clean and disinfect floors and other surfaces in hospitals, scrubbing with water, detergents and sanitizers or disinfectants is sufficient. Mops should be washed and dried thoroughly each day to reduce contamination.

5. Hospital Personnel

Hospital staff are the potential sources of pathogens that are frequently antibiotic resistant. All hospital staff attending patients must be free from infections such as boils, respiratory infections.

All hospital staff and medical students should receive general health protection. Hepatitis B vaccine should be given to those at special risk.

6. Monitoring

Samples may be taken from various surfaces of the hospital to isolate and identify the microorganisms prevalent in hospital environment.

Microbiological screening of staff may be undertaken to detect carriers in critical areas such as dialysis units or for specific purposes such as before cardiac surgery, to eliminate *Staphylococcus aureus* from carriage sites.

7. Isolation

Isolation is the separation of a patient from other people and the care of the patient in an isolated environment.

Isolation is effective control method to prevent the spread of pathogens among patients, staff and visitors.

"**Barrier nursing**" is a term used to describe the attempts to "isolate" a patient when strict physical segregation is not possible. The patient is nursed in the same multi-bedded ward as other patients, but is protected by the strict aseptic precautions against the transmission of infections.

In Reverse isolation, the patient is protected from acquiring infections.

8. Universal Blood and Body fluid precautions

To minimise the risk that a health care worker might transmit HIV or HBV to a patient, the following measures were recommended by the centers for disease control.

1. Use of barrier protection-Gloves should be worn when treating bleeding patients, when drawing blood, and for procedures involving contact with mucous membranes or potentially infectious material. Gloves should be changed after contact with each patient.

   Masks protective eye-wear, face shields and gowns should be worn during procedures that may generate splashes or droplets of blood or other body fluids.
2. Hands and skin should be washed immediately and thoroughly, after removing gloves, and always before taking care of another patient.
3. Prevent injuries caused by needles, scalpels, and the other sharp instruments. Needles should never be recapped, removed from disposable syringes, or bent or broken by hand. All sharp items should be placed in a puncture-resistant container, located as close as possible to the user, for disposal.
4. Minimize mouth to mouth resuscitation, always use a protective device.
5. Health care workers with exudative lesions or weeping dermatitis should refrain from all direct patient care and from handling patient care equipment until the condition resolves.
6. Pregnant health care workers must be familiar with and must strictly adhere to precautions. The infant is also at risk of infection if the mother is infected.
7. All health care workers who are exposed to blood should receive HBV vaccine.

9. Laundry

The washing of linen can be manual by "dhobies" or mechanical by washing machines. Special care is necessary when washing is done by dhobies. The linen used by the patients, doctors, paramedical staff may be "clean contaminated" or "contaminated" when soiled with blood, pus, urine feces or any other bodyfluids.

The contaminated linen must be disinfected before giving to 'dhobies' for washing. The disinfection can be done by chemical disinfectant or by boiling or autoclaving at low pressure of steam.

Both the "clean contaminated" and "contaminated" linen should be transported to laundry separately in thick polythene bags of different colors.

10. Dietetics Service

Food can be a source of infection to hospitalised patients. All necessary precautions should be taken from procurement of food material to supply of cooked food so that no patient gets any type of infection due to consumption of food prepared and supplied in the hospital.

Special care should be taken in transporting the cooked food from kitchen to the ward No uncovered food should be transported. All the uncooked food should be washed thoroughly preferably using mild disinfectants like potassium permanganate.

The food handlers should be examined from time to time for carriage of pathogenic organisms causing food and water borne diseases.

11. Instrumental Procedures

Surgery, catheterization and other invasive procedures may introduce organisms into the tissues. Anaesthetic machines and respirators may facilitate the spread of organisms from patient to patient. Incubators can be a source of opportunistic organisms and may infect premature babies. Hence diagnostic and treatment procedures must be carried out with greatest care and all apparatus must be free from organisms. Instruments used to penetrate the body must be sterile.

12. Hospital Building And Ward Design

The movement of personnel and apparatus within wards of special units may affect the rate of infection. Good ward design with adequate space, ventilation, air flow which maintains the rest and quiet of the patient will reduce the rate of cross-infection. Wards and outpatient departments including dressing stations must be designed to facilitate unidirectional traffic and the flow of material from the "clean" to the "dirty" sides of a unit, with a minimum crossing of paths.

13. Antibiotic Policy

Antibiotics may act as selective agents in the hospital environment by encouraging the emergence and spread of antibiotic-resistant and opportunistic bacteria and increases the incidence, toxic-side effects and the cost of treatment. A rational antibiotic policy plays an important role in infection control.

One policy is complete withdrawal of one or two or more antibiotics from clinical use, which may reduce the emergence of resistance to these drugs. Another policy that may be helpful is the rotational use of different sets of antibiotics for successive periods.

14. Surveillance

Surveillance is the systematic observation and recording of cases of transmissible diseases, which forms the basis for an effective control program. The data collected continuously must be tabulated, analyzed and reviewed. There should be one full-time person for every 300 to 500 beds to ensure adequate surveillance, investigation of infections and infection-control activities. This person is normally a pathologist, an epidemiologist, a microbiologist or a nurse and is usually called an Infection-control officer (ICO).

15. Infection Control Program

To prevent and control nosocomial infections an effective infection control program must be established by administration by combining hospital policy-making committee, infection-control committee, Microbiology laboratory and infection-control officer.

ORGANIZATION OF INFECTION-CONTROL PROGRAM
Hospital Policy-Making Committee (develop policies for control of nosocomial infection)
⇅
Infection-Control Committee (develop guidelines for patient care; monitor effectiveness of control program)

↓↑

Microbiology Laboratory

–isolate and identify organisms;

–identify source of organisms;

–monitor disinfection and sterilization procedures.

↓↑

Infection-Control Officer

(Pathologist or Microbiologist or epidemiologist or nurse)

–implement infection-control practices

–surveillance and investigation of infections in patients and personnel (staff)

–maintain a continuing education program

QUESTIONS

Long Essay

1. Define Nosocomial infection. Describe the sources, transmission of nosocomial infections. Add a note on prevention, control and management of Hospital infections.

Short Essays

1. Define hospital infection. Mention two organisms causing it.
2. Nosocomial infections.
3. Control of hospital infection.
4. Asepsis.
5. Isolation.
6. Universal blood and body fluid precautions.
7. Hospital infection control policy/program.

20

Microbial Pathogenicity

- *Pathogenicity*
- *Virulence*
- *Exaltation*
- *Attenuation*
- *Factors determining virulence/pathogenicity*
  - *Communicability of transmissibility*
  - *Adhesion or colonization*
  - *Invasiveness/Aggressiveness*
  - *Toxigenicity/Bacterial toxins*
    - *Exotoxins*
    - *Endotoxins*
      - *LAL assay*
      - *Biological effects/Endotoxic shock*
  - *Extracellular enzymes*
  - *Resistance to phagocytosis*
  - *Survival within phagocytes*
  - *Infective dose*
  - *Routes of infection*
  - *Plasmids*
  - *Bacteriophages*

PATHOGENICITY

Pathogenicity is defined as the capacity of a microbial species to produce disease. *e.g., Mycobacterium tuberculosis*, *Salmonella typhi* are referred to as pathogenic.

VIRULENCE

Virulence is defined as the degree or intensity of pathogenicity in a strain or clone of microorganism. *e.g.,* The species *Mycobacterium tuberculosis* may contain several strains with varying degrees of virulence.

The term virulence is often expressed in relation to host-parasite relationship. The virulence property of an organism is variable. Pathogenicity is therefore a qualitative term and virulence a quantitative one.

EXALTATION

Enhancement of virulence is known as **"exaltation"**, which can be achieved by serial passage in favourable and susceptible hosts.

ATTENUATION

Reduction in virulence is known as **"attenuation"**, which can be achieved by following means

(*i*) by serial passage through unfavourable host (other than natural host)

(*ii*) by repeated subcultures

(*iii*) by growth under high temperature

(*iv*) by growth in the presence of weak antiseptics

(*v*) by prolonged storage in cultures

(*vi*) by desiccation

(*vii*) by mutations.

e.g., Sabin's oral polio vaccine (OPV) is a live attenuated strain (a mutant); BCG (Bacillus Calmette-Guerin) is a live attenuated vaccine, attenuated by 239 serial subcultures over a period of 13 years in a glycerine-bile-potato medium.

FACTORS DETERMINING VIRULENCE/PATHOGENICITY

In order to cause infectious disease, a pathogen must be able to

1. infect the host
2. adhere to, colonize or invade the host
3. grow and multiply in the host tissues
4. resist host defence mechanisms
5. damage the host.

There are several factors, which contribute to or determine virulence, known as virulence determinants or aggressins.

Communicability or Transmissibility

The ability of a parasite to spread from one host to another is known as communicability, which determines the survival and distribution of a parasite in a community.

The means of communicability is direct contact or indirect contact by fomites, air, water, food, soil and vectors etc. The infections in which the pathogen is shed in oral or nasal secretions as in respiratory infections and in feces as in intestinal infections, are highly communicable. Some times human infection represents a dead-end, preventing communicability of the pathogen *e.g.,* Rabies, hydatid disease.

Adhesion and Colonization

After being transmitted to host, the pathogen must be able to adhere to and colonize host cells and tissues. Adhesion involves specific surface interactions between adherence factors on the bacterial surface and complementary receptor sites on the host's cell surface. Microorganisms adhere with a high degree of specificity to particular tissues, with various kinds of adhensins.

e.g., Fimbriae or pili, glycocalyx or capsule, slime or biofilms, hemagglutinin, teichoic and lipoteichoic acids in Gram positive bacteria, adherence proteins such as ligands, mucus gel, colonisation factors, IgA protease, fibronectin.

Hemagglutinin adhesins may be – filamentous *e.g., Bordetella pertussis*; mannose-resistant *e.g., Salmonella typhimurium*; fibrillar *e.g., Helicobacter pylori*. *Streptococcus mutans* produces polysaccharide which anchors the bacterium to tooth surface; coagulase negative Staphylococci produce *polysaccharide* slime which attaches bacterium to prosthetic devices and catheters. IgA protease is produced by *Neisseria gonorrhoeae* and *Hemophilus influenzae*.

Fibronectin is a glycoprotein found in plasma and on mucosal surfaces. *Streptococcus pyogenes*, *Staphylococcus aureus* and *Treponema pallidum* etc. attach themselves to the fibronectin.

Adhesins are antigenic. Specific immunisation with adhesins has been attempted as a method of prophylaxis in some infections.

Invasiveness/Aggressiveness

It refers to the ability of a pathogen to spread or invade and multiply in healthy tissues, usually by producing lytic substances or passively through disrupted skin and mucosal surfaces.

Examples

I. Trauma – wounds, lesions, ulcers, breaks, abrasions, burns, needle sticks, insect bites.

II. Inhalation – smoking, noxious gases

III. Implantation of medical devices

IV. Child birth

V. Other diseases – malignancies, diabetes, repeated infections

VI. Alcoholism

VII. Overuse of antibiotics.

Highly invasive pathogens produce generalised or spreading type of lesions *e.g.,* streptococcal septicemia following wound infections; whereas less invasive pathogens cause more localised lesions *e.g.,* Staphylococcal abscess. Some pathogens are non-invasive but can cause fatal diseases *e.g.,* tetanus by *Clostridium tetani.*

Toxigenicity/Bacterial Toxins

Some microorganisms produce poisonous substances known as "Toxins". They are of two types.

I. Exotoxins – excreted into the surrounding medium.

II. Endotoxins – retained within the cell as an integral part of cell wall.

Exotoxins

1. Proteins (polypeptides) with a mol. wt. 10,000 – 900,000.
2. Heat labile, can be inactivated by heating at 60–80°C.
3. Soluble.
4. Excreted (secreted) from the microbial cells into the surroundings (into the culture medium or into the circulatory system and tissues of a host).
5. Do not require cell lysis or bacterial death for their release. Toxins can be separated from cultures by physical methods such as filtration.
6. Possess enzymatic action.
7. Associated with specific diseases.
8. Possess specific pharmacological effects.
9. Possess specific tissue affinities.
10. Most lethal substances known; highly potent.
11. Active in very minute doses and possess very high toxicity. Active in micrograms or less for laboratory animals.

12. It can be inactivated by formaldehyde, phenol, acids, betapropiolactone, iodine, heat into antigenic **"toxoids",** which can be used for immunisation *e.g.,* tetanus toxoid, diphtheria toxoid.
13. Strongly antigenic (immunogenic), both toxins and toxoids stimulate the formation of antibodies, known as "antitoxins".
14. Antitoxins can neutralise toxins specifically, *e.g.,* Tetanus antitoxin (ATS), diphtheria antitoxin.
15. Cannot produce fever in the host (not pyrogenic).
16. Cannot produce shock.
17. Often given the name of the disease they proudce. *e.g.,* cholera toxin, diphtheria toxin, tetanus toxin.
18. Produced mainly by Gram positive bacteria and by some Gram negative bacteria.
19. Production may be under the control of genetic or plasmid or phage DNA.

Table 20.1 Control of toxin production

Toxin	*Genetic Control*
Cholera toxin Pertussis toxin Shiga toxin	Chromosomal
Tetanus toxin *E.coli* enterotoxins (LT) Anthrax toxin	Plasmid DNA
Diphtheria toxin Botulinum toxin	Phage DNA (Prophage)

20. categorised as neutrotoxins, cytotoxins or enterotoxins according to their mechanism of action.

Table 20.2 Exotoxins and their site of action

Exotoxin	*Site affected*	*Bacterial examples*
Neurotoxin	Nervous tissue	*Clostridium botulinum* *Clostridium tetani*
Enterotoxin	Intestinal mucosa	*Staphylococcus aureus* *Bacillus cereus* *Vibrio cholerae* *E. coli* *Salmonella* sp. *Klebsiella* sp. *Clostridium welchii*
Cytotoxin	General tissues	*Shigella* sp. *Vibrio parahemolyticus* *Staphylococcus aureus* *Clostridium difficle*

21. Exotoxins exert their effect in a variety of ways

(*i*) inhibition of protein synthesis. *e.g.,* diphtheria toxin, shiga toxin

(*ii*) inhibition of nerve synapse function. *e.g., Clostridium botulinum* toxin

(*iii*) disruption of membrane transport

(*iv*) damage to plasma membrane.

22. Some well known diseases caused by bacteria that produce exotoxins, are listed here below:

Table 20.3 Diseases caused by toxins

Pathogen	*Disease*	*Toxin*	*Toxin activity in vivo*
1. *Clostridium botulinum*	Botulism	Botulinum toxin	Neurotoxin, muscle paralysis
2. *Clostridium tetani*	Tetanus	Tetanospasmin	Neurotoxin, spasmodic muscle contraction
3. *Corynebacterium diphtheriae*	Diphtheria	Diphtheria toxin	Nerve paralysis; heart damage
4. *Vibrio cholerae*	Cholera	Cholera toxin	Loss of fluid from small intestine; vomiting
5. *Bordetella pertussis*	Whooping cough	Pertussis toxin	Paroxysmal coughing, vomiting
6. *Shigella dysenteriae*	Bacillary dysentery	Shiga toxin	Neurological disturbances; diarrhoea
7. *Staphylococcus aureus*	Staphylococcal food-poisoning	enterotoxin	Nausea, vomiting, diarrhoea
8. *Escherichia coli*	Diarrhoea	Enterotoxin	Loss of fluid from small intestine

23. Botulinum type A toxin is used to treat strabismus, blepharospasm and hemifacial spasm.

24. Exotoxins may occur in many forms, but the "AB structural model" is common. Each toxin is composed of two subunits –

(*i*) Fragment 'B' or binding subunit – binds to target cells but are nontoxic and biologically inactive. The B subunit binds to specific receptors on target **cells** or tissues such as the gangliosides GM_1 for cholera toxin, GT_1 and/or GD_1 for tetanus toxin, and GD_1 for botulinum toxin.

(*ii*) Fragment 'A' or active subunit – responsible for enzymatic, toxic effect inside the host cell. A subunit enters the cell through a pore in the plasma membrane caused by B fragment or by endocytosis.

Endotoxins

1. Lipopolysaccharides (LPS).
2. Relatively heat stable, can withstand heat over 60°C for many hours.
3. They form an integral part of the outer membranes of cell wall, as a component of somatic antigen (O-antigen).
4. They are released upon cell lysis or cell death only.
5. Do not possess enzymatic action.
6. Do not possess specific pharmacological effects.
7. Do not possess specific tissue affinities.

8. Action is common to all endotoxins; non-specific.
9. Less potent than exotoxins; active in very large doses only.
10. Weakly antigenic.
11. Cannot stimulate the formation of antitoxins; can stimulate the formation of antibodies to polysaccharide moiety (somatic or O-antigen).
12. Cannot be rendered nontoxic when combined with homologous antibody.
13. Cannot be converted to toxoids.
14. Pyrogenic; often produce fever in host.
15. Can produce shock, known as endotoxic shock.
16. Present in Gram negative bacteria *e.g., Salmonella, Shigella, Escherichia, Neisseria* etc.
17. Biological activity or toxicity of endotoxins, is largely due to lipid A.
18. **Limulus amoebocyte lysate (LAL) assay** can detect small amounts of endotoxin in various body fluids, which is helpful in the laboratory diagnosis of infections caused by Gram negative bacteria.

    Limulus polyphemus is the atlantic coast horseshoe crab, and the hemolymph (blood) of this crab contains a single type of white cells called amoebocytes. Each amoebocyte is packed with proteins responsible for clotting. When the crab blood comes in contact with endotoxin, either in a purified form or as a component of Gram negative bacteria, the clotting proteins of the amoebocytes are released and the blood forms a gel or clot. The LAL test is sensitive at the nanogram level. This clotting reaction is advantageous to the crab because it localizes an infection in a walled-off area and prevents blood loss.
19. Some Gram negative bacteria such as *Yersinia pestis* and *Bordetella pertussis* produce toxins in addition to their LPS endotoxins.
20. Bacteria containing LPS along with O-antigen form Smooth (S) colonies on agar media, whereas loss of O-antigen results in the formation of Rough (R) colonies and this phenomenon is called smooth to Rough ($S \rightarrow R$) variation.
21. ***Biological effects of endotoxins or endotoxic shock*** are as follows :

    Pyrogenicity, lethal action, hypotension, activation of complement, leucopenia, clotting of limulus lysate, polyclonal activation of B-lymphocytes, local Shwartzmann reaction, macrophage migration inhibition, stimulates natural killer (NK) cells, stimulates macrophages to produce cytokines such as inter-leukin-1, tumour necrosis factor (TNF), and colony stimulating factor (CSF), disseminated intravascular coagulation, induction of prostaglandins and leucotrienes, stimulates non-specific resistance to infections.

Endotoxins initially activate blood clotting factor XII (Hageman factor), which in turn activates four humoral systems – coagulation, complement, fibrinolytic and kininogen systems.

Septicemia by Gram negative bacteria cause the syndrome of endotoxic shock, characterised by fever, leucopenia, thrombocytopenia, decrease in blood pressure, circulatory collapse and bloody diarrhoea leading to death.

The pyrogenic effect of fluids such as normal saline and dextrose used for intravenous administration is usually due to the presence in them of endotoxins from contaminant bacteria.

Table 20.4 Differences between exotoxins and endotoxins

Exotoxins	*Endotoxins*
1. Proteins (polypeptides) with a molecular weight of 10,000-900,000	Lipopolysaccharides
2. Heat labile; can be inactivated by heating at 60–80°C	Relatively heat stable; can withstand heat over 60°C for many hours
3. Excreted (secreted) from the microbial cells into the surroundings (into the culture medium or into the circulatory system and tissues of a host)	They form an integral part of the outer membranes of cell wall as a component of somatic antigen (O-antigen)
4. Do not require cell lysis or bacterial death for their release; toxins can be separated from cultures by physical methods such as filtration	They are released upon cell lysis or cell death only
5. Possess enzymatic action	Do not possess enzymatic action
6. Possess specific pharmacological effects	Do not possess specific pharmacological effects
7. Possess specific tissue affinities	Do not possess specific tissue affinities
8. Highly potent; active in very minute doses only	Less potent than exotoxins; active in very large doses only
9. Strongly antigenic	Weakly antigenic
10. Can be converted to antigenic toxoids by inactivation with formaldehyde, betapropiolactene, iodine, phenol, acids and heat; which can be used for immunisation	Cannot be converted to toxoids
11. Both toxins and toxoids stimulate the formation of antibodies known an "antitoxins".	Cannot stimulate the formation of antitoxins; can stimulate the formation of antibodies to polysaccharide moiety (somatic antigen or O-antigen)
12. Antitoxins can neutralise toxins specifically	Cannot be rendered non-toxic when combined with homologous antibody.
13. Cannot produce fever in the host (not pyrogenic)	Pyrogenic; often produce fever in the host
14. Cannot produce shock	Can produce shock, known as endotoxic shock
15. Produced mainly by Gram positive bacteria and by some Gram negative bacteria *e.g.*, Clostridium tetani, *Clostridium botulinum*, *Corynebacterium diphtheriae*, *Vibrio cholerae*	Present in Gram negative bacteria only *e.g.*, *Salmonella*, *Shigella*, *Escherichia*, *Neisseria* etc.

Extracellular enzymes

Some bacterial products enhance virulence by promoting invasiveness into the tissue and by inhibiting host's resistance.

Table 20.5 Bacterial enzymes

Enzyme	*Action*	*Example*
Hyaluronidase	Hydrolyzes hyaluronic acid in tissue; invasive factor	Staphylococci, Streptococci, Clostridia
Coagulase	Clots plasma; useful in identification	*Staphylococcus aureus*
Lecithinase	Hydrolyzes membrane lipids	*Clostridium welchii*
Collagenase	Hydrolyzes collagen in tissue; invasive factor	*Clostridium perfringens*
Leucocidin	Kills leucocytes	*Staphylococcus aureus*
Hemolysin	Lyses RBC; invasive factor	Staphylococci, Streptococci, Clostridia
Streptokinase	Lyses fibrin	*Streptococcus pyogenes*

Hyaluronidase hydrolyzes hyaluronic acid, an intercellular cement substance and helps the pathogen to penetrate the tissues. Hence, it is called "Spreading factor". *Staphylococcus aureus, Streptococcus pyogenes* and *Clostridium welchii* etc. produce hyaluronidase.

Lecithinase destroys membrane lipids and collagenase collagen, a tissue fiber found in muscles; produced by *Clostridium welchii* and responsible for its virulence.

Fibrinolysin (streptokinase) produced by *Streptococcus pyogenes* breaks down fibrin barrier and promote spreading of streptococcal lesions.

Depolymerizing enzymes such as mucinase, lipases, proteases, nucleases, neuraminidase etc. may contribute to virulence.

Staphylococcus aureus produces coagulase enzyme which converts fibrinogen into fibrin; which is deposited around the lesion, and protects bacteria from host phagocytes.

Hemolysins are substances that lyse RBC, releasing their hemoglobin known as **hemolysis.** Hemolytic strains are generally more virulent than non-hemolytic strains of the same species. Bacterial hemolysins from various species differ in their chemical nature and mode of action.

Some hemolysins on blood agar plates produce visible changes. When colonies are surrounded by a clear, colorless, transparent zone, where RBC have been lysed completely is known as β-hemolysis *e.g.*, group A Streptococci (*Streptococcus pyogenes*). Some bacterial hemolysins reduce the hemoglobin to methemoglobin, which results in the formation of a greenish zone around the colonies. This is called α-hemolysis, *e.g.*, *Streptococcus viridans*, pneumococci. Some bacteria cannot produce hemolysis, called γ-hemolysis or non-hemolytic, *e.g.*, *Enterococci*.

Resistance to Phagocytosis

Presence or absence of capsules influences virulence. Capsules inhibit phagocytosis thereby promote virulence. Capsulated bacteria such as Pneumococci, *Klebsiella pneumoniae*, *Hemophilus influenzae* are highly virulent. When they lose capsules (by mutations), they become avirulent.

Some bacterial surface antigens such as Vi antigen of *Salmonella typhi* and K antigens of *E.coli* promote virulence of bacteria by inhibiting phagocytosis and lytic activity of complement.

Protein A of *Staphylococcus aureus* and M proteins of *Streptococcus pyogenes* can prevent complement activity and thereby promote virulence.

Survival Within Phagocytes

Intracellular pathogens use different strategies to resist intracellular killing mechanisms of macrophages and other phagocytes and may multiply intracellularly.

Some methods adopted by bacteria to avoid intracellular killing are as follows:

Mycobacterium tuberculosis	– Prevents phagosome - lysosome fusion.
Salmonella typhi, Yersinia enterocolitica	– Fail to stimulate O_2–dependent killing
Staphylococcus aureus, Neisseria gonorrhoeae	– Produce catalase to negate effect of toxic O_2 radicals
Legionella pneumophila	– Inhibits phagolysosome acidification

Infective dose

Virulence is estimated in terms of the number or weight of microorganisms or micrograms of toxin required to kill a particular species of animal. This is called Minimum lethal dose (MLD). Minimum Infecting Dose (MID) is the minimum number of bacteria required to produce clinical disease or death, in a susceptible animal under standard conditions. As different animals exhibit differences in susceptibility to various microorganisms, these doses are more accurately expressed as LD 50 and ID 50, which is defined as the dose required to infect or kill 50 per cent of the animals tested under standard conditions.

Routes of Infection

Bacteria can survive and multiply only when introduced by optimal routes and related to the modes by which different bacteria are able to initiate tissue damage and establish themselves. For example, cholera vibrios are infective orally but cannot cause infection when introduced subcutaneously. Some bacteria, such as Streptococci can initiate infection, whatever be the mode of entry.

Plasmids

Plasmid mediated factors are associated with virulence. In *E.coli* both enterotoxin genes and colonisation factor genes are coded for by plasmids. R factors increase the severity of clinical disease by conferring multiple drug resistance on bacteria.

Bacteriophages

Phage directed virulence is characteristically seen in *Corynebacterium diphtheriae* and *Clostridium botulinum.* The diphtheria bacilli are harmless by themselves; but when it is infected with β-phage (corynephage), the phage DNA (prophage) codes for the synthesis of diphtheria toxin, which is responsible for the clinical manifestations of diphtheria disease. Similarly *Clostridium botulinum* (types C and D) produces toxin, coded by Tox^+ bacteriophages.

QUESTIONS

Essay Type Questions

1. Describe the factors determining microbial pathogenicity and virulence.

   Or

   Describe bacterial virulence factors.

   Or

   Write a note on virulence factors in bacteria .
2. Describe bacterial toxins.

Short Notes

1. Differentiate pathogenicity from virulence.
2. Virulence.
3. Attenuation.
4. Virulence factors.
5. Bacterial toxins.
6. Exotoxins.
7. Endotoxins.
8. Toxoids.
9. LAL assay.
10. Endotoxic shock.
11. Name any four extracellular enzymes produced by bacteria.
12. What is the difference between attenuation and exaltation ?
13. Name any two bacterial appendages that offer resistance to phagocytosis.
14. Define MLD and MID.
15. Define LD 50 and ID 50.
16. Name two phages which code for the synthesis of bacterial toxins. What diseases they cause ?
17. Hemolysins.
18. Hemolysis.
19. Name any four bacteria that produce toxins and the diseases caused by them.

21

Normal Microbial Flora of The Human Body

INTRODUCTION

The term "**normal microbial flora**" refers to the microbial population that inhabit the internal and external surfaces of healthy normal humans and animals.

The human fetus is sterile under normal conditions, but is exposed to a variety of microorganisms at birth. Microbial colonization of the neonate begins as the child passes through the birth canal and is exposed to the vaginal flora of the mother. The neonate is then exposed to microorganisms in the environment and to those that colonize hospital personnel and other individuals. Within a short time, the infant develops its own indigenous normal microbial flora. The normal flora of any individual undergoes constant change in accordance with changes in life-style and environment. The normal microbial flora is more or less constant for each species and broadly divided into Resident flora and Transient flora.

RESIDENT FLORA

It consists of relatively fixed types of microorganisms constantly found in a given area, at a given age. If disturbed, it promptly re-establishes itself. They prevent colonisation by other microorganisms.

TRANSIENT FLORA

It consists of either nonpathogenic or pathogenic microorganisms that inhabit the skin or mucus membranes for hours, days or weeks. It varies from time to time, derived from the environment, does not establish itself permanently. If the resident flora is disturbed, transient microflora may colonize, proliferate and produce disease.

ROLE OF NORMAL MICROBIAL FLORA

The normal microbial flora plays a very important beneficial role in the human body.

(1) The microbial flora of intestine synthesizes B-complex vitamins and vitamin-K, which may be absorbed. Thus, they supply some nutritional needs of the host.

(2) They prevent or interfere with colonization or invasion of the body by pathogens through bacterial interference.

(3) Normal microflora raises the overall immune status of the host against pathogens having related or shared antigens.

(4) Normal microflora may produce antibiotic like substances called bacteriocins (*e.g.,* colicins, pyocines etc.) which may kill or inhibit the growth of pathogens.

(5) Normal flora may liberate endotoxins, which may activate alternate complement pathway and help the defense mechanisms of the body.

Normal microflora may have some harmful effects.

(1) When host immunity decreases, they may become opportunistic pathogens and cause disease.

(2) Penicillinase producing microorganisms can aggravate infection by conferring drug resistance against antibiotics.

(3) They cause confusion in diagnosis due to their ubiquitous presence in the body, and their morphological similarity with some pathogens.

(4) Certain alpha hemolytic streptococci, that live as commensals in the mouth may cause dental caries.

NORMAL FLORA OF THE SKIN

The human skin is constantly exposed to environment and contains largely transient flora.

The normal resident flora of the skin differs in different anatomic sites by secretions, habitual wearing of clothing, occupation and environment and proximity to the mucous membranes such as mouth, nose and perineum.

Profuse sweating, washing and bathing cannot eliminate resident flora, whereas transient flora is eliminated from the skin by low pH, fatty acids in sebaceous secretions and the presence of lysozyme.

The normal resident flora of skin includes *Staphylococcus epidermidis (albus), Staphylococcus aureus, Propionibacterium acnes*, Diphtheroids, *Candida* sp, *Pityrosporum.*

NORMAL FLORA OF CONJUNCTIVA (EYE)

The conjunctival flora is normally held in check by the mechanical action of blinking, flow of tears, which contain an antibacterial lysozyme.

The normal flora of eye includes *Staphylococcus epidermidis, Staphylococcus aureus*, diphtheroids *(Corynebacterium xerosis), Neisseria* sp, *Moraxella* sp, *Haemophilus parainfluenzae.*

NORMAL FLORA OF MOUTH AND UPPER RESPIRATORY TRACT

The mouth and upper respiratory tract contains a wide range of microorganisms-*Staph epidermidis, Staph. aureus*, alpha hemolytic streptococci (viridans streptococci), *Streptococcus pneumoniae,*

Corynebacterium sp. (diphtheroides), *Neisseria* sp, *Branhamella* sp, *Haemophilus* sp, *Micrococcus* sp.

The lower respiratory tract (trachea, bronchi) do not have a normal flora, because of the efficient mechanical removal of microorganisms by an upward movement of cilia-driven mucus. A few bacteria, which enter alveoli are engulfed by phagocytes.

Viridans Streptococci are the primary microbes in the oral cavity.

The normal flora associated with tongue and buccal mucosa are Viridan streptococci (*Strept. mitior, Strept. salivarius*), *Streptococcus* sp, *Neisseria* sp, *Veillonella* sp, *Actinomyces* sp, *Lactobacillus* sp, Yeasts (*Candida* sp).

The normal flora associated with teeth and gingival crevices are *Bacteroides* sp. *Fusobacterium* sp. alpha hemolytic streptococci (*Strept. Sanguis, Strept. mutans*), *Streptococcus* sp, *Actinomyces* sp, *Lactobacillus* sp, *Porphyromonas gingivalis, Prevotella* sp, Spirochaetes (*Treponema denticola*), *Wolinella* sp, *Selenomonas* sp, *Trichomonas tenax*.

The teeth themselves can become areas for microbial adherence. *Streptococcus mutans* is associated with tooth surface and cause **dental caries** (tooth decay). *Streptococcus mutans* produces glucan, a sticky polymer of glucose that acts like a cement and binds the bacterial cells together and to the tooth surface. This glucan is formed in the presence of disaccharide sucrose (the sugar found in confections), through a process catalyzed by an enzyme located on the surface of cocci; which splits sucrose into monosaccharides glucose and fructose. The enzymes then links the glucose molecules together to form glucan, while the fructose is fermented by the streptococci into Lactic acid. This lactic acid can etch the surface of the teeth, enhancing microbial adherence. Although *Streptococcus mutans* initiates dental caries, other bacteria such as *Lactobacillus* and *Actinomyces* may act as secondary invaders. The aggregation of bacteria and organic matter on the surface of the teeth is termed "**dental plaque**", which contains very high number of bacteria, about 10^8 cells per mg.

NORMAL FLORA OF NOSE, NASOPHARYNX AND ACCESSORY SINUSES

Nares, nasopharynx and accessory sinuses are heavily colonized by bacteria trapped from inhaled air by infiltration through the nasopharynx. The normal flora includes Viridans Streptococci, *Staphylococcus epidermidis, Neisseria* sp, *Corynebacterium* sp, *Moraxella lacunata*.

High doses of antibiotics may eradicate normal flora and results in colonization by Gram negative bacilli such as *E.coli, Klebsiella, Proteus* and *Pseudomonas* sp.

Nasopharynx frequently carries pathogenic bacteria such as *Streptococcus pyogenes, Streptococcus pneumoniae, Neisseria meningitidis, Staphylococcus aureus, Bordetella pertussis, Haemophilus influenzae* and *Corynebacterium diphtheriae*.

NORMAL FLORA OF THE GASTROINTESTINAL TRACT

Gastrointestinal tract is the most heavily colonized portion of the body.

Stomach consists of *Lactobacillus* sp and yeasts such as *Candida* sp. Administration of cimetidine in peptic ulcer leads to a great increase in microbial flora of the stomach.

Small Intestine consists of Enterococci, Lactobacilli, Corynebacteria, *Candida* sp., *Bacteroides* sp, *E. coli*.

Large intestine or colon has the largest microbial population, around 10^{11} organisms per gram wet weight, which means that about 25% of feces is made up of microorganisms. Over 300 different bacterial species have been isolated from human feces. It has been calculated that an adult excretes 3×10^3 bacterial cells daily through defecation.

There are about 300 times as many anaerobic bacteria as facultatively anaerobic bacteria.

The normal flora of large intestine includes *Escherichia coli, Proteus* sp, *Klebsiellae* sp, *Enterobacter* sp, *Bacteroides* sp, *Fusobacterium* sp, *Bifidobacterium* sp, *Eubacterium* sp, *Lactobacillus* sp, *Clostridium* sp, and protozoans such as *Trichomonas hominis, Entamoeba histolytica, Endolimax* sp and *Iodamoeba* sp.

IMPLANTATION OF LACTOBACILLI

The oral administration of the Gram positive bacterium *Lactobacillus acidophilus* may cure some intestinal disorders. The principle is that ingestion of large numbers of the lactobacilli may result in replacement of undesirable organisms by harmless or beneficial organisms in the intestine. The implantation of Lactobacilli depends on ingestion of large number of the organisms and on supplying lactose that can be readily utilized by the microorganism. Several commercial products containing lactobacilli are available for therapeutic use.

NORMAL FLORA OF THE UROGENITAL TRACT

The urogential tract is sterile in the upper portions (*i.e.,* upper urethra, urinary bladder, kidneys, testes, ovaries), but it may contain large numbers of microorganisms in the lower urethra, meatus, vagina and vulva. *Staphylococcus epidermidis*, nonhemolytic streptococci and diphtheroids are predominant in the distal portions of male and female urethras.

Mycobacterium smegmatis, a saprophyte is commonly present in urethral secretions of both males and females.

The vagina of new born is colonized by Lactobacilli due to glycogen deposition in vaginal epithelial cells as a result of estrogen passively transferred from the mother. The pH is acidic due to lactic acid produced by fermentation of glycogen by lactobacilli and may remain for a few days. Once the estrogen is eliminated, the pH becomes neutral or slightly alkaline and remains so till puberty. This causes a change in normal flora to alpha hemolytic Streptococci, nonhemolytic Streptococci, Micrococci, diphtheroids and coliforms.

The adult female genital tract has a very complex normal flora. From puberty to menopause, the pH of vagina becomes acidic 4.4 to 4.6. It is because the estrogen causes glycogen deposition in vaginal epithelial cells. As a result, lactobacilli that are acidophilic colonize vagina and ferment glycogen to produce lactic acid.

The normal adult vaginal flora, often comprises–*Lactobacillus* (Dodderlein's bacilli), *Staphylococcus epidermidis*, Peptococci, Peptostreptococci, *Clostridium* sp, Diphtheroids, *Gardnerella* sp, *Ureaplasma*, *Enterococci, Neisseria* sp, Group B Streptococci (*Strept. agalactiae*), Streptococci and *Candida* sp.

BACTERIA IN BLOOD AND TISSUES

Blood and internal tissues are sterile but there may be a transient bactermia following brushing teeth, bowel movement and catheterization.

QUESTIONS

Essay Question

1. Describe the normal flora of the human body.

Short Notes

1. Normal flora of genitourinary tract.
2. What is the importance of normal flora?
3. What is the difference between resident and transient flora?
4. Normal flora of intestine.
5. What sites in the body are free from microorganisms?
6. Why is there not a normal flora in the lower respiratory tract.
7. Lactobacillus acidophilus.

22

Collection and Transport of Specimens for Laboratory Investigation/Diagnosis

The laboratory diagnosis of infectious diseases begins with the collection of a clinical specimen for examination. The general principles to be followed, while collecting the sample are as follows. (Fig. 1).

- Wash hands before and after collection of sample.
- Collect the sample before the administration of antibiotics.
- Strict aseptic techniques must be practiced while collecting the sample.
- Collect the specimen at right time in relation to patient's symptoms.
- The specimen collected must be representative of the infectious process. For example, in a case of pneumonia sputum should be collected but not the saliva.
- The specimen should be collected in an adequate amount.
- The specimen should not be contaminated by organisms from outside source.
- Specimen should be collected in sterile containers and sealed and properly labelled with patient's name, age sex, hospital no., clinical history and treatment given.
- The specimen should be transported immediately without any delay to the laboratory.
- If necessary, transport media may be used for preserving any organisms which may present in the sample.
- The specimens should be immediately processed.

The commonly collected specimens for bacteriological examination are:

Throat swabs, sputum, nasal swabs, ear swabs, eye (conjunctival) swabs, wound swabs, blood, pus, feces, urine, CSF, aspirations–pleural, ascitic, synovial fluids, vaginal swabs and rectal swabs.

When viral diseases are suspected, several different specimens may be taken in special transport media supplied by virology laboratories. The specimens should be refrigerated at 4°C or should be delivered to the laboratory within one hour. The specimens collected in viral infections are as follows:

CNS diseases – CSF, brain, blood, feces, throat swabs or throat washings.

Respiratory diseases – Sputum, throat swabs or throat washings.

Eye diseases – conjunctival swabs or scrapings.

Skin lesions – Vesicle or pustule fluid in capillary tubes, air-dried slides from scrapings of macules or papules.

For serological tests two blood samples (paired sera) are collected, the first taken as soon as possible after the onset of illness, the second 2-3 weeks later so that antibody titres can be compared to demonstrate a rise. Alternatively, diagnosis may be based on the demonstration of specific IgM antibody in a single, early blood sample.

Specimens collected in fungal diseases include skin scrapings, nails, hair and other specimens in the same way as for bacteriological examination.

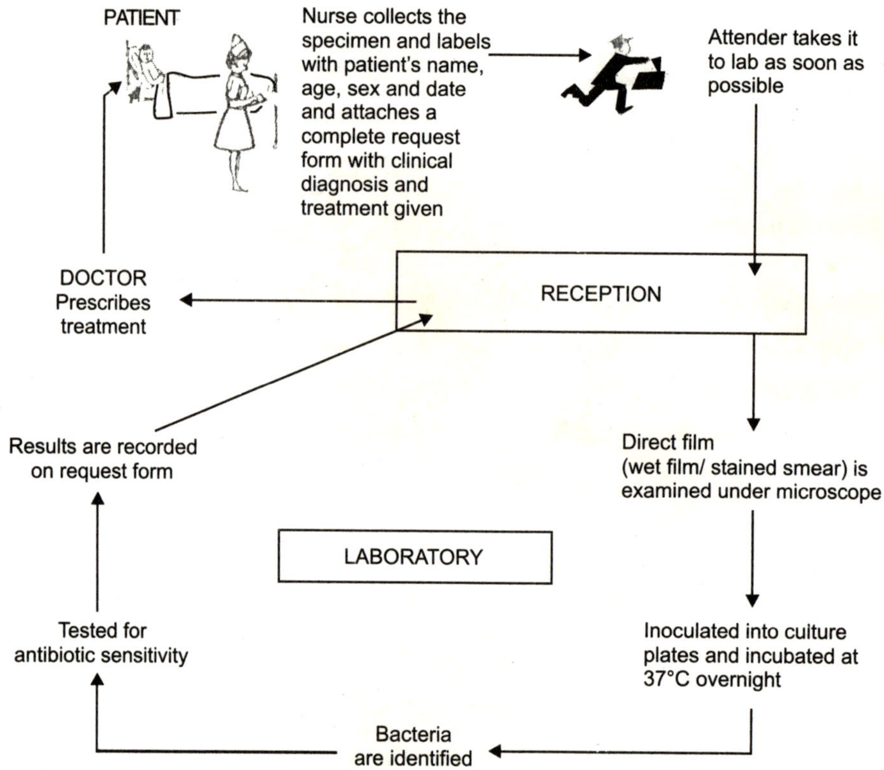

Fig. 22.1. The sequence of laboratory identification of bacteria from infectious material.

23

Uses of Experimental Animals

- *Rabbits*
- *Infant rabbits*
- *Adult mice*
- *Suckling mice*
- *Nude mice*
- *NZB (New Zealand Black Strain) mice*
- *Rats*
- *Guinea pigs*
- *Hamsters and infant hamsters*
- *Sheep*
- *Goats*
- *Marmoset*
- *Ferrets*
- *Armadillos*
- *Chimpanzees*
- *Rhesus monkeys*
- *Germ-free animals (Gnotobiotic animals)*

RABBITS

Adult rabbits are widely used in medical microbiology

– for pathogenicity and virulence testing, *e.g.,* Pneumococci (*Streptococcus pneumoniae*)

– for production of antisera, *e.g.,* Amboceptor.

– for maintenance of Nichol's strain of *Treponema pallidum* in rabbit testes.

– for testing enterotoxin (ST, SL) production by rabbit illeal loop test.

– for demonstration of *Listeria monocytogenes* by Anton's test.

– for differentiation of *Mycobacterium tuberculosis* from *Mycobacterium bovis.*

– to demonstrate Arthus Reaction (type III hypersensitivity).

– for pyrogen testing.

– Rabbit serum is used as a source of complement (C) in cytotoxicity test of HLA typing.

INFANT RABBITS

Infant rabbits are used

(*a*) for testing enterotoxins of enterotoxigenic bacteria (ETEC) by infant rabbit bowel test.

(*b*) as animal model for *Vibrio cholerae.*

ADULT MICE

Adult mice are used in clinical microbiology for various experiments

- for toxigenicity testing of *Clostridium tetani, Clostridium welchii* and *Clostridium botulinum.*
- *Mycobacterium leprae* can be maintained in the foot pads of mice.
- for isolation and cultivation of *Toxoplasma gondii.*
- for isolation of causative agents such as – *Borrelia recurrentis*, *Borrelia duttoni*, *Rickettsia tsutsugamushi*, *Chlamydia psittaci*, rabies virus and *Histoplasma capsulatum* etc.
- for pathogenicity and virulence testing of pneumococci, *Cryptococcus neoformans, Bordetella pertussis*, HSV encephalitis, lymphocytic choriomeningitis virus.
- for production of hybridomas.

SUCKLING MICE

Suckling mice are used

1. for isolation and cultivation of viruses, *e.g.,* Arboviruses, Coxsackie viruses A and B.
2. in preparation of vaccines, *e.g.,* Infant mouse brain vaccine for rabies, 17 D vaccine for yellow fever, Japanese B encephalitis vaccine.
3. for testing heal stable (ST) enterotoxin of enterotoxigenic *E.coli* by infant mouse intragastric test.

NUDE MICE

A mouse, in which cell mediated Immunity is suppressed either by thymectomy or by administration of antilymphocyte serum is known as nude mouse.

Nude mice are used as experimental animals in leprosy to produce generalised infection, resembling lepromatous leprosy.

NZB (NEW ZEALAND BLACK STRAIN) MOUSE

A genetically inbred strain of mice in which autoimmune disease resembling systemic lupus erythematosus develops spontaneously.

RATS

Rats are used as experimental animals

- for isolation of causative agents – *Yersinia pestis*, *Trypanosoma brucei.*
- for pathogenicity and virulence testing of *Bacillus anthracis*, *Yersinia pestis, Entamoeba histolytica* and *Blastomyces dermatitidis*.

GUINEA PIGS

Guinea pigs are used widely in clinical microbiology

1. for isolation of causative organisms of various diseases such as *Mycobacterium tuberculosis*, *Mycobacterium bovis*, *Brucella* sp., *Leptospira* sp., *Rickettsia* sp., *Chlamydia* sp., *Toxoplasma gondii*, *Trypanosoma* sp. etc.

2. for toxigenicity testing of *Corynebacterium diphtheriae*, *Clostridium tetani*, *Clostridium welchii*, *Clostridium botulinum* etc.
3. for pathogenicity and virulence testing of *Listeria monocytogenes, Bacillus anthracis, Clostridium welchii, Entamoeba histolytica* and *Cryptococcus neoformans* etc.
4. for standardisation of toxins and antitoxins, *e.g., Corynebacterium diphtheriae, Clostridium tetani.*
5. for testing invasiveness of enteroinvasive *E.coli* by Sereny's test.
6. to obtain serum as a source of complement for CFT.
7. to obtain peritoneal macrophages for testing migration inhibition factor (MIF).
8. to differentiate epidemic typhus (*Rickettsia prowazeki*) from endemic typhus (*Rickettsia mooseri*) by Neill-Mooser reaction or Tunica reaction.

HAMSTER

Hamsters are used as experimental

1. for isolation of causative organisms – *Leptospira* sp., *Toxoplasma gondii* etc.
2. for pathogenicity testing – *Bacillus anthracis*, *Leishmania donovani* (in Chinese hamster), *Leishmonia tropica* (in syrian hamster).
3. for production of hepatitis by *Entamoeba histolytica.*
4. for maintenance of viruence of *Entamoeba histolytica.*
5. for testing drugs efficacy against *Leishmania donovani.*

Infant Hamster is used for testing tumor potential of adenoviruses.

SHEEP

Sheep is used

1. to obtain blood for preparation of bacteriological media such as blood agar.
2. to obtain RBC for serological tests, *e.g.,* Paul-Bunnel test.

GOATS

Goats are used

1. serum used for tissue culture.
2. used for the production of antisera.

MARMOSET

Marmoset used for cultivation of Hepatitis A virus (HAV).

FERRETS

Ferrets used as animal model for Influenza viruses.

ARMADILLO

The nine-banded armadillo (*Dasypus novemcinctus*) is highly susceptible to infection with leprae bacilli and used for the cultivation of *Mycobacterium leprae*.

CHIMPANZEE

Chimpanzee is used

1. for cultivation of hepatitis viruses.
2. as animal model for gonococcal urethritis.

RHESUS MONKEYS

Rhesus monkeys are widely used in clinical virology as experimental animals

1. to prepare monkey kidney tissue culture for the cultivation of viruses.
2. for pathogenicity testing of polio viruses.
3. monkey RBC are used for hemagglutinating (HA) activity of measles virus.
4. *Autos triviroatus* monkeys are used for cultivation of *Plasmodium falciparum*.

GERM-FREE ANIMALS (GNOTOBIOTIC ANIMALS)

James A. Reyniers (1928) developed techniques and equipment for rearing germ-free animals (chickens), in the absence of microorganisms, though the first attempt to raise germ-free chickens was made by Pasteur (1897).

Germ-free animals (rats, mice, guinea pigs, rabbits etc.) can be obtained by cesarian section, performed under sterile conditions in a special germ-free chamber. New-born animals are introduced into a sterile rearing cage and provided with sterile air, water and food. Once established, a colony of germ-free animals can be maintained by natural reproduction under germ-free conditions.

Germ-free animals living in association with one or more known microorganisms are called "Gnotobiotic" (Greek, gnoto = known; biota = flora and fauna). A gnotobiotic system is one in which the composition of the microflora is known.

When compared with normal animals, germ-free animals have underdeveloped immune system making them highly susceptible to infections. They lack antibodies to normal flora antigens (which confer partial protection against pathogens).

Germ-free animals are used as important practical tools in biology and medicine.

1. By comparing the properties of germ-free animals with those of normal animals, the functions of normal flora can be found out. For example, germ-free animals require high levels of vitamins B and K, which normal animals do not require in their diet, indicating the role of normal flora in producing these vitamins.

2. Gnotobiotic animals can be used to assess the effect of one particular species or several known species of microorganisms.
3. They also help us to understand the interactions between microorganisms and their hosts.

QUESTIONS

Short Notes

1. Uses of Rabbits
2. Suckling mice
3. Nude mice
4. Uses of Guinea pigs
5. Germ-free animals (Gnotobiotic animals)

24

Bacteriology of Milk, Water and Air

BACTERIOLOGY OF MILK

Introduction

Milk is the normal secretion of mammary glands of mammals. It is the "most nearly complete" food for humans, and is an excellent medium for many microbial species.

Milk serves as a carrier of several diseases. Pathogenic organisms of both bovine and human origin have been isolated from milk.

Several diseases of cattle including staphylococcal and streptococcal infections, tuberculosis, brucellosis, salmonellosis, Q fever, foot and mouth disease may be transmitted to man. These organisms may get into the milk either directly from the udder or indirectly from infected body discharges, which may drop, splash or be blown into the milk.

Some of the important diseases of human origin that have been transmitted by milk are typhoid fever, shigellosis, *E.coli* diarrhea, cholera, diphtheria, tuberculosis, staphylococcal and streptococcal infections and poliomyelitis.

Bacteriological Examination of Milk

Sampling Milk

If the milk is contained in retail bottles or packets, one unopened bottle or packet may be used as sample. If the milk is in a bulk container, it is mixed thoroughly, and sample is collected with a sterile dipper from the depth aseptically.

Tests

The methods commonly employed for enumerating microbial population of milk are as follows:

1. Rapid platform test
   (*a*) Organoleptic test
   (*b*) Clot on boiling test
   (*c*) sediment test
   (*d*) pH
   (*e*) Alcohol test/Alcohol-alizarin test
   (*f*) Titrable acidity
2. Direct microscopic count (DMC) – Breed's method
3. Standard plate count (SPC)
4. Dye reduction tests or reductase tests
   (*a*) Methylene blue reduction test (MBRT)
   (*b*) Resazurin test
5. Phosphatase test
6. Special techniques for specific types of microorganisms.

Rapid Platform Tests

In dairy units some rapid platform tests are done to check the bacteriological quality of milk, supplied by different vendors.

(*a*) ***Organoleptic test.*** It involves examination of color, taste, odor of milk. The normal cow's milk is yellow and buffalow milk is white in color and a little sweetish in taste. Any other color or bitter taste or abnormal smell may be due to bacterial growth and should be rejected.

(*b*) ***Clot on boiling (COB) test.*** Take 10 ml of milk in a test tube and boil it for 5 min. The formation of clot or flakes or coagulation is a positive test and is due to developed acidity (Lactic acid) by contaminating microorganisms and should be rejected.

(*c*) ***Sediment test.*** It is done to judge the cleanliness of milk. Measured quantity of milk is filtered or centrifuged and checked for sediment. A good quantity milk gives no visible dirt, whereas poor quality milk shows a dark or blackish deposit on the filter pad. The milk is accepted or rejected by referring the following chart.

Table 24.1 ISI Standards chart

Sediment (mg)	*Grade*
0.0	Excellent
0.2	Good
0.5	Fair
1.0	Poor
2.0	Very poor

(*d*) ***pH.*** The normal milk has a pH of 6.5 - 6.8. Any deviation from this may be due to disease of animal or contamination of milk and should be rejected.

(*e*) ***Alcohol test/alcohol-alizarin test.*** Take 5 ml of milk in a test tube and alcohol or a mixture of alcohol-alizarin solution is added along the sides. The formation of flakes or clot is indicative of contamination and constitutes a positive test and the milk should be rejected.

This test is used to know the suitability of milk for high heat treatment (sterilization) and keeping quality.

(*f*) ***Titrable acidity.*** Normal fresh milk has a pH of 6.5 - 6.8, slightly acidic. The "natural or apparent acidity" (0.13 to 0.15 % lactic acid) of milk is due to the presence of casein, acid phosphates and citrates etc. When milk is contaminated by bacteria, they cause breakdown of lactose and produce lactic acid (90%) and other acids (10%) which leads to an increase in the acidity, known as "**Read or developed acidity**". The sum total of these two is known as "**Total or titrable acidity**" and is expressed as "per cent lactic acid (LA)."

It is measured by the amount of alkali required to change the pH of milk from its initial value (6.5 – 6.8) to pH of color change of phenolphthalein indicator in milk.

1 ml of phenolphthalein is added to 10 ml of milk and is titrated against N/9 NaOH till a pink color appears. The volume of N/9 NaOH used is recorded and per cent lactic acid (% LA) is calculated as follows:

$$\% \text{ LA} = \frac{9 \times \text{normality of NaOH} \times \text{Volume of NaOH used}}{\text{Volume of milk}}$$

Direct Microscopic Count (DMC) or Breed's Method

The microbial content of milk can be determined by the direct microscopic examination of known volume of milk in a fixed smear. The method is performed as follows:

A square cm (cm^2) area is marked on a clean, grease-free glass side. 0.01 ml of milk is spread uniformly over this area by means of a special pipette (Breed's pipette) or syringe. The smear is air-dried and stained with a methylene blue solution. The slide (5-10 fields) is examined under oil-immersion objective, and the number of microorganisms per field is determined.

In order to express the final count quantitatively, the area of the microscopic field must be known.

The diameter of oil-immersion lens (field) = 0.16 mm

The area seen in the oil-immersion field = πr^2

$= 3.14 \times 0.08 \times 0.08$

$= 0.02$ sq mm (mm^2)

One square cm (the area over which the sample was spread) is 100 sq mm.

Thus, there would be 100/0.02 = 5000 microscopic fields in one sq cm.

The average count per field is multiplied by the total number of microscopic fields. This will give the number of organisms in 0.01 ml of sample.

The advantages of DMC are:

1. The test is more rapid and results are obtained on the spot within 15 minutes.

2. More samples can be examined as less work is required.

3. Less expensive as the amount of equipment required is much less.

4. The slides may be preserved as a permanent record and examined whenever the occasion arises.

5. Different morphological types can be distinquished. This information is of great value for determining the source and nature of the contamination.

The disadvantages of DMC are:

1. The microscopic method may be the source of error unless the milk contains a high count. This is because a large factor is used for converting the number of organisms per field to the number per ml of milk.

2. The method does not differentiate dead from living organisms.

3. The method is less useful for pasteurized milk because most of the organisms are dead.

Standard Plate Count (SPC) or Viable Count or Colony Count or Pour Plate Method

This is an agar plate method, commonly used for the estimation of the number of bacteria in milk.

The milk sample is diluted several times (serial dilutions) and a small volume (usually 1 ml) of the diluted sample is mixed with agar medium in test tubes that is molten and cooled to 45°C, and the mixtures are shaken or rolled between the palms (as in shake cultures) and poured immediately into sterile petriplates. After the agar is hardened, each cell is fixed in place and forms an individual colony upon incubation. Plates may be incubated at 35–37°C for 48 hrs. for routine work; at 5–7°C for 7–10 days to enumerate psychrophiles; or at 55°C for 48 hrs. to enumerate thermophiles.

The colonies can be seen trapped deep inside the medium. The total number of colonies equals the viable microorganisms in the diluted sample. The visible colonies can be counted with naked eye or in a colony counter and the number of colonies per ml of the sample is reported as the standard plate count

(SPC) per ml.

$$\text{Number of cells per ml} = \frac{\text{Number of colonies}}{\text{Amount inoculated} \times \text{Dilution}}$$

SPC has several advantages – 1. it counts viable bacteria only, 2. differential counts can be determined, 3. it can be used to determine quality of milk samples with low bacterial count, pasteurised milk and high grade raw milk.

SPC also has several disadvantages. The count obtained does not represent all the viable organisms present in milk. There are many reasons for this discrepancy – 1. for each cell to produce a colony, the bacteria would have to be well separated. In milk there are chains, packets and clumps, each containing two to many cells, which would form only one colony, 2. not all kinds of bacteria will grow in a particular physical environment and on the nutrients supplied in the piating medium, 3. some rapidly growing species inhibit the growth of other species.

Dye reduction Tests (Reductase Tests)

Milk, after it leaves the cow, becomes exposed and mixed with air, acquires an oxidation-reduction (O/R) potential of about + 300 mV. As bacteria grow in the milk, they consume oxygen and produce reducing substances that lower the O/R potential to a negative value. The rate of shift in O/R potential depends on the number and kinds of bacteria and the rate of their metabolism. This change in redox potential can be detected by adding an appropriate indicator to a sample of milk and incubating under specified conditions.

This dye reduction test is based on the bacterial dehydrogenase activity. Dehydrogenases are flavin enzymes which transfer hydrogen atoms from a substrate to biological acceptors or redox dyes, which undergo a color change.

Methylene blue and resazurin are two O/R indicators useful for the reductase test. The color transformations which occur between the oxidized and reduced forms of these compounds are:

Oxidized form in milk	– Methylene blue (blue color)
	– Resazurin (slate blue color)
Reduced form in milk	– Leucomethylene blue (colorless)
	– Resorufin (pink)
	– Dihydroresorufin (colorless)

The results of these tests are reported in terms of the time required for the reduction of the indicators. In general, the reduction time is inversely proportional to the initial bacterial content of the sample.

Limitations of the reductase test – 1. the rate of decolorization of the dye is influenced by the kinds of microorganisms present, 2. the conditions under which the test is performed are more favorable for the growth of mesophiles than for either psychrophiles or thermophiles.

Methylene blue reduction test (MBRT)

The test depends on the principle that the dye is colored when oxidized, but becomes colorless when reduced.

10 ml of milk sample is added into a sterile test tube and 1 ml of methylene blue solution is added and gently mixed. The tube is closed and incubated in a water bath at 35 to 37°C. The tube is observed for 30 min., 1 hour and later until the blue color disappears. The negative control included consists of 10 ml of boiled milk to which 1 ml methylene blue is added.

The result of the test is reported in terms of the time required for the reduction of methylene blue. Milk may be classified on the basis of the methylene blue reduction time as follows:

1. Class I – Excellent milk; not decolorized in 8 hrs.
2. Class II – Good milk; decolorized in less than 8 hrs, but less than 6 hrs.
3. Class III – Fair milk; decolorized in less than 6 hrs, but not less than 2 hrs.
4. Class IV – Poor milk, decolorised in less than 2 hrs.

MBRT is used for 1. assessing the hygienic quality of milk, 2. evaluation of the quality of raw milk, 3. detection of post-pasteurization contamination.

Resazurin test

It is another reduction test which employs resazurin dye in place of methylene blue. Resazurin undergoes a series of color changes, slate blue to pink to colorless, depending upon O/R changes, whereas methylene blue changes only from blue to colorless. Resazurin, therefore permits readings of degrees of reduction at shorter intervals than does methylene blue.

The test is performed by mixing 1 ml of resazurin (1:20,000 dil) with 10 ml of milk sample in a sterile tube. The tube is placed in water bath at 35 to 37°C and examined at regular intervals. The color of the milk, which is initially blue is compared with a series of standard disks prepared for the purpose. Either Lovibond comparator or special resazurin disks can be used.

If the color remains blue (disks 6 or 5) for 1 hr, the milk is normal in microbial content; if mauve or mauve-pink (disk less than 5), the microbial content is high and the milk is regarded as abnormal; if disk number is less than 3 is obtained in 30 minutes, the milk is grossly abnormal; if the color is completely reduced (disk 0) in 1 hr or less, the milk contains many pus cells and probably pathogenic organisms. High grade milk requires atleast 3 hrs to reach the pink color.

Phosphatase test

The test is performed on pasteurized milk to determine whether pasteurisation has been successful. Alkaline phosphatase is a thermolabile enzyme present in raw milk and in many tissues, which is inactivated by adequate pasteurization.

The test is based on the property of the enzyme, to liberate phenol from phenyl phosphoric ester (disodium phenyl phosphate) added to a sample of milk. The amount of phenol liberated is estimated by the addition of dichloroquinonechloramide, which turns blue in the presence of phenol.

$$\text{Disodium phenyl phosphate} \xrightarrow{\text{Phosphatase}} \text{Phosphate + phenol}$$

$$\downarrow + \text{ Dichloroquinonechloramide}$$

Blue color

Phenol is converted into indophenol blue. The indophenol blue is extracted by shaking with butyl alcohol and the concentration determined quantitatively by comparing with a series of color standards in a colorimeter.

When the milk is heated at 62°C or above for 30 min, all the enzyme present is destroyed. The presence of enzyme indicates that milk has been underheated.

Special Techniques for Specific Types of Microorganisms

The DMC, SPC and reductase tests are performed to obtain an estimate of the total population.

Occasionally it is necessary to examine milk or dairy products for specific types of microorganisms, such as coliforms, thermodurics or pathogens. Special procedures are required for this.

1. Thermoduric bacteria – Milk sample is heated at 61.7 to 62.8°C for 30 min and then plated as for SPC.

2. Psychrophilic bacteria – Procedure for SPC is followed, but plates are incubated at 5°C for 7 days.

3. Thermophilic bacteria – SPC method is followed but incubated at 55°C.

4. Coliform bacteria – Selective and differential media are inoculated as for bacteriological analysis of water.

5. Proteolytic bacteria – SPC procedure is followed, but 5% skim milk is added to medium so that medium becomes opaque. Proteolytic bacteria will digest casein and show clear zones around colonies.

6. Betahemolytic streptococci – Milk sample is inoculated into blood agar medium, inoculated and observed for colonies showing betahemolytic zones; Gram's stain may be done from colonies to identify streptococci.

7. Yeasts and Molds – Milk sample is inoculated on to potatodextrose agar (PDA) or Martin's rose Bengal Agar (MRBA) medium with acidic pH and incubated at room temperature (20–25°C) for 5 days.

Milk ring test for Brucellosis

The milk sample is mixed with a drop of the stained *Brucella* antigen (killed *Brucella abortus* stained with hematoxylin) in a test tube and incubated in a water bath at 70°C for 40-50 minutes. If antibodies are present in the milk, the bacilli are agglutinated and rise with the cream to form a blue ring at the top, leaving the milk unstained. If antibodies are absent, no colored ring is formed and the milk remains uniformly blue.

Whey agglutination test can also be used to detect the antibodies in milk.

BACTERIOLOGY OF WATER

Most of the water bodies in India and the world are being polluted in diversified manner due to increasing industrialization, urbanization, agricultural and various other human activities. Drinking water supplies contaminated with sewage or excreta from humans and animals may cause various diseases.

Water-borne diseases

Bacterial
- *Salmonella* gastroenteritis (typhoid and paratyphoid fevers)
- Cholera
- Shigellosis (bacillary dysentery)
- *Campylobacter* and *Helicobacter* infections
- *Vibrio parahemolyticus* gastroenteritis
- *Yersinia enterocolitica* gastroenteritis
- Traveller's diarrhoea (*E.coli*)
- *Clostridium perfringens* gastroenteritis
- Listeriosis

Viral
- Poliomyelitis

– Rotavirus diarrhea
– Norwalk gastroenteritis
– Type A hepatitis

Protozoan – Amoebiasis
– Giardiasis
– Balantidiasis

Helminthic – Tape worm infections
– Trichinosis
– Pin worm infections
– Whip worm infections
– Round worm infections

Biochemical Oxygen Demand (BOD)

BOD may be defined as that quantity of oxygen required to decompose organic and inorganic matter by aerobic biological action. BOD is a way of expressing the amount of organic compounds in waste waters or sewage as measured by the volume of dissolved oxygen required by microorganisms to metabolize it under aerobic conditions. The more oxidizable organic material present, the higher the BOD, that is, the more oxygen will be utilized by bacteria to degrade it.

BOD is a good index of organic pollution. High BOD values mean that a high level of organic material is present; whereas low values mean that little oxidizable material is present.

Dissolved oxygen (DO) of water is of paramount importance to all living organisms. The presence of DO in water is mainly due to, 1. direct diffusion from air, 2. photosynthetic evolution by aquatic autotrophs. The first one is purely a physical process and depends on the solubility of the oxygen under the influence of temperature, salinity, water movements etc., whereas the latter is a biological process and depends on the availability of light and the rate of metabolic processes resulting in diurnal fluctuations.

The BOD of a water sample is measured by incubating the sample at 20°C for 5 days in the dark under aerobic coditions (BOD_5 20°C). In tropical and subtropical kelts, where the temperature, and rate of metabolic activities are higher, the incubation should preferably be done at 27°C for 3 days (BOD_3 27°C). Since nitrification consumes oxygen significantly, thereby resulting in overestimation of BOD and must be checked by adding 1 ml of 0.05% solution of allylthiourea. In the water samples where more than 70% of the initial oxygen consumed, it is necessary to aerate/oxygenate and/or dilute the sample with BOD free water to avoid oxygen stress.

Chemical Oxygen Demand (COD)

In recent times with the increase of industrial pollution by discharging large amounts of various chemically oxidizable organic substances of different nature entering into aquatic systems, BOD alone does not give a clear picture of the organic matter content of the water sample. In addition, the presence of various toxicants in the sample may severely affect the validity of the BOD test. Hence, COD is a better estimate of the organic matter, which needs no sophistication and time saving. However, COD *i.e.,* the oxygen consumed does not differentiate the stable organic matter from the unstable form. Therefore, the COD values are not directly comparable to that of BOD.

The amount of organic matter in water is estimated by their oxidability by chemical oxidant such as potassium permanganate or potassium dichromate (the constituent carbon and hydrogen are oxidized and not the nitrogen). In the permanganate method, the organic matter is first oxidized with a known volume of $KMnO_4$ and then the excess of oxygen is allowed to react with potassium iodide to liberate iodine in amounts equal to the excess oxygen, which is estimated titrimetrically with sodium thiosulphate solution using starch as an indicator.

Total Carbon Content (TOC)

As COD cannot give a direct value of the oxygen demand of the waste and several organic compounds present in wastes from refineries, petrochemical complexes, and similar industries another test known as "TOC" is employed.

The TOC of a sample, which represents all the organic compounds present in the waste water is determined by combustion of the organic compounds and by estimating the total CO_2 produced.

In practice, BOD and COD tests are more frequently used as they are simple, relatively inexpensive and can easily be conducted in a laboratory.

BACTERIOLOGICAL EXAMINATION (ANALYSIS) OF WATER

Bacterial Indicators

Certain bacteria, particularly *E.coli* and related coliforms, fecal streptococci and *Clostridium perfringens* are normal inhabitants of the large intestine of humans and animals and are constantly present in feces. Thus the presence of any of these bacterial species in water is evidence of fecal pollution of human or animal origin. If these organisms are present, the pathogens are also expected, since they too occur in feces. The examination of water for pathogens is usually not recommended because – they enter into water sporadically, and do not survive for long periods of time, hence their detection may be missed, because of their small number in water. On the other hand, the coliform bacilli are excreted in feces in large numbers remain viable longer in water than intestinal pathogens, and can be easily detected even in high dilutions. The coliform group of bacteria has universally been used for more than 80 years as prime indicator to assess the microbial quality of raw as well as treated drinking water. Fecal Streptococci and *Clostridium perfringens* are used as indicators when the coliform bacilli, the prime indicators fail to indicate the fecal contamination in water.

Tests. The routine test generally used in bacteriological examination of water are:

1. Multiple tube dilution technique -- It consists of
   (*a*) Presumptive coliform test or MPN technique
   (*b*) Confirmed test
   (*c*) Completed test
2. Eijkman test
3. SPC (Plate count or colony count)
4. Membrane filter method
5. Examination for fecal streptococci
6. Presence-Absence (P-A test)

Collection of Water Samples

1. Sample must be collected in a sterile bottle.

2. Contamination of the sample must be avoided during and after sampling.
3. Sample must be a true representative of the water supply (river, lake, pond or well etc.) from which it is taken.
4. The sample should be tested as immediately as possible after collection.
5. If there is any delay in examination, the sample should be stored at a temperature between 0° and 6°C.

Presumptive Coliform Count (Multiple Tube Dilution Method or Mean (Most) Probable Number (MPN) Method)

An estimation of the number of coliform bacilli in a water supply is usually made by adding varying quantities of water sample (from 0. ml to 50 ml) to lactose broth or **bile salt lactose peptone water** or **MacConkey broth** or **lauryl tryptose broth** of adequate 0.1 strength with an indicator of acidity (*e.g.*, neutral red, bromocresol purple), contained in bottles with durham tubes to show the formation of gas.

This method requires examination by culture of several samples of several different quantities of the water so that an average result, called "**Mean probable number**" can be stated. It has been shown that if one 50 ml, five 10 ml and five 1 ml volume of samples or five 10 ml, five 1 ml and five 0.1 ml volume of samples are tested. This range of quantities may be altered according to the likely condition of the water examined. Thus 50 ml quantity is included when testing filtered or chlorinated water, where the number of bacteria are likely to be less, and in this case it is not necessary to examine 0.1 ml volumes. This 0.1 ml amount of sample (1 ml of sample diluted 1 in 10) is tested only when the water supply is suspected of being highly contaminated. The culture tubes or bottles are incubated at 37°C and examined after 24 hrs. Those that show acid and gas are considered to be "**presumptive positive**', as a result of growth of coliform bacilli. Negative cultures, if any, are incubated for further 24 hrs, and if acid and gas develop they too are regarded as being presumptive positive.

In reporting the results, combination of positive and negative results can be referred to McCrady's probability tables and the mean probable number (MPN) of coliform bacilli can be computed per 100 ml of water.

Table 24.2a, b, c Probability tables

Table 24.2 a

Quantity of water	50ml	10ml	1ml	
No. of samples of each quantity tested	1	5	5	
	0	0	0	0
	0	0	1	1
	0	0	2	2
	0	1	0	1
	0	1	1	2
	0	1	2	3
	0	2	0	2
	0	2	1	3
	0	2	2	4
	0	3	0	3

Table 24.2 b

Quantity of water	10ml	1ml	0.1ml	
No. of samples of each quantity tested	5	5	5	
	0	0	0	0
	0	0	1	2
	0	0	2	4
	0	1	0	2
	0	1	1	4
	0	1	2	6
	0	2	0	4
	0	2	1	6
	0	3	0	6

Number giving positive reaction (acid and gas)				Probable number of coliform bacilli In 100 ml of water
	0	3	1	5
	0	4	0	5
	1	0	0	1
	1	0	1	3
	1	0	2	4
	1	0	3	6
	1	1	0	3
	1	1	1	5
1	1	2	7	
	1	1	3	9
	1	2	0	5
	1	2	1	7
	1	2	2	10
	1	2	3	12
	1	3	0	8
	1	3	1	11
1	3	2	14	
	1	3	3	18
	1	3	4	20
	1	4	0	13
	1	4	1	17
	1	4	2	20
	1	4	3	30
	1	4	4	35
	1	4	5	40
	1	5	0	25
	1	5	1	35
	1	5	2	50
	1	5	3	90
	1	5	4	160
	1	5	5	180+

Number giving positive reaction (acid and gas)				Probable number of coliform bacilli In 100 ml of water
	1	0	0	2
	1	0	1	4
	1	0	2	6
	1	0	3	8
	1	1	0	4
	1	1	1	6
	1	1	2	8
	1	2	0	6
	1	2	1	8
	1	2	2	10
	1	3	0	8
	1	3	1	10
	1	4	0	11
	2	0	0	5
	2	0	1	7
	2	0	2	9
	2	0	3	12
2	1	0	7	
	2	1	1	9
	2	1	2	12
	2	2	0	9
	2	2	1	12
	2	2	2	14
	2	3	0	12
	2	3	1	14
	2	4	0	15
	3	0	0	8
	3	0	1	11
	3	0	2	13
	3	1	0	11
	3	1	1	14
	3	1	2	17
	3	1	3	20
	3	2	0	14
	3	2	1	17
	3	2	3	20
	3	3	0	17
	3	3	1	20
	3	4	0	20
	3	4	1	25
	3	5	0	25

Table 24.2c

Quantity of water	10ml	1 ml	0.1ml	
No. of samples of each quantity tested	1	5	5	
Number giving positive reaction (acid and gas)				Probable number of coliform bacilli in 100 of water
	4	0	0	13
	4	0	1	17
	4	0	2	20
	4	0	3	25
	4	1	0	17
	4	1	1	20
	4	1	2	25
	4	2	0	20
	4	2	1	25
	4	2	2	30
	4	3	0	25
	4	3	1	35
	4	3	2	40
	4	4	0	35
	4	4	1	40
	4	4	2	45
	4	5	0	40
	4	5	1	50
	4	5	2	55
	5	0	0	25
	5	0	1	30
	5	0	2	45
	5	0	3	60
	5	0	4	75
	5	1	0	35
	5	1	1	45
	5	1	2	65
	5	1	3	85
	5	1	4	115
	5	2	0	50
	5	2	1	70

	5	2	2	95
	5	2	3	120
	5	2	4	150
	5	2	5	175
	5	3	0	80
	5	3	1	110
	5	3	2	140
	5	3	3	175
	5	3	4	200
	5	3	5	250
	5	4	0	130
	5	4	1	170
	5	4	2	225
	5	4	3	275
	5	4	4	350
	5	4	5	425
	5	5	0	250
	5	5	1	350
	5	5	2	550
	5	5	3	900
	5	5	4	1600
	5	5	5	1800+

False Positive Presumptive Tests

A positive test does not necessarily mean that coliforms are present. Bacteria such as *Pseudomonas maltophila*, *Serratia liquefaciens*, *Hafnia alvei* and *Bacillus* strains may give positive results. False positives occur –

1. due to the presence of aerobic or facultatively anaerobic, spore-forming, gas producing bacteria.
2. due to synergetic fermentation of lactose by gas producing "symbionts", usually when a Gram positive and Gram negative organisms growing together.
3. by the presence of oxidase positive bacteria capable of producing gas from lactose.

False positive test can be eliminated by inhibiting the growth non-coliform orgnanisms. This can be achieved by adding triphenylmethane stain in the fermentatiion medium.

Confirmed Test

Fermentation tubes showing any amount of gas are subjected to confirmed test. Gently shake the presumptive positive tubes showing gas and transfer a loopful of culture to the **brilliant green lactose bile broth (BGLB)** tubes. Incubate all the inoculated tubes at 35°C for 48 hours.

If gas produced – coliform group confirmed.

If no gas produced – test negative – coliform group absent.

All the tubes showing gas production in confirmed test are subjected to the completed test as follows.

Completed Test

Streak the **Eosin-methylene blue (EMB) agar** or **Endo agar** plates with a loopful of culture from positive confirmed test tubes. Invert the plates and incubate at 35°C for 24 hours.

Typical colonies – Nucleated, with or without metallic sheen

Atypical colonies – Opaque, nonnucleated, mucoid, pink after 24 hrs of incubation

Negative colonies – All other colonies except those described above.

If typical or atypical colonies are present, smears are prepared and Gram's staining is done to confirm the morphological characteristics of coliforms. Colonies are also inoculated into lactose broth fermentation tubes and incubated at 35°C for 48 hrs. The formation of gas in fermentation tubes and demonstration of Gram negative, non-sporulating bacilli constitute completed test for coliform group.

Table 24.3 Differences between *E.coli* and *Enterobacter*

	Indole	M.R.	V.P.	Citrate
E.coli	+	+	–	–
Enterobacter aerogenes	–	–	+	+

Differential Coliform Test or Eijkman Test

The Eijkman test is done to find out whether the coliform bacilli detected in the presumptive test are *E.coli* from human origin or animal origin. Subcultures are made from presumptive positive tubes into **Brilliant green lactose broth (BGLB)** or **lauryl tryptone broth** or **lactose broth** or MacConkey's broth and incubated at 44°C and 37°C in a thermostatically controlled water bath.

The formation of acid and gas at 44°C confirms the presence of *E.coli* of human origin and at 37°C indicates coliform group.

Standard Plate Count (SPC)

Plating is same as for milk examination.

Membrane Filter Method

The bacteriological examination of water by membrane filter method consists of following steps:

1. A sterile filter disk (cellulose acetate membrane filter or millipore) is placed in a filtration unit and sterilized.

2. A known volume of water is drawn through this filter disk into a suction flask. The bacteria are retained on the surface of the membrane filter.

3. The membrane filter disk is placed on the surface of an agar medium in petridish of suitable size and incubated.

4. Upon incubation, colonies develop on the filter disk wherever bacteria were trapped during filtration, and can be easily counted.

This method possesses several distinct advantages:

1. It permits the examination of bacteria from a large volume of water. No dilutions are, therefore, required. Colony count is more accurate and reliable.

2. The filter disk can be transferred to any desired medium. This permits the isolation of any organism on a differential medium.

3. It provides a more rapid examination of water than the standard procedure.

4. It requries much less equipment and, therefore, the examination can be done in the field.

The disadvantage of this method is it cannot be used, if water contains considerable amount of algae, colloidal or other materials which are likely to clog the filter, Secondly, if water samples are heavily contaminated with non-coliforms, the growth of coliforms will be inhibited.

Examination for Fecal Streptococci

Tests for fecal streptococci may be of value when there is a difficulty in interpretation as when presumptive coliforms are present, but E.coli are absent or where there is a question concerning the sanitary significance of coliforms isolated from a water sample. In some parts of the world, fecal streptococci, rather than coliforms, are used as indicators of fecal pollution of water. The normal habitat of these organisms is the intestine of humans and animals and they are not found in nature in the absence of fecal contamination. On the other hand, some believe that the coliforms do not always represent fecal pollution because the organisms may persist in soil and water for long periods of time and occasionally multiply outside the human or animal body.

Subcultures from presumptive positive tubes are made into **Glucose azide broth** or **Lactose broth** in which **sodium azide** is incorporated and incubated at 45°C for overnight or prolonged for 48 hrs. The presence of fecal streptococci is indicated by the formation of acid and should be plated on Mac Conkey agar for confirmation. Fecal streptococci produce characteristic minute pink or red colonies.

Membrane filter method can also be used for the detection of fecal streptococci from water samples.

Presence-Absence Test (P-A Test)

The presence-absence test is a simple modification of multiple tube method. This test is recommended for use on routine water samples. One large test sample (100 ml) in a single culture bottle is used to obtain qualitative information for the presence or absence of indicator bacteria. Further, the quantitaitve analysis can be done by mulitple tube or membrane filtration methods. Thus, for routine qualitative analysis, P-A test is much convenient, economic and time saving.

Inoculate 100 ml of water sample to be analysed into P-A culture bottle containing Lactose broth. After mixing thoroughly the bottle is incubated at 35°C for 48 hrs. Examine the bottle after 2 hrs and 48 hrs for acidity (color change). If gas is produced, it will result in foaming, when the bottle is gently shaken. The culture is then transferred to Brilliant green Lactose kile broth (BGLB) and incubated at 35°C for 24 or 48 hrs. Formation of BGLB broth confirms the presence of coliform bacilli. The P–A test result is reported as positive or negative for coliforms per 100 ml of sample.

Bacteriological Standards of Drinking Water

The following standards are laid down by ICMR for treated and untreated water.

Treated water

1. Coliform bacilli should be absent in 100 ml of water sample and the MPN should be less than 10 per 100 ml. This is for 90% samples examined throughout the month.

2. No sample should show an MPN in excess of 10 per 100 ml.

3. An MPN coliform bacteria of 8 to 10 per 100 ml should not occur in consecutive samples.

4. Repeat the sampling at the same point every day until the MPN of coliform bacteria is less than 8 to 10 per 100 ml.

Untreated water

1. Throughout any month none of the samples should show an MPN of coliform bacteria more than 8 to 10 per 100 ml.

2. An MPN of 20 per 100 ml may be permitted occasionally, if E.coli is absent.

3. If the MPN of coliform bacteria is consistently 20 or more, water supply should be treated.

Table 24.4 Classification of drinking water according to bacteriological tests.

	Presumptive coliform count	*E.coli count per 100 ml*
Class I Excellent	0	0
Class II Satisfactory	1–3	0
Class III Suspicious	4–10	0
Class IV Unsatisfactory	More than 10	0, 1 or more

BACTERIOLOGY OF AIR

Introduction

The microbial population of air is transient and variable. Air is not a medium in which microorganisms grow, but it is a carrier of dust and droplets that may be laden with microorganisms.

Microorganisms may be carried on dust particles, in large droplets that settle out quickly, and in the droplet nuclei, that remain when small liquid droplets evaporate.

Organisms introduced into the air may be transported a few feet or many kilometres. Some air-borne microorganisms die in a matter of seconds; others survive for weeks, months or longer. The fate of air-borne microorganisms depends upon humidity, temperature, sunlight and the size of particles bearing microorganisms and the nature of microorganisms. For example, spores and cysts survive for longer periods in air.

Algae, protozoa, yeasts, molds and bacteria have been isolated from the air near the earth's surface. Whereas bacteria and fungal spores have been found at high altitudes above the earth's surface.

Enumeration of Microorganisms in Air or Sampling Devices for Trapping Microorganisms in Air

There are several methods which require special devices, designed for enumeration of microorganisms in air –

1. Liquid impingement devices
   - Bead bubbler device
   - Lemon's sampler
   - Porton impinger and preimpinger

2. Solid impingement devices
   - Settling plate technique or sedimentation
   - Sieve device
   - Slit sampler
   - Andersen's air sampler
   - Funnel device
3. Filtration
4. Centrifugation
   - Wells air centrifuge
   - Cylindrical sampler
5. Electrostatic precipitation
6. Thermal precipitation.

Impingement in Liquids

The air is drawn through a very small opening or a capillary tube and bubbled through the liquid. The organisms get trapped in the liquid medium. Samples of the liquid are then plated to determine its microbial content.

Bead Bubbler Device **or** ***Capillary Impinger (Fig 24.1)***

It consists of a suction flask containing broth, glass beads and a gas bubbler. The air is drawn through capillary tube and bubbled through the broth so that organisms are trapped in the broth due to mechanical action between glass beads and air bubbles.

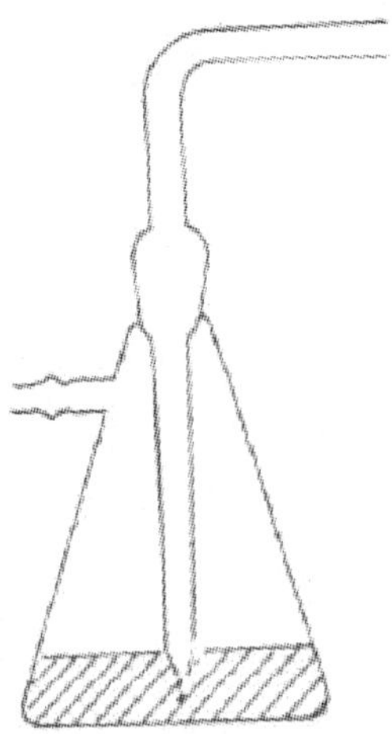

Fig. 24.1 Capillary impinger

Lemon's Device/Apparatus (Fig. 24.1)

The lemon sampler consists of a glass folin aeration tube with a bulb at one end perforated by 6 holes. The tube is passed through a two-hole rubber stopper, and the bulb centred near the bottom of the containing test tube. The Kjeldahl trap with square glass baffle is shortened at both ends for convenience, and a slight bend made in the intake so that this may be inserted into the remaining hole of the stopper. A small flow meter measures the rate of air flow entering the upper open end of the folin tube. An air pump is attached to the exhaust end of Kjeldahl trap.

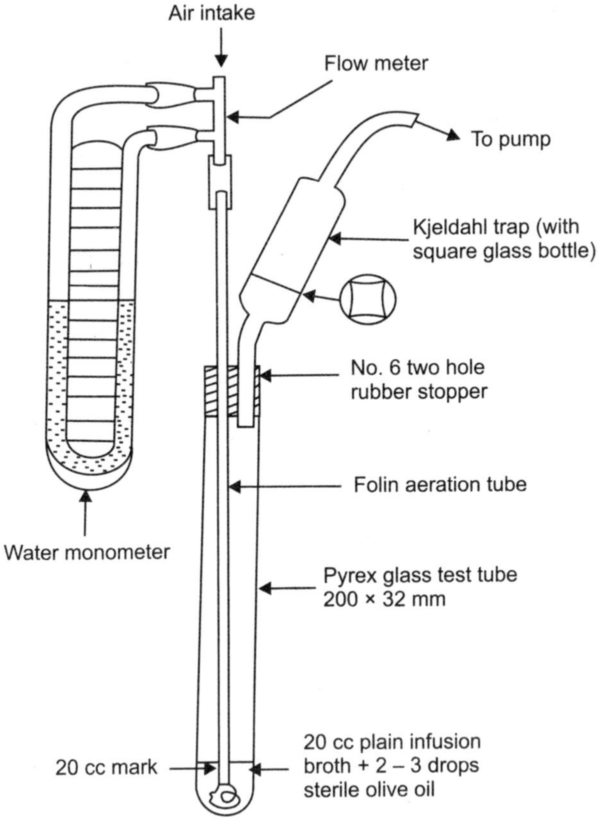

Fig. 24.2 Lemon's device

The entire bubbler should be sterilized by autoclaving or rinsing with 70% alcohol and drying. Air drawn in at the rate of 25 to 30 lit. per minute is dispersed through 20 ml of broth containing 2 or 3 drops of olive oil to prevent foaming.

The Porton Impinger and Pre-Impinger

The porton impinger consists of a narrow glass flask with a ground glass neck into which fits a hollow ground glass stopper. The stopper bears a side arm to which suction is applied. The intake tube terminates below in a jet in which air flows with maximum velocity with suction, so that particles as small as 0.5 to 1 μm diameter (size of bacterial cells) are trapped.

The pre-impinger comprises a glass bulb which is half-filled with broth medium. The neck and intake hole are connected to a proton impinger. Particles upto 4 μm diameter can penetrate the pre-impinger fluid.

Impingement on Solid Surfaces

Settling-Plate Technique or *Sedimentation*

One technique for the bacteriological sampling of air is simply to expose a petridish containing an agar medium to the air for a designated period of time 30 min to one hour. When the petridish is incubated, microorganisms that have settled on the agar surface grow into colonies. When fastidious pathogens such as streptococci are to be demonstrated blood agar plates can be used.

This method gives a rough approximation of the numbers and kinds of air-borne microorganisms and specially used for bacteriological examination of air in hospital wards and operation theatres. It is one of the simplest procedures used for air examination.

The settling plate technique has certain limitations. It does not indicate the number of organisms present in a given volume of air and is of no value from a quantitative stand point.

Slit Sampler or Slit Device (Fig. 24.3)

The air is drawn through a very narrow slit on to a petridish containing agar medium. The slit is approximately the length of the petridish. The petridish is rotated mechanically at a particular speed, so that the organisms are evenly distributed on it.

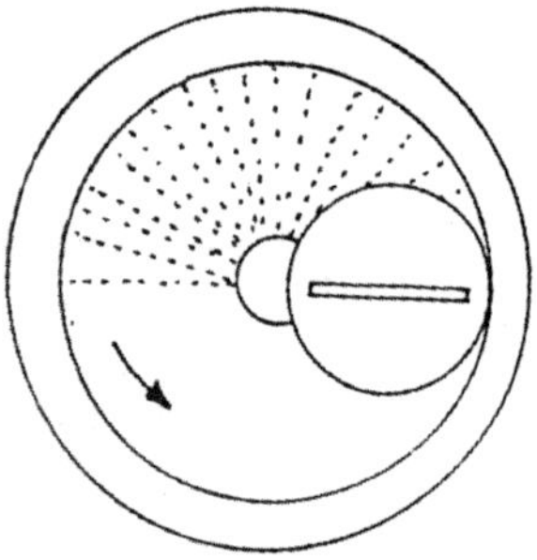

Fig. 24.3 Slit sampler

Sieve Device or *Sieve Sampler (Fig. 24.4)*

It has a large number of small holes in a metal cover, under which is located a petridish containing an agar medium.

Air is drawn through small holes in the metal cover. As air-borne microorganisms pass through holes they impinge on the surface of agar medium. When the agar medium is incubated, the organisms multiply and form colonies, which then can be counted.

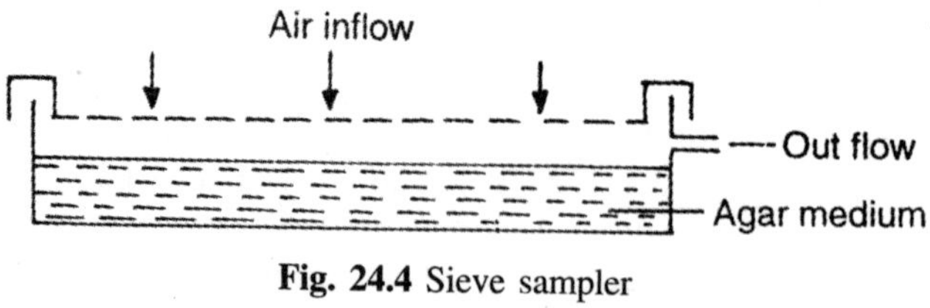

Fig. 24.4 Sieve sampler

Andersen's Air Sampler

In this device, air is drawn through a circular orifice and then through a succession of six circular plates, each perforated with 400 holes. The air passes through the perforations and the particles get impacted on to sterile medium in petridishes. The succession of plates has progressively smaller holes so that the largest particles are impacted on to the first dish and the smallest on the sixth.

Thus, the sampler automatically separates air particles into six aerodynamic sizes which indicate respiratory tract penetration and hazard. It is a device for size grading of air-borne particles on solid culture media, which are incubated and viable count is estimated.

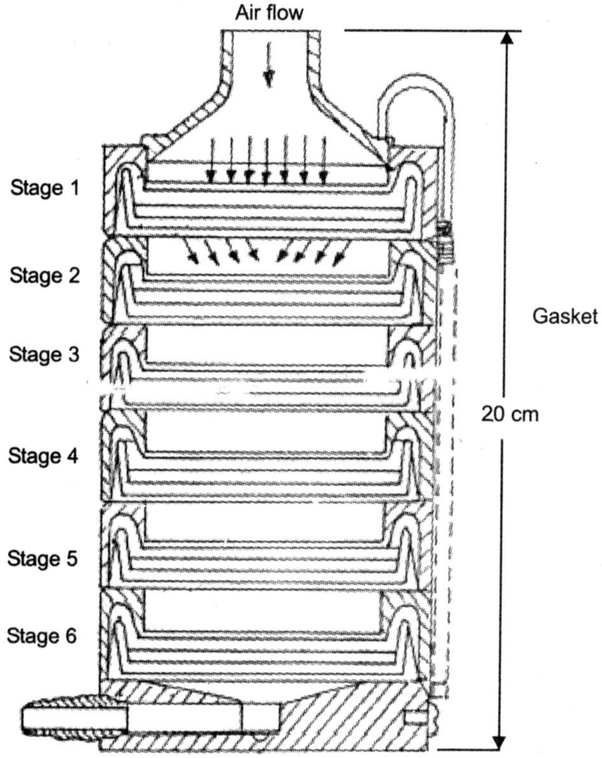

Fig. 24.5 Andersen's air sampler

Funnel Device **or** ***Hollanender and Dalla Valle Sampler***

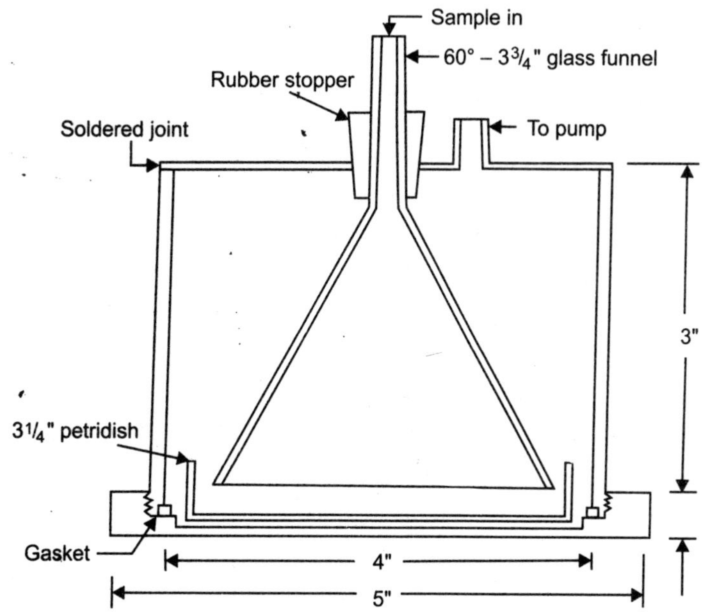

Fig. 24.6 Funnel device

It consists of a brass container with a removable bottom. The container is fitted with an inverted glass funnel which sits approximately half inch from the bottom of a petridish. The petridish is placed in the lower portion of the container before use, then screwed tightly against the gasket. The inside of the funnel and rim are swabbed with alcohol before use. The air passes through funnel stem, and the air-borne organisms are impinged upon the agar medium. The air is drawn by means of a pump in series with a flow meter. The method is simple, portable and efficient and all testing is carried out in one operation.

Filtration

The membrane filter devices can be used for direct sampling of microorganisms by filtration of air. Polypore type of filters and millipore membrane filters are used for removal of organisms from air by filtration. After filtration, the membrane is agitated in a broth to disperse the particles, then samples of the suspension are mixed with melted agar and incubated and counts determined. The counts may be higher than the actual number of viable particles, because clumps of organisms may be fragmented during agitation of the sample.

Centrifugation

Sampler of this type employ centrifugal force for propulsion of air particles to the collecting surface. When air moves in a circular direction at high speed, the suspended aerosols are impacted on the collecting surface by a force proportional to the particle velocity and mass.

In one type of centrifuge, the sampler remains stationary while the aerosol travels in a circular path, the larger prticles being collected at the bottom. In another type, the collecting vessel and aerosols rotate at high velocity resulting in the impaction of particles on the walls.

Well's Air Centrifuge

It utilizes the principle of centrifuging particles from the air on to culture medium. Well's air centrifuge consists of a head assembly with exhaust fan, air inlet tube and chamber to contain the sample tube. The variable-speed motor is mounted in an aluminium housing. The head assembly fan and sample chamber are driven by the motor through a hub on which rests the sample tube. The air inlet tube is suspended from the case top by means of a rubber disk and clamp.

The molten agar medium is poured into the sample tube, which is inserted in the centrifuge and switched on. The incoming air is mixed with the agar and the medium is spread as a thin film on the wall of the sample tube by the centrifugal force of rotation. The organisms are deposited in the agar film, and after incubation may be counted.

The Well's air centrifuge is simple to operate, quickly manipulated and portable, all testing is carried out in one step.

Cylindrical Sampler

Borzani and Vairo recommended a sampler composed of aluminium alloy in cylinder form. The cylinder contains a certain volume of air and a solid culture medium at the bottom. It is centrifuged, the time and rate being predetermined. The suspended cells are deposited on the surface of the medium, and after incubation the colonies are counted.

Electrostatic Precipitation

Electrostatic air samplers collect particles by drawing air over an electrically charged surface. The sampler holds two petridishes in separate plastic units over positive and negative electrodes. A small electrically operated blower draws air at equal rates through the two units. Both positively and negatively charged organisms exist in air simultaneously. Those having a positive charge are collected on the petridish placed over the negative electrode; those negatively charged are collected on the petridish placed over the positive electrode.

Thermal Precipitation

Samplers of this type collect particles on surfaces by means of thermal gradients. Air-borne particles are repelled by hot surfaces and deposited on colder surfaces by forces proportional to the temperature gradient.

Since such samplers require careful adjustment and the air sampling rates are quite low, they are not commonly used.

Samplers to Trap Fungal Spores and Pollen

Rotorod, Hirst trap, cascade impactor, vertical cylinder trap, Bukard trap and several other samplers are used to trap fungal spores, pollen from air samples.

QUESTIONS

Essays Type Questions

1. Describe bacteriological analysis of water.
2. Give an account of bacteriological examination of milk.
3. Describe various sampling devices to trap microorganisms from air.

Short Notes

1. DMC or Breed's count.
2. Standard plate count or colony count or viable count or pour plate method.
3. Melthylene blue reduction test.
4. Resazurin test.
5. Phosphatase test.
6. Milk ring test.
7. Multiple tube dilution technique.
8. Presumptive coliform count or MPN.
9. BOD.
10. Indicators of water pollution.
11. Eijkman test.
12. Membrane filter method.
13. Fecal streptococci as indicators of water pollution.
14. Settling plate technique.
15. Andersen's sampler.

25

Biomedical Waste (Hospital Waste) Management

Biomedical waste or hospital waste is the waste that is generated during the process of patient care.

Safe handling of biomedical waste is a matter of serious concern. Thousands of tonnes of biomedical waste originating from hospitals, nursing homes and clinics in the form of cotton swabs and bandages infected with blood, IV fluid bags, needles, catheters, human tissues and body parts etc. continue to be dumped in open garbage bins on the roads. This improper disposal of waste is one of the prime reasons for the spread of infectious diseases. The Govt. of India has published a Gazette notification on 20th July 1998, titled Biomedical waste (handling and management) Rules, making all persons who generate, collect, receive, store transport, treat, dispose or handle medical waste in any form responsible for handling the medical waste without any adverse effect to human health and environment. It is mandatory for various hospital and health care institutions to implement these rules.

The hospital wastes are segregated preferably at the point of generation into infectious waste and non-infectious waste, which should be collected in appropriate containers.

Infectious wastes include discard cultures, microbiological wastes, blood and body fluids, contaminated laboratory wastes, used syringes and needles, pathological wastes such as clinical specimens and tissues, bedding and other wastes like bandages and used cotton swabs, and animal carcasses used in laboratory experiments. Chemical waste is also hazardous. Covered containers can be used for segregation of waste. Black plastic bags are used for non-infectious general waste, whereas yellow and red plastic bags are used for infectious waste. Blue or white colored rigid, puncture proof containers are used for syringes, needles, lancets and other invasive instruments. This type of segregation helps in safe handling and transportation of waste and accordingly their treatment.

The treatment of biomedical waste can be done by incineration, autoclaving and chemical treatment.

Incineration—is an efficient method for the sterilization and disposal of hazardous infectious hospital waste. Soiled dressings, pathological materials, animal carcasses, infected linen/bedding, sharp needles and other clinical wastes are literally burned to ashes at temperature of 870-980°C in an incinerator by electricity. Plastics such as disposable syringes, rubber catheters, culture plates and specimen containers made of polyvinylchloride (PVC) and polyethylene may emit dense black smoke when incinerated. They can be autoclaved before disposal. Toxic air emissions during incineration and heavy metals in ash may constitute health hazard.

Autoclaving—is used for microbiological waste, blood and blood products, body fluids and used syringes and needles. Autoclaved material is usually land-filled. Autoclaving is not recommended for pathological waste.

Chemical treatment—ensures disinfection. One percent hypochlorite or any suitable disinfectant may be used.

Infectious waste after treatment can be disposed of by land-filling or deep burial. Liquid waste can be disposed into sewage drains.

QUESTIONS

Essay Question

1. Describe the importance and procedures of hospital waste management.

Short Notes

1. Hospital waste management (or) management of biomedical waste.
2. Incineration.

26

Biological Weapons

Biological weapons or bioweapons are major potential means of mass destruction used in biological warfare. Bioweapons may be defined as microorganisms or their products (toxins) that infect and grow in the target host producing a clinical disease that kills or incapacities the target host. Biological weapons are relatively easy to make. Scientists are busy to design and produce weapons loaded with deadly microbes or their toxins.

The pathogens commonly used biological warfare are as follows:

Bacteria

(*i*) *Bacillus anthracis* (anthrax)

(*ii*) *Yersinia pestis* (plague)

(*iii*) *Franciselle tularensis* (tularemia)

(*iv*) *Coxiella burnetii* (Q fever)

(*v*) *Vibrio cholerae* (cholera)

(*vi*) *Clostridium botulinum* (botulism)

Viruses

(*i*) Variola virus (small pox)

(*ii*) Influenza virus (Influenza)

(*iii*) Ebola-influenza hybrid

Toxins

(*i*) Botulinum toxin

(*ii*) Aflatoxin

(*iii*) Ricin (a lethal toxin extracted from castor bean)

(*iv*) Saxitoxin (an alkaloid neurotoxin produced by dinoflagellates, when consumed through contaminated food such as shell fish causes paralysis and death)

(*v*) RNAi (Interference RNA tailored to latch on to specific mRNA sequences thus virtually silencing any gene).

Index

B